59.25

D1555955

Pediatric Thrombotic Disorders

Pediatric Thrombotic Disorders

Edited by

Neil A. Goldenberg, MD, PhD
Associate Professor of Pediatrics, Johns Hopkins University School of Medicine, and Chief Research Officer and Director, Thrombosis Program,
All Children's Hospital, Johns Hopkins Medicine, St Petersburg, FL, USA

Marilyn J. Manco-Johnson, MD
Director of the Hemophilia and Thrombosis Center and Professor of Pediatrics at the University of Colorado, Aurora, CO, USA

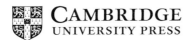

CAMBRIDGE
UNIVERSITY PRESS

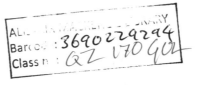

CAMBRIDGE
UNIVERSITY PRESS

University Printing House, Cambridge CB2 8BS, United Kingdom

Cambridge University Press is part of the University of Cambridge.

It furthers the University's mission by disseminating knowledge in the pursuit of
education, learning and research at the highest international levels of excellence.

www.cambridge.org
Information on this title: www.cambridge.org/9781107014541

First published 2015

Printed in the United Kingdom by TJ International Ltd, Padstow, Cornwall

A catalog record for this publication is available from the British Library

Library of Congress Cataloging in Publication data
Pediatric thrombotic disorders / edited by Neil A. Goldenberg, Marilyn J. Manco-Johnson.
  p. ; cm.
Includes bibliographical references and index.
ISBN 978-1-107-01454-1 (hardback : alk. paper)
I. Goldenberg, Neil A., 1971– , editor.   II. Manco-Johnson, Marilyn J., editor.
[DNLM: 1. Thrombosis.   2. Blood Platelet Disorders.   3. Child.   4. Infant.
5. Thromboembolism.   QZ 170]
RC394.T5
616.1350083–dc23
                                                            2014025975

ISBN 978-1-107-01454-1 Hardback

....

Every effort has been made in preparing this book to provide accurate and
up-to-date information which is in accord with accepted standards and
practice at the time of publication. Although case histories are drawn from
actual cases, every effort has been made to disguise the identities of the
individuals involved. Nevertheless, the authors, editors, and publishers can
make no warranties that the information contained herein is totally free from
error, not least because clinical standards are constantly changing through
research and regulation. The authors, editors, and publishers therefore
disclaim all liability for direct or consequential damages resulting from the use
of material contained in this book. Readers are strongly advised to pay careful
attention to information provided by the manufacturer of any drugs or
equipment that they plan to use.

Contents

Contributors

Catherine M. Amlie-Lefond, MD
Associate Professor of Neurology and Director,
Pediatric Vascular Neurology Program,
University of Washington, Seattle Children's Hospital,
Seattle, WA, USA

Uma Athale, MD
Associate Professor of Pediatrics, Division of
Hematology/Oncology, McMaster Children's
Hospital, McMaster University, Hamilton, ON,
Canada

Timothy J. Bernard, MD
Associate Professor of Pediatrics, Neurology and
Child Neurology and Director, Pediatric Stroke
Program, Children's Hospital Colorado,
University of Colorado School of Medicine, Aurora,
CO, USA

Brian R. Branchford, MD
Instructor, Section of Hematology/Oncology/Bone
Marrow Transplantation, Department of Pediatrics,
University of Colorado–Anschutz Medical Campus &
Children's Hospital Colorado, Aurora, CO, USA

Leonardo R. Brandao, MD, MSc
Assistant Professor of Pediatrics, Division of
Hematology/Oncology, The Hospital for Sick
Children, Toronto, ON, Canada

Anthony K.C. Chan, MD
Division of Hematology/Oncology, McMaster
University Health Sciences Center, Hamilton, ON,
Canada

Meera Chitlur, MD
Barnhart-Lusher Hemostasis Research Endowed
Chair, Director, Hemophilia Treatment Center and
Hemostasis Program, Director, Special Coagulation
Laboratory, and Associate Professor of Pediatrics,
Wayne State University, Division of Hematology/
Oncology, Children's Hospital of Michigan, Detroit,
MI, USA

Neil A. Goldenberg, MD, PhD
Associate Professor of Pediatrics, Departments of
Pediatrics and Medicine, Johns Hopkins University
School of Medicine, Baltimore, MD, USA; All
Children's Research Institute, All Children's Hospital,
Johns Hopkins Medicine, St Petersburg, FL, USA

Gili Kenet, MD
Director, Thrombosis Unit, National Hemophilia
Center, Sheba Medical Center, Tel-Hashomer, Israel

Peter H. Lin, MD
Chief of Vascular Surgery, Baylor College of Medicine,
Houston, TX, USA

Courtney A. Lyle, MD, MAS
Department of Pediatrics, Division of
Hematology/Oncology, Billings Clinic, Billings,
MT, USA

Christoph Male, MD, MSc
Department of Pediatrics, Division of Hematology,
Medical University of Vienna, Vienna, Austria

Marilyn J. Manco-Johnson, MD
Director of the Hemophilia and Thrombosis Center
Professor of Pediatrics, Section of Hematology/
Oncology/Bone Marrow Transplantation,
University of Colorado–Anschutz Medical
Campus & Children's Hospital Colorado, Aurora,
CO, USA

Mahendranath Moharir MD, MSc, FRACP
Assistant Professor, University of Toronto, and Staff
Pediatric Neurologist, Division of Neurology,
Department of Pediatrics, The Hospital for Sick
Children, Toronto, ON, Canada

Paul Monagle, MD
Department of Paediatrics,
University of Melbourne, Department of
Haematology, Royal Children's Hospital,
Melbourne, VIC, Australia

Ulrike Nowak-Göttl, MD
Thrombosis and Hemostasis Unit, Department of Clinical Chemistry, University Hospital of Kiel & Lübeck, Germany

Leslie Raffini, MD, MSCE
Associate Professor of Pediatrics, Division of Hematology, Children's Hospital of Philadelphia, University of Pennsylvania Perlman School of Medicine, Philadelphia, PA, USA

Madhvi Rajpurkar, MD
Assistant Professor of Pediatrics, Chief, Division of Hematology and Thrombosis Service, Children's Hospital of Michigan and Wayne State University, Detroit, MI, USA

Shoshana Revel-Vilk, MD, MSc
Director, Pediatric Hematology Center, Pediatric Hematology/Oncology Department, Hadassah Medical Center, Jerusalem, Israel

Anjali A. Sharathkumar, MD, MS
Assistant Professor of Pediatrics, Hematology, Oncology and Stem Cell Transplantation, Hemophilia and Thrombosis Program, Ann & Robert H. Lurie Children's Hospital, Chicago, IL, USA

Robert Francis Sidonio Jr., MD, MSc
Assistant Professor of Pediatrics, Hemostasis/ Thrombosis, Aflec Cancer and Blood Disorders Center, Emory University, Atlanta, GA, USA

Mindy L. Simpson, MD
Assistant Professor of Pediatrics, Hematology/Oncology, Rush University Medical Center, Chicago, IL, USA

Courtney D. Thornburg, MD
Department of Pediatrics, University of California San Diego and Rady Children's Hospital, San Diego, CA, USA

Cameron C. Trenor III, MD
Attending Physician in Pediatric Hematology–Oncology, Boston Children's Hospital, Dana-Farber Cancer Institute, Co-Director, Cerebrovascular Disorders and Stroke Program, Director of Clinical Research, Vascular Anomalies Center, and Instructor in Pediatrics, Harvard Medical School, Boston, MA, USA

Michael Wang, MD
Associate Professor of Pediatrics, Clinical Director, Hemophilia & Thrombosis Center, University of Colorado–Anschutz Medical Campus and Children's Hospital Colorado, Aurora, CO, USA

Suzan Williams, MD, MSc
The Hospital for Sick Children, University of Toronto, Toronto, ON, Canada

Donald L. Yee, MD
Associate Professor of Pediatrics, Baylor College of Medicine, and Attending Physician, Texas Children's Hospital, Houston, TX, USA

Guy Young, MD
Director, Hemostasis and Thrombosis Center, Children's Hospital Los Angeles, and Associate Professor of Pediatrics, University of Southern California, Keck School of Medicine, Los Angeles, CA, USA

Preface

Over the past few decades, thrombotic disorders have become increasingly recognized as an important problem in pediatrics, affecting neonates through teens and young adults. These thrombotic disorders include both venous and arterial thromboembolism, as well as peripheral vascular, central vascular, cardiac, or cerebrovascular events. Accordingly, their optimal diagnosis and acute and chronic management often requires the ongoing expertise of diverse pediatric specialists, from hematologists to radiologists, emergentologists, intensivists, cardiologists, and neurologists, among others – all of whom can benefit from the collective work of a broad panel of experts brought together to produce this comprehensive text, *Pediatric Thrombotic Disorders*.

The chapters of this book are designed to provide up-to-date coverage of many of the most salient and topical issues in pediatric thrombotic disorders, including: thrombophilia evaluation, thrombolysis, heparin-induced thrombocytopenia/thrombosis, pulmonary embolism, arterial ischemic stroke, and new antithrombotic agents. In addition, this text contains chapters seldom addressed by other books or special issues devoted to thromboembolism or pediatric hematology/

oncology, such as: gastrointestinal and visceral thromboses, infection-associated venous thromboembolism, and severe thrombophilias.

One of our greatest rewards is the opportunity to mentor and teach students, residents, fellows, and junior faculty. Accordingly, we and our coauthor colleagues have striven in this book to develop content that is suitable and of interest across a broad range of readers and "learners," among which last category we include ourselves. We hope you share our perspective that every chapter in this text offers knowledge and perspectives from which each reader – whether coming from a background of pediatric hematology or another discipline, and whether a medical student or a professor emeritus – may benefit... and we welcome your feedback and ideas for improving upon it in future editions.

We dedicate this book to the pediatric patients with thrombotic disorders for whom we have had the privilege of caring, and who have taught us so much clinically, in research, and in our own lives.

Neil A. Goldenberg, MD, PhD
Marilyn J. Manco-Johnson, MD

Acknowledgments

The editors are sincerely grateful to Nisha Doshi, Jane Seakins, and Beata Mako of Cambridge University Press, as well as to Laurel McDevitt of All Children's Hospital, Johns Hopkins Medicine, for their editorial and production expertise and tireless support throughout the development of this text.

Extremity and caval deep venous thrombosis

Madhvi Rajpurkar and Shoshana Revel-Vilk

Introduction

Advances in supportive care have changed the landscape of clinical pediatrics from acute life-threatening conditions to more chronic diseases. Venous thromboembolism (VTE), comprising of deep venous and thrombosis (DVT) and pulmonary embolism (PE), traditionally considered as an acute and chronic disease of the elderly, is increasingly recognized in hospitalized children and has emerged as a significant public health burden. Although the incidence of pediatric thrombosis is lower than that in adults, over the last few decades it has been recognized that pediatric thrombosis has become a substantial health hazard and may be associated with significant morbidity and mortality. Additionally, the health-care burden of VTE may be particularly high for affected children, given the additional impact imposed on the child's family members and by the much greater life expectancy compared with affected elderly adults. Evidence-based recommendations for management of pediatric thrombosis are still lacking, due to lack of large carefully conducted clinical trials and most recommendations are either directly extrapolated from adults or are based on consensus or expert opinions [1]. As the incidence of pediatric thrombosis increases and newer anticoagulant drugs make their way into the clinical field, investigators have felt the necessity for improved diagnostic testing, risk adapted treatment regimens and better definitions of outcome measures after pediatric thrombosis [2]. This chapter focuses on recent knowledge and current advances in pediatric extremity and caval thrombosis.

Epidemiology

Over the last two decades, pediatric VTE has become required as an increasingly frequent complication. The estimated incidence from the Canadian Childhood Thrombophilia registry as originally reported in 1994 was 0.07/10,000 children per year as compared to 5.6–16 cases/10,000 adults per year [3]. However, it is now estimated that pediatric VTE is approximately ten-fold more common than the initial estimates from the Canadian registries. The population prevalence of pediatric VTE in the USA is estimated to be 0.6–1.1 per 10,000 and recent epidemiologic analysis of both the Kid's Inpatient Database (KID) and the Pediatric Health Information System (PHIS) have estimated the incidence to be as high as 42–58/10,000 hospital admissions [4–6]. The analysis of the KID has also demonstrated that the majority of childhood VTE events occur in a tertiary care inpatient setting as compared to community hospitals caring for children (40.2/10,000 vs. 7.8/10,000 admissions). This increasing trend is attributable to the increasing use of central venous catheters (CVCs) for supportive care of children, better imaging techniques for thrombus detection, increasing awareness of the problem and thus lower threshold for screening survival, and improvement in incidence of critically sick children.

Pediatric VTE shows a bimodal age pattern. The highest incidence of pediatric VTE is seen in neonates and infants with a second peak seen in adolescents, particularly teenage girls either in relation to pregnancy or the use of hormonals [7]. Another study demonstrated that the highest VTE risk for non-hospitalized children was in children > 11 years of age as compared to the hospitalized children, where the highest incidence is seen ages < 1 years and > 11 years [8].

Upper and lower extremity and superior and inferior vena caval (SVC, IVC) DVT are the most common sites for thrombosis in children. According to the analysis of the PHIS database, of the specific sites identified, the proportion of VTE cases represented by upper extremity DVT was 15.7%, lower extremity DVT 21% and vena caval thrombosis 18.3% [6].

Pediatric Thrombotic Disorders, ed. Neil A. Goldenberg and Marilyn J. Manco-Johnson. Published by Cambridge University Press. © Cambridge University Press 2015.

From an analysis of the Health Cost and Utilization Project using KID in 2006, the occurrence of lower extremity DVT was estimated to be 29.5% [9].

Etiology and risk factors

Pediatric VTE is a multifactorial disease with a higher incidence in children with chronic or complex medical conditions. The etiopathogenesis of VTE is best explained by the Virchow's triad. In 1845, Virchow postulated that three factors were important in the development of thrombosis: (1) impairment of normal laminar blood flow, (2) endothelial or vascular injury and (3) alterations of the blood (hypercoagulability). Common risk factors for pediatric VTE are listed in Table 1.1. Many of the conditions listed in Table 1.1 may cause thrombosis by affecting more than one factor of the Virchow's triad mentioned above. Venous thromboembolism can be classified as provoked or non-provoked (also called spontaneous) depending on the presence of a proximate identifiable triggering risk factor such as surgery, presence of a CVC, initiation of hormonal contraception, etc. Such events may occur with or without an underlying prothrombotic condition (e.g., genetic or acquired thrombophilia, chronic

Table 1.1 Risk factors for pediatric venous thrombosis (Virchow's triad)

1. **Endothelial damage**
   a. Central venous catheters, ventricular atrial shunts, etc.
   b. Sepsis
   c. Antiphospholipid antibodies
   d. Trauma
   e. Inflammatory conditions (e.g., systemic lupus erythematous, inflammatory bowel disease)

2. **Disruption of the laminar blood flow or stasis**
   a. Post-operative state
   b. Immobility
   c. Anatomical variants (e.g., May–Thurner anomaly, Paget–Schroetter syndrome)
   d. Complex congenital heart disease or cardiomyopathy
   e. Total parenteral nutrition (TPN)

3. **Hypercoagulable state**
   a. Inherited
      Deficiency of protein C, S, antithrombin III
      Factor V Leiden, prothrombin gene mutation
      Elevated homocysteine

   b. Acquired
      Antiphospholid antibodies
      Pregnancy or hormonal supplementation
      Nephrotic syndrome
      Medications (e.g., asparaginase chemotherapy)
      Infections (e.g., varicella)
      Malignancy

inflammatory disease) and may have an additive effect on the risk of thrombosis imparted by an underlying prothrombotic condition. However, all children with a proximate triggering event may have an underlying prothrombotic condition and thus it is important to note the subtle difference in terminology. A VTE may be provoked but not have an underlying prothrombotic condition. On the other hand, a child with underlying prothrombotic condition (e.g., a potent inherited thrombophilia trait, such as homozygous factor V Leiden) may present without a proximate triggering factor (unprovoked DVT). True idiopathic DVT, which implies an absence of either a provoking risk factor or an underlying prothrombotic condition, can also exist but is rare in children. In children, the majority of VTE is associated with an underlying associated disorder (76.2% according to a recent analysis of the KID database) [9]. This is in contrast to VTE in adults, where up to 40% of episodes may be idiopathic. Other studies have reported the proportion of VTE represented by idiopathic cases to be approximately 5% in children and < 1% in neonates [7]. The presence of a CVC is the most common provoking risk factor for the development of DVT in children. It is estimated that approximately 60% of the cases of DVT in children and > 90% of cases in neonates are associated with CVC. According to an analysis of the KID database, the most common complex medical conditions associated with VTE were cardiovascular conditions (18.4%), malignancies (15.7%) and neuromuscular conditions (9.9%) [9]. These rates are similar to those reported by other epidemiologic studies [6,10]. The reader is referred to other chapters for a detailed discussion of pediatric evidence of VTE clinical risk factors and the risk for VTE associated with inherited and acquired laboratory thrombophilias.

Central venous catheters

Since the limitations of peripheral intravenous catheters have become apparent, the frequency of insertion of CVCs has increased. These catheters can be placed in the umbilical vein (UVC) in the neonates or in large central vessels (Hickman or Portacath®, and peripherally inserted central catheter, PICC). As mentioned above, the presence of a CVC is the most common triggering risk for the development of DVT in children. This also explains the difference in the most common site of DVT in adults compared with children. In adults, lower extremity DVT is more common. In children, upper extremity or more proximal (including superior vena caval) DVT is more common because most CVCs in children are inserted into the upper venous system.

CVCs are critical for supportive care of sick children and have contributed to the significant improvement in outcomes of such children. However, the insertion of a CVC can cause thrombosis by directly disrupting the vascular endothelium, by altering the blood flow and by alteration of the local milieu due to infusion of hypertonic solutions such as total parenteral nutrition (TPN) infusions. The risk of thrombosis with a CVC varies depending not only on catheter and individual patient-related risk factors but also on the reasons/underlying conditions for which the CVC is inserted.

Catheter-related risk factors may be related to the caliber of the CVC in relation to the vessel size, catheter composition, infusate, site, and frequency of access and duration of use. Although there are no well-designed clinical trials that compare the thrombotic risk of differing catheter materials, one study revealed increased risk with polyethylene catheters (70%) as compared to silicone catheters (20%) and polyurethane catheters (17%) [11]. Other studies have confirmed that polyethylene catheters are the most thrombogenic, but found no significant differences between silicone, polyurethane and polyvinylchloride catheters [12–14]. The use of heparin-bonded catheters has been demonstrated to prolong catheter patency (i.e., function), but has not been shown to reduce the risk of thrombosis [15]. In one study that evaluated the risk of VTE in infants with CVC, it was found that catheters in the femoral vein and multiple-lumen catheters were associated with a higher risk [16]. In another multicenter prospective study that evaluated the risk of catheter-associated symptomatic VTE, femoral and subclavian vein CVC were shown to have the highest risk [17]. This study also demonstrated that the incidence of VTE was independent of CVC type (PICC, untunneled CVC, tunneled exteriorized CVC and subcutaneous ports) and CVC size [17]. Some studies have indicated that the risk of thrombosis is also related to the duration of catheter dwell *in situ*. The use of UVC or PICC for > 6 days was associated with a higher risk of thrombosis. In one study, duration of non-tunneled femoral CVC > 14 days was associated with a higher risk of DVT, while another study did not demonstrate this [17,18].

Among children with CVC, neonates are at heightened risk for DVT. Some evidence suggests that, within this subgroup, VTE risk factors include small for gestational age with < 1250 g birth weight, hematocrit > 55% and maternal history of pre-eclampsia [19]. More generally among all children, sepsis and infection appear to be risk factors for CVC-associated DVT [19]. The incidence is highly variable depending on the diagnostic modality and approach (e.g., universal screening identifies more cases than diagnostic evaluation of symptomatic patients). In addition to the physical risk factors for thrombosis, infusion of hypertonic solutions, presence of calcium and high levels of dextrose are additional risk factors. In children on long-term TPN, CVC-related DVT is a significant issue. Retrospective studies have shown the incidence to be 0.2–0.4 per 1,000 catheter days or 20–75% [20]. It is also thought that patients with short bowel syndrome may have a higher incidence of thrombosis as compared to other children on TPN due to high frequency of intraluminal bacterial overgrowth due to dysmotility, which may predispose to a higher risk of catheter infection – a risk factor for development of thrombi [21,22].

Cardiac diseases

Complex congenital heart conditions with or without associated extracorporeal membrane oxygenation (ECMO) are independent risk factors for the development of thrombosis in children. In one prospective observational study, the cumulative incidence of VTE was found to be 3.8% of all children with cardiac disorders admitted to the pediatric intensive care unit (PICU) [23]. In this study, the most common risk factor for thrombosis was the presence of a CVC (in 41% of patients). Other risk factors associated with an increased VTE incidence were unscheduled PICU admissions, age < 6 months, use of ECMO, increased CVC duration with complicated hospital course and single ventricle cardiac lesions. Interestingly, 32% of imaging studies that detected VTE were ordered for symptoms other than those directly attributable to VTE. The role of inherited thrombophilia in children with cardiac conditions and thrombosis has also been investigated. One study found heterozygous factor V Leiden (FVL) mutation in 17.3%, methylenetetrahydrofolate reductase (MTHFR) 677C-T mutation in 28.8% and prothrombin G20210A mutation (PT) in 5.8% of patients [24], while another study found that the overall frequency of FVL and/or PT was 22% in children with cardiac disease and thrombosis [25].

Cancer

In adults, the presence of a malignant disorder greatly increases the risk of thrombosis. In children with cancer, extremity and vena caval thrombosis are the most common sites of DVT due to the presence of a CVC [26], but cerebral sinovenous thrombosis may also be seen, especially in patients with acute lymphoblastic leukemia treated with asparaginase chemotherapy. According to the analysis of the PHIS database, coexistent malignant disorders were seen in 11% of children with VTE [6]. In another study, VTE occurred in 5.3% of adolescents and young adults with cancer [27]. This study also showed that patients with leukemia and sarcomas were at a higher risk of VTE than other malignant disorders. A single-center retrospective study in children revealed the cumulative incidence was as high as 2.1%, with highest occurrence seen in hematological malignancies such as acute leukemia and in teenagers [26]. In a multicenter prospective study in children with cancer, the risk of CVC-related DVT was 4.6% [28]. The pathogenesis of thrombosis in malignant disorders is multifactorial. The risk may be related to the presence of a CVC, type of cancer, chemotherapy medications such as L-asparaginase and dexamethasone and other complications such as sepsis. The reader is referred to other chapters for detailed discussion on cancer-related thrombosis.

Anatomical causes

Although there is a rapidly growing literature on risk factors such as CVCs and cancer in the pathogenesis of pediatric VTE, there is a paucity of data on VTE due to anatomical causes. The development of the venous circulation is complex and many anatomic variants are possible and are found in approximately 1% of adults [29]. Interrupted or absent IVC have also been described in association with DVT [29]. For example, absent IVC was found in 0.3% of healthy individuals and up to 2% of patients with other cardiovascular anomalies [29]. A high index for suspicion should be maintained for anatomical abnormalities or local compression when children present with DVT without a specific provoking factor.

Iliac vein compression syndrome was originally described by May and Thurner in 1957 by using autopsy studies. The May–Thurner syndrome is caused by the compression of the left common iliac vein between the overlying right common iliac artery and an underlying vertebral body. Chronic compression along with the pulsations of the overlying artery may lead to vascular intimal damage and formation of venous "spurs" resulting in acute or chronic venous thrombosis [30]. It is important to identify this anatomical anomaly, which has been described in up to 22–32% of 430 autopsies, as treatment with anticoagulation may not be adequate. Without thrombectomy and endovascular treatment, such as stent placement, individuals with the May–Thurner anomaly may be at increased risk for recurrent thrombosis. Similar "May–Thurner-like physiology" may be seen when the compression occurs due to local lesions such as tumors, lymphadenopathy or ectopic kidney.

Paget–Schroetter syndrome or effort-induced thrombosis of the upper extremity may be seen with involvement of the axillary and subclavian veins as a consequence of strenuous activity involving the arms and chest, as a complication of thoracic outlet syndrome or with a presentation of spontaneous thrombosis in the absence of identifiable thrombosis risk factors. Thoracic outlet syndrome refers to the compression of the neurovascular bundle (brachial plexus, subclavian artery and vein) as it exits the thoracic outlet. The cause of Paget–Schroetter syndrome is usually secondary to an underlying anatomic abnormality at the thoracic outlet such as a cervical rib, musculofascial band or first rib anomalies, but can also simply result from a congenitally narrow course of the subclavian vein between the first rib, clavicle and subclavius muscle – often exacerbated by subclavius muscle hypertrophy in the setting of effort-induced thrombosis. Repeated compression of the subclavian vein leading to venous stasis combined with perivascular fibrosis and endothelial damage due to venous stretching leads to DVT. Anticoagulation alone with or without thrombolysis may lead to high rate of recurrence. Endovascular treatment along with removal of local compression such as cervical rib resection may be necessary to prevent recurrent events [31].

Presentation

Children may present with local pain, swelling or redness of the involved extremity. CVC-related thrombosis is associated with CVC-associated blood stream infection, and therefore a level of suspicion for thrombosis should be maintained in children with CVC-associated blood stream infections, particularly when the latter are refractory/recurrent despite appropriate antibiotic therapy. When thrombosis is associated with a CVC, CVC dysfunction may be an early sign. It is recommended to investigate for DVT in a case of occluded CVC if the catheter fails to function after two local instillations of a thrombolytic agent [1,32]. Frequently, CVC-related DVT is asymptomatic in children, and may be detected during routine screening or imaging for other procedures. By contrast, patients with CVC-associated thrombosis (sometimes with only a remote history of CVC placement) can develop SVC thrombosis that, when sufficiently occlusive, may present with SVC syndrome characterized by facial and neck swelling and dilatation of superficial collateral venous circulation of the arms, neck and chest, all due to impaired deep venous return in the upper venous system. Children with effort-induced thrombosis of the upper extremity may present after significant use of that arm, e.g., in baseball or basketball practice [31]. Neonates with acute VTE may present with new-onset thrombocytopenia. It is important to note that in patients with a previous history of thrombosis, ruling out a recurrent thrombotic event is warranted if progressive or new symptoms develop. An unequivocal change in the extent of thrombosis, compared with the previous ultrasound scan, might be indicative of new ipsilateral DVT [33].

Diagnosis

Radiologic studies

Compression ultrasound (CUS) with Doppler remains the most common technique for diagnosis of extremity DVT, particularly at and above the level of the popliteal vein in the leg. Advantages of CUS are that it is inexpensive, portable, readily available, requires no sedation and conveys no radiation exposure. The deep veins can be evaluated in transverse and longitudinal scans. The compressibility of the vein can be assessed and failure of the vein to collapse is indicative of the presence of a thrombus. Bulging of the vein also suggests that a thrombus is present. Additionally, color flow and Doppler images should be obtained. Flow deficits can be detected on color flow Doppler [34]. Lack of tissue density on imaging ultrasound with concomitant lack of Doppler flow suggests a fresh or non-echogenic clot. However, several factors such as small diameter of blood vessels, lower pulse pressure in children and the presence of a CVC may interfere with the diagnosis of thrombosis by ultrasound. If clinical suspicion for thrombosis is high, then other diagnostic modalities such as conventional venography, magnetic resonance venography (MRV)

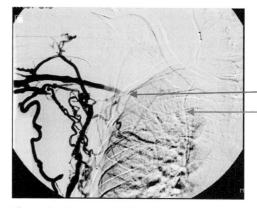

Figure 1.1 Venogram of right upper extremity complete obstruction of the distal subclavian vein (upper arrow) and superior vena cava with extensive collaterals. A central venous catheter (CVC) can also be seen (lower arrow).

or computerized tomography venography (CTV), may be performed after discussion with the radiologist. The CUS technique has also been used for the diagnosis of DVT of the upper extremity and jugular, axillary and distal subclavian veins. However, ultrasound has poor sensitivity for DVT in the proximal subclavian, innominate or SVC. Diagnostic sensitivity of CUS is greatly dependent upon amenability of the vein to compression maneuver, and veins underlying bony structures (e.g., chest wall) are not amenable to compression. 2D echo cardiography can image the heart chambers and often the proximal SVC, and can be used in conjunction with CUS of the distal subclavian and upper extremity veins for a full evaluation of the upper venous system. Alternatively, MRV or CTV may be used for DVT diagnosis in the chest and other central veins, although MRV is more subject to motion artifacts of respiration as well as flow artifacts. Contrast venography (Figure 1.1) is the historical gold standard for the diagnosis of extremity and caval DVT in adults but is infrequently used outside of settings of suspected May–Thurner anomaly, Pagett–Schroetter syndrome or periprocedurally for thrombolytic interventions, due to the invasive technique, requirement for contrast and radiation exposure. Interestingly, the Prophylactic Antithrombin Replacement in Kids with Acute Lymphoblastic Leukemia Treated with Asparaginase (PARKAA) study showed that CUS was relatively insensitive in the diagnosis of SVC and proximal subclavian DVT, while venography was insensitive to the diagnosis of internal jugular DVT [35]. Thus it is necessary to tailor the diagnostic modality to the suspected site of thrombosis to accurately diagnose DVT. The MRV and CTV techniques are being used often in many pediatric tertiary care centers for diagnosis of caval, abdominal/pelvic and proximal upper venous system DVT.

Particular attention should be paid to spontaneous DVT. As mentioned above, spontaneous DVT in children is rare. In upper extremity DVT, an anatomical variant such as a cervical rib or a functional thoracic inlet syndrome should be considered in the absence of an obvious predisposing factor. In case of left iliac vein DVT, the diagnosis of May–Thurner syndrome or other anatomical abnormalities should be entertained and appropriate studies should be obtained [29]. Venography is the gold standard for diagnosis of such anatomical variants but, due to limitations mentioned above, may not be feasible in all patients. Positioning of the upper extremity (abduction of at least 30°) is important in demonstration of Paget–Schroetter syndrome [36]. The CTV or MRV methods may be used for diagnosis and should be performed after consultation with the radiologist.

D-dimer

In adults, an elevated D-dimer has been used as a screening test for prediction of VTE. In a patient who has a low clinical index of suspicion for VTE based on history, signs and symptoms, a negative D-dimer can reliably exclude VTE, particularly in the setting of "rule-out" PE. Conversely, in a patient with a high index of suspicion for VTE (particularly PE), a positive D-dimer should prompt diagnostic imaging. However systematic data in children are scarce. One retrospective study in patients < 21 years of age found that the D-dimer test was sensitive (92%) but only moderately specific (57%) for diagnosis of VTE [37]. However, interpretation of D-dimer values need to be made with caution as there are significant age-related differences in the normal range of D-dimer levels [38]. Larger studies are needed to evaluate the role of D-dimer in the diagnosis of pediatric VTE. Given the low incidence of VTE in children in general, D-dimer is likely to play a stronger prognostic than diagnostic role, wherein the latter remains guided by clinical index of suspicion.

Management

Most of the recommendations cited in this chapter are based on extrapolation from adult evidence and on expert opinion [1,32,34]. Children with DVT are in most cases treated with anticoagulation. The aims of anticoagulation in children, based on evidence from adult literature, are to reduce the risk of thrombosis extension or embolization, reduce the incidence of recurrent thrombosis and maintain vessel patency, where clinically relevant. In rare cases, thrombolysis/thrombectomy may be used in an effort to preserve life, limb or organ function, or reduce the incidence/severity of post-thrombotic syndrome (PTS). High-quality evidence is lacking for this last indication, and a large randomized controlled clinical trial of catheter-directed thrombolysis in adult iliofemoral DVT (the ATTRACT trial, NCT 00790335) is ongoing.

Where possible, it is recommended that pediatric hematologists with experience in the field of thrombosis and hemostasis should manage children with DVT [1]. When this is not possible, a combination of a pediatrician and adult hematologist supported by consultation with an experienced pediatric hematologist is suggested. This recommendation is based on the known differences in the use of anticoagulant drugs in children compared to adult and on the limited evidenced-based data on the management of thrombotic events in children [1].

Anticoagulation

Currently, the routine anticoagulant agents used in children are unfractionated heparin (UFH), low molecular weight heparin (LMWH) and vitamin K antagonists (VKA). The mechanism of action, pharmacokinetics, therapeutic ranges and monitoring of these anticoagulation methods have been reviewed [1]. The main advantages of UFH are its short half-life and reversal with protamine, both enabling rapid normalization of coagulation in case of bleeding and/or prior to urgent invasive procedures. Thus, in children with DVT who are at higher risk of bleeding or in possible need of an invasive procedure, UFH would be the drug of choice [32].

Initial treatment with UFH or LMWH is recommended for at least 6 days for children with a first DVT [1,32]. For ongoing therapy, the use of either LMWH or VKA (target NR of 2–3) is recommended. For children in whom clinicians will subsequently prescribe VKAs, it is recommended to begin oral therapy as early as day 1 and discontinue UFH/LMWH on day 7 or later than day 7 if the INR is < 2.0 [1].

The LMWHs have become the anticoagulant of choice in children beyond the acute period of DVT (e.g., for outpatient therapy), as well as the anticoagulant of choice for non-critically ill children presenting with acute thrombosis and normal renal function. The potential advantages of LMWH are reduced need for therapeutic monitoring, lack of interference by other drugs or diet, reduced risk of heparin-induced thrombocytopenia relative to UFH and hypothesized reduced risk of osteoporosis relative to UFH.

The subcutaneous doses required to achieve therapeutic peak anti-factor Xa levels of 0.5–1 IU/ml for enoxaparin, reviparin, dalteparin, tinzaparin and nadroparin in children have been reviewed [1]. In most studies of children with DVT, the LMWH used was enoxaparin. The dose of enoxaparin for children > 2 months of age is 1 to 1.25 mg/kg/dose twice daily and adjusted to achieve the recommended therapeutic levels. In order to decrease the inconvenience associated with twice daily dosing, a once daily enoxaparin regimen of 1.5 mg/kg is sometimes used in adults. A study that evaluated whether a once-daily dosing enoxaparin regimen would be feasible in children showed that in almost half of children the median 24-hour level was below the lower limit of the desired trough range of 0.1 IU/ml anti-Xa activity [39]. In an open-label pilot safety study, 80 children with DVT were treated with enoxaparin with a 4 h post-dose target anti-Xa activity of 0.5–0.8 IU/mL. Following the acute treatment period (7–14 days) children were stratified to receive once daily or twice daily doses. No significant differences were found between the two groups in the occurrence of PTS, VTE recurrence, bleeding and therapy-related death [40].

The safety and efficacy of LMWH in children was summarized in a systematic review and meta-analysis of single-arm studies [41]. The rates of new thrombotic events on LWMH during the acute phase of treatment and the rates of recurrent VTE events on secondary prophylaxis therapy were 2.5% and 3.9%, respectively. The rates of clinically relevant bleeding and minor bleeding were 2.9% and 11.4%, respectively. Safety and efficacy were not associated with age or publication year. The only published multicenter randomized study of anticoagulation for VTE in children used reviparin [42]. The REVIVE (Reviparin in Venous Thromboembolism) trial randomized children with a first VTE to receive either UFH followed by VKAs (target international normalized ratio [INR], 2.5) for 3 months or reviparin (target anti-Xa range, 0.5 to 1.0 units/ml) for 3 months. The study was closed early because of slow accrual. As a

result, comparative efficacy and safety between the two regimens remains unclear.

Point of care monitors and educational programs can contribute to the efficacy and safety of, as well as adherence to, VKA therapy in children [43,44]. While no study in children has definitively compared the efficacy and safety of LMWH vs. VKA, meta-analysis data in adults show a statistically non-significant reduction in the risk of major bleeding (OR 0.45; 95% CI: 0.18–1.11) in favor of LMWH [45]. In children, LMWH is often administered through an indwelling catheter (Insuflon™); however, this therapy may be associated with development of hematomas at the site of multiple injections, and theoretically could affect consistency of drug absorption. In spite of this, and due to the relatively difficult management of VKA in children (frequent monitoring, food and drug interaction, etc.), many pediatric hematologists suggest the use of LMWH over VKA, especially for short-term therapy (< 6 months). Longer use of LMWH may be associated with osteoporosis [46], a potential concern that is raised from the much more robust data on the high rate of bone demineralization with pathologic fractures that is associated with the no-longer-recommended long-term use of unfractionated heparin [1]. The VKA may also have a deleterious effect on bone mineralization although data are conflicting.

The decision to use LMWH versus VKA as subacute anticoagulation should be made collaboratively with the patient and family, after weighing pros and cons, in order to achieve optimal adherence and outcome. Use of LMWH may be preferable in infants under 1 year of age [32]. For children with cancer who experience a DVT, LMWH is the preferred anticoagulant because of the relative ease of administering anticoagulation around the usual frequent procedures [1], and due to adult trial findings on LMWH for this indication (e.g., the CLOT and ONCENOX trials) [47–49].

The duration of anticoagulation in children with DVT depends on the clinical circumstance, and is not based upon high-quality pediatric evidence – rather, it is largely extrapolated from adult trials. Clinical experience has indicated that not all pediatric DVT have the same potential for progression or recurrence and that therapy may be based upon risk factors for good or poor thrombotic outcome [34]. For children with unprovoked DVT it is recommended to continue anticoagulation for at least 6 to 12 months. The decision to continue therapy beyond 6 to 12 months may be based on family and physician preference to avoid the unknown risk of recurrence. The inconvenience of therapy, potential impact of therapy on growth and development and bleeding risk associated with anticoagulation should be taken into consideration in the discussion of anticoagulation duration. In children with recurrent unprovoked DVT, indefinite treatment with VKA is recommended.

For children with provoked DVT (sometimes also called "secondary," but not to be confused with "recurrent" [i.e., second or more] episodes of DVT) in whom the risk factors have resolved, it is recommended to administer anticoagulation therapy for 3 months. If the potentially reversible risk factor has not resolved or been controlled (e.g., ongoing use of CVC, asparaginase therapy, active nephrotic syndrome, etc.), anticoagulation is often continued in either therapeutic or prophylactic doses until the risk factor has resolved. Patients with underlying prothombotic conditions characterized by intermittent symptomatic acute flares of the disease in whom DVT develops during such a flare are often managed, after an initial 3-month course, with episodic secondary prophylaxis during subsequent episodes of symptomatic flare. (Systemic lupus erythematosus is somtimes an exception to the aforementioned paradigm of episodic secondary prophylaxis, wherein an unusually high risk of recurrent VTE may be perceived in this disorder.) Episodic DVT prophylaxis requires that patients are reliable and capable to promptly contact their provider and/ or seek medical attention during flares. In patients who experienced asparaginase-associated TE complications, the administration of anticoagulation as secondary prophylaxis for a transient period following subsequent asparaginase doses has enabled this important anti-neoplastic agent to be safely and effectively continued [50,51]. In children with recurrent DVT with an existing reversible risk, anticoagulation is recommended until resolution of the precipitating factor, but for a minimum of 3 months.

In children with CVC-related DVT, management is dependent upon the requirement to maintain the CVC. If the CVC is no longer required, or is not functioning, the CVC should be removed after 3–5 days of therapeutic anticoagulation [1]. If the CVC is required and the CVC is still functioning, it is suggested to keep the CVC and give anticoagulation for 3 months at therapeutic doses. After the initial 3 months, prophylactic doses of VKAs or LMWH are typically maintained until the CVC is removed

(Table 1.1). If recurrent DVT occurs while the patient is receiving prophylactic therapy, it is suggested to increase to therapeutic dosing and maintain this regimen for a minimum of 3 months following recurrence and until the CVC is removed [1].

There is no direct evidence to guide the optimal antithrombotic management, including intensity and duration of therapy, for DVT in children with laboratory evidence of thrombophilia. Thus, universal thrombophilia testing after a first episode of DVT in children is not cost-effective when used solely to determine anticoagulation duration [52]. However, some inherited thrombophilias have been associated with increased VTE recurrence risk, and the extrapolated indication of anticoagulation in children is the prevention of recurrent VTE; therefore, evaluation for thrombophilia is not unreasonable in order to inform therapeutic discussions and decision-making with patients/parents, in the absence of RCT-derived evidence on optimal duration of anticoagulation. Nevertheless, according to current guidelines the treatment of DVT in children should not be influenced by the presence or absence of laboratory thrombophilia [1]. An exception to this recommendation may be considered for select case scenarios, such as children with unprovoked DVT who are diagnosed with persistent (positive twice, at least 12 weeks apart) antiphospholipid antibodies (APLA), who should remain on long-term anticoagulation [32,53]. Optimal duration of anticoagulation in children with provoked VTE who meet criteria for antiphospholipid antibody syndrome is less clearly defined. For further detail on considerations for diagnostic evaluation of inherited and acquired thrombophilia in children, the reader is referred to other chapters.

Progression of DVT on therapeutic anticoagulation is a relatively uncommon, but clinically challenging, concern in children. If progression occurs on VKA therapy despite a therapeutic target INR range of 2 to 3, it is recommended to resume UFH or LMWH. Subsequently, therapeutic options include treatment with LMWH at usual therapeutic doses, or switching to VKA using a higher therapeutic INR of 3 to 4 or addition of aspirin to VKA therapy [1]. If progression occurs on LMWH, increasing the dose of LMWH to a higher targeted anti-factor Xa activity can be considered. Severe thrombophilia, such as a high titer APLA or severe deficiency of protein C, protein S or antithrombin, should be considered in children who develop progressive or recurrent thrombosis while on therapeutic anticoagulation. For further details on the diagnosis and management of children with severe thrombophilia, the reader is referred to other chapters.

Ancillary treatments: thrombolysis and IVC filters

Thrombolytic therapy offers the possibility of achieving more rapid resolution of vessel occlusion than is achieved with conventional anticoagulant therapy but is associated with an increased risk of bleeding. Thrombolysis can be given systemically, catheter-directed or in combination with mechanical thrombectomy. The role of thrombolysis for treating occlusive proximal limb DVT in children is controversial [54]. The UK guidelines recommend considering the use of thrombolytic therapy in children with extensive DVT, particularly those involving the pelvic veins, SVC, IVC and intracardiac sites [32]. Others have suggested systemic thrombolytic therapy for occlusive SVC, IVC and iliac DVT if symptoms are present for no more than 14 days and catheter-directed thrombectomy/ thrombolysis if symptoms are present for more than 14 days or there is no recanalization after 24–48 hours of systemic thrombolytic therapy [34]. As the potential bleeding risk associated with thrombolytic therapy is not negligible, when thrombolytic therapy is being considered, management decisions should be made with a multidisciplinary team including pediatric hematologists, interventional radiologists with pediatric experience, pediatric pharmacists and pediatric intensivists [55]. Percutaneous or surgical intervention may be needed for management of DVT secondary to vascular structural abnormalities such as thoracic outlet syndrome, interrupted duplex vena cava, etc. [56]. For children with recurrent DVT secondary to structural venous abnormalities, it is recommended to treat with indefinite anticoagulation unless successful percutaneous or surgical intervention can be performed [1]. For a detailed discussion of thrombolytic modalities and evidence, the reader is referred to other chapters.

The most important indication for the use of IVC filter in both adults and children is the prevention of pulmonary embolism (PE) in patients with lower limb, pelvic, or IVC DVT in whom systemic anticoagulation is contraindicated either on a temporary or long-term basis [32]. Progression of lower limb DVT on adequate anticoagulation therapy may also be an indication for an IVC filter [1]. Prophylactic IVC filter placement may be considered before endovascular thrombolysis for lower extremity DVT. Retrievable filters should be used in children for appropriate indications [57]. Size is a significant limitation and thus an IVC filter would not be suitable for children < 10 kg. The filter should be removed as soon as possible if thrombosis is not present in the basket of the filter and when contraindication to anticoagulation is resolved [1]. A summary of retrospective reports of 61 children (age 7–12 years), who underwent IVC filter placement, found that all reported IVC filter placements were technically successful without any complications [57–59]. Filter retrieval was successful in 22 of 28 attempted (79%) at 1–115 days post-insertion [57,58]. Complications during retrieval included IVC stenosis, successfully treated with angioplasty and contained IVC perforation. Successful insertion and retrieval of IVC filter was reported in three young children (2–3 years of age) [60].

Outcomes

Death

The mortality rate of children with DVT is largely attributed to their underlying disease. In the Canadian Childhood Thrombophilia Registry, the all-cause mortality was 16%, while the mortality rate directly attributable to the DVT event was 2.2% [61]. Similarly, in the Netherlands Registry, the mortality rate directly attributable to DVT was 2% [62].

Thrombus resolution

Vascular recanalization after DVT is believed to possibly help prevent recurrent thrombosis and the development of PTS [63]. Nevertheless, the extent to which thrombus resolution or decrease in thrombus extent is relevant to clinical outcomes remains unclear, both in children and adults. Hence, historically these measures have not been included among the main efficacy outcomes in registration trials of new anticoagulants seeking an indication for VTE treatment.

A series of 160 children consecutively treated for a non-cerebral VTE using enoxaparin for at least 5 consecutive days showed a complete thrombus resolution rate of 48% [64]. The rate of resolution was lower for occlusive compared to non-occlusive thrombus. Age at time of event (neonates vs. non-neonates), location, initial treatment (UFH vs. LMWH) and dose of enoxaparin were not related to outcome [64]. In children who developed thrombosis during cardiac surgery, the rate of resolution at last follow-up (at least 2 years after surgery) was 62% [65]. Factors associated with thrombus resolution were location (intrathoracic, 75%; extrathoracic arterial, 89%; extrathoracic venous, 60%), non-occlusive thrombi, older age at surgery, higher white blood cell count and lower fibrinogen after surgery. In a series of children with cancer and DVT, the rate of complete thrombus resolution was 67% [49]. Achievement of therapeutic anti-Xa activity was not related to outcome.

Bleeding

Bleeding as a complication of antithrombotic therapy is an important morbidity in VTE patients. The reported bleeding risk in the Netherlands Registry was around 7% [62]. The risk for bleeding depends on patient-related factors (i.e., underlying disease, concomitant therapies, etc.) and antithrombotic therapy-related factors (i.e., type of therapy, dose and duration). Bleeding is estimated to occur in 20% of children during a therapeutic course of oral vitamin K antagonists and 17% receiving LMWH; using standard definitions "major" hemorrhage occurs in 2–4% [1]. The recommended management of antithrombotic therapy-induced bleeding depends on the type of therapy and severity and extent of bleeding [1].

VTE recurrence

The rate of DVT recurrence in children has been reported at 3.5% to 8% [41,61,62] at variable follow-up periods. In the Canadian registry the rate of recurrence was higher in older children [61]. In a single-center study, neither duration of enoxaparin therapy, nor quality of therapy (i.e., time of recommended anti-Xa levels of 0.5–1 IU/ml), were protective against recurrent DVT [66]. The impact of inherited thrombophilia on the risk of DVT recurrence in children was summarized in a systematic meta-analysis [67]. Recurrence was associated with all inherited thrombophilia traits except the factor V variant and elevated lipoprotein(a). Elevated D-dimer and factor VIII levels have also been associated with the development of a composite measure of poor outcome following VTE in children, in which recurrent VTE was a key component [73].

Post-thrombotic syndrome

Post-thrombotic syndrome is a syndrome of chronic venous insufficiency following DVT secondary to venous hypertension that develops as a result of venous valvular reflux, thrombotic veno-occlusion, or other causes of impaired venous return [68,69]. In a systematic review, the frequency of PTS following upper or lower extremity DVT was 26% (95% CI: 23–28%) among a total of nearly 1,000 children studied [70]. Individual studies have suggested that younger age, obesity, lack of thrombus resolution, number of vessels involved in the initial DVT, delayed initiation of anticoagulation, and elevated D-dimer and factor VIII levels are associated with development of PTS in children [70–73].

Adults who developed PTS had significantly worse quality of life (QoL) compared to those who did not develop PTS [74]. The QoL of patients with PTS was worse than in patients with other chronic diseases (e.g., chronic respiratory conditions and angina) and worse in patients with more severe PTS. No QoL data are available in children with PTS. Development of PTS in adults has been associated with an increased economic burden [75]. Again no pediatric data exist, but one might assume that this burden is even greater when PTS has earlier onset – i.e., in childhood.

Symptoms of PTS include persistent or intermittent swelling, aching pain, heaviness, cramps, itching or tingling in the affected limb and fatigue with exertion. Symptoms in the lower extremities may be aggravated by standing or walking and improve with resting, leg elevation and supine position [68]. Physical findings of PTS in the lower limb include edema, dilated superficial collateral veins, perimalleolar or more extensive telangiectasia, secondary varicose veins, brownish pigmentation of stasis dermatitis and venous eczema. Lipodermatosclerosis, brawny tender thickening of the subcutaneous tissues of the medial lower limb, may occur. In severe cases, venous leg ulcers, which can be precipitated by minor trauma, can occur and are generally chronic, painful and slow to heal. In the upper extremity, there may be dilation of the superficial veins of the upper arm and chest wall and dependent cyanosis of the arm.

The diagnosis of PTS is based on the development of characteristic symptoms and signs in a patient with prior DVT. Two main clinical scales for diagnosing and grading PTS were developed for children – the modified Villalta scale and the Manco-Johnson instrument [69,72]. In the modified Villalta scale, individual symptoms and signs are graded on a scale of 0–2. The symptom and sign scores are added together to provide a final numerical score that is categorized as mild, moderate or severe PTS [72]. The Manco-Johnson instrument includes physical examination findings (basic Clinical–Etiologic–Anatomic–Pathologic [CEAP] assessment) and assessment of pain-related functional limitations using the Wong–Baker "faces" pain scale at rest, in activities of daily living and during age-appropriate aerobic physical activity [69].

Currently, there is insufficient justification to advocate for use of one measure over the other for the assessment of PTS after lower and upper DVT [76,77]. While both scales are feasible for clinical use, each scale has its strengths and weaknesses. The modified Villalta scale that reports graded severity of PTS and was used in cohorts from different institutions, was never internally validated. The Manco-Johnson instrument that reports functional limitation and was internally validated was only used in a few institutions [76]. Both scales lack assessment of PTS-related QoL and loss of venous access, an important measure especially for PTS in the upper venous system [77]. Whenever feasible, both instruments should be administered in clinical investigation of childhood PTS. A training video has been developed for the administration of the Manco-Johnson instrument [78] and for the original (adult) Villalta score [38].

To minimize confounding by acute thrombotic veno-occlusion, diagnosis of PTS should be deferred until at least 6 months following the acute DVT event [76]. The Subcommittee of the International Society on Thrombosis and Haemostasis (ISTH) Scientific and Standardization Committee has advocated for a time point of 6 months post-event as constituting "possible PTS" and 12 or more months as indicating "definitive PTS," restricted by confirmation on two independent PTS evaluations performed at least 3 months apart [76]. In a single center cohort study, the severity of PTS fluctuated in 11/33 (33%) children over a median interval of 12 months from the diagnosis of DVT [63]. Still, in another cohort study, all cases of PTS at 2 years following diagnosis of DVT had been detected already at 1 year post-DVT [73]. Whether the fluctuation observed over approximately the initial year post-DVT in the former study is due to natural history of PTS or to limitations in inter- and intrarater reliability of a given instrument, or both, is not yet clear.

With regard to DVT case identification, in a patient with clinical manifestations compatible with PTS, with no definitive prior history of DVT, further investigations such as CUS are useful to detect a previously undiagnosed DVT. Although by definition, PTS cannot be diagnosed without an antecedent venous thrombosis, the Working Group for definition of PTS in children recognized the importance of vessel injury secondary to the use of CVCs, and of CVC-related asymptomatic thrombosis [77]. Indeed, physical and functional findings similar to those reported in PTS have been reported secondary to the use of CVCs [79–82]. Treatment of PTS is limited. In adults, the cornerstone of managing PTS is compression therapy, primarily using elastic compression stockings (ECSs) [83]. There are no published controlled studies on the effectiveness of ECSs in children with PTS. A successful use of ECS in a 6-year-old child with PTS was reported [84]. In adults, venoactive medications, such as aescin (horse chestnut extract) or rutosides, may offer short-term improvement of PTS symptoms [85]. Exercise training was associated with improved PTS-related QoL and reduced severity of PTS [86]. Mechanical options that reduce edema and improve symptoms such as intermittent pneumatic compression units and a VenoWave device have also been used with some success [87]. Surgical and endovascular treatment of moderate to severe PTS was shown to have some potential in adults when medical treatments have failed [88]. Unfortunately, no published data are available for the use of venoactive medications, exercise training, mechanical and/or surgical treatments in children. Most experts will suggest using ECSs as reasonable first-line approach for children with PTS, as there may be symptomatic benefit, and unlikely harm. Exercise and reduction in excess body weight, when appropriate, are also reasonable choices. Other options of treatment should be considered on a case-by-case basis. Surgical treatments of venous disease have been largely unsuccessful due to low flow in the venous system and surgical venous bypass has been complicated by a high rate of early venous reocclusion. If considered, surgical attempts may be deferred in a small child until full growth of the venous system has been achieved. Future multicenter studies are needed for assessing the efficacy of the different treatment options in children with PTS. Given the limited treatment options, VTE primary and secondary prevention (albeit with limited evidence on primary prevention in children – see also other chapters on VTE prevention) remain the principal means for PTS prevention. Once a DVT has occurred, prompt initiation of appropriate anticoagulation, consideration of thrombolysis in selected cases as noted above, use of ECSs, and prevention of recurrent ipsilateral DVT by appropriate intensity and duration of anticoagulation therapy could be protective regarding the risk and severity of PTS. The use of knee-high ECSs 30–40 mmHg for up to 2 years post-DVT was suggested to prevent PTS in adults [89], although the conclusiveness of such studies has been debated. The efficacy of ECSs for PTS prevention in children with DVT has not been studied. Experience shows that children and families often resist the use of ECSs because of discomfort, concerns regarding physical appearance, peer acceptance and stigma, and expense. The need for an adequately fitted garment requires a garment fitter with pediatric experience, and reassessment/replacement with wear and patient growth.

Conclusions

Although DVT has become an increasingly recognized complication in children, most of the recommendations for diagnosis and management of DVT in children are based on extrapolations from adults. Nevertheless, anticoagulation is the standard of care. Future studies are needed to establish evidence for the standard of care, systematically evaluate long-term outcomes, and investigate the role and performance of newer antithrombotic approaches.

References

1. Monagle P, Chan AK, Goldenberg NA, Ichord RN, Journeycake JM, Nowak-Gottl U, et al. Antithrombotic therapy in neonates and children: Antithrombotic Therapy and Prevention of Thrombosis, 9th ed: American College of Chest Physicians Evidence-Based Clinical Practice Guidelines. Chest 2012;141(2 Suppl): e737S–801S.

2. Mitchell LG, Goldenberg NA, Male C, Kenet G, Monagle P, Nowak-Gottl U. Definition of clinical efficacy and safety outcomes for clinical trials in deep venous thrombosis and pulmonary embolism in children. J Thromb Haemostasis 2011;9(9):1856–8.

3. Andrew M, David M, Adams M, Ali K, Anderson R, Barnard D, et al. Venous thromboembolic complications (VTE) in children: first analyses of the Canadian Registry of VTE. Blood 1994;83(5):1251–7.

4. Setty BA, O'Brien SH, Kerlin BA. Pediatric venous thromboembolism in the United States: A tertiary care complication of chronic diseases. Pediatr Blood Cancer 2012;59(2):258–64.

5. Kerlin BA. Current and future management of pediatric venous thromboembolism. Am J Hematol 2012;87(Suppl 1):S68–74.

6. Raffini L, Huang YS, Witmer C, Feudtner C. Dramatic increase in venous thromboembolism in children's hospitals in the United States from 2001 to 2007. Pediatrics 2009;124(4):1001–8.

7. Spentzouris G, Scriven RJ, Lee TK, Labropoulos N. Pediatric venous thromboembolism in relation to adults. J Vasc Surg 2012;55(6):1785–93.

8. Sandoval JA, Sheehan MP, Stonerock CE, Shafique S, Rescorla FJ, Dalsing MC. Incidence, risk factors, and treatment patterns for deep venous thrombosis in hospitalized children: an increasing population at risk. J Vasc Surg 2008;47(4):837–43.

9. Setty BA, O'Brien SH, Kerlin BA. Pediatric venous thromboembolism in the United States: a tertiary care complication of chronic diseases. Pediatr Blood Cancer 2012;59(2):258–64.

10. Chalmers EA. Epidemiology of venous thromboembolism in neonates and children. Thromb Res 2006;118(1):3–12.

11. Pottecher T, Forrler M, Picardat P, Krause D, Bellocq JP, Otteni JC. Thrombogenicity of central venous catheters: prospective study of polyethylene, silicone and polyurethane catheters with phlebography or post-mortem examination. European Journal of Anaesthesiology 1984;1(4):361–5.

12. Bennegard K, Curelaru I, Gustavsson B, Linder LE, Zachrisson BF. Material thrombogenicity in central venous catheterization. I. A comparison between uncoated and heparin-coated, long antebrachial, polyethylene catheters. Acta Anaesthesiol Scand 1982;26(2):112–20.

13. Curelaru I, Gustavsson B, Hultman E, Jondmundsson E, Linder LE, Stefansson T, et al. Material thrombogenicity in central venous catheterization III. A comparison between soft polyvinylchloride and soft polyurethane elastomer, long, antebrachial catheters. Acta Anaesthesiol Scand 1984;28(2):204–8.

14. Linder LE, Curelaru I, Gustavsson B, Hansson HA, Stenqvist O, Wojciechowski J. Material thrombogenicity in central venous catheterization: a comparison between soft, antebrachial catheters of silicone elastomer and polyurethane. J Parenter Enteral Nutr 1984;8(4):399–406.

15. Anton N, Cox PN, Massicotte MP, Chait P, Yasui Y, Dinyari PM, et al. Heparin-bonded central venous catheters do not reduce thrombosis in infants with congenital heart disease: a blinded randomized, controlled trial. Pediatrics 2009;123(3):e453–8.

16. Gray BW, Gonzalez R, Warrier KS, Stephens LA, Drongowski RA, Pipe SW, et al. Characterization of

central venous catheter-associated deep venous thrombosis in infants. J Pediatr Surg 2012;**47**(6):1159–66.

17. Male C, Julian JA, Massicotte P, Gent M, Mitchell L. Significant association with location of central venous line placement and risk of venous thrombosis in children. Thromb Haemost 2005;**94**(3):516–21.

18. Aiyagari R, Song JY, Donohue JE, Yu S, Gaies MG. Central venous catheter-associated complications in infants with single ventricle: Comparison of umbilical and femoral venous access routes. Pediatr Crit Care Med 2012;**13**(5):549–53.

19. Revel-Vilk S, Ergaz Z. Diagnosis and management of central-line-associated thrombosis in newborns and infants. Semin Fetal Neonatal Med 2011;**16**(6):340–4.

20. van Ommen CH, Tabbers MM. Catheter-related thrombosis in children with intestinal failure and long-term parenteral nutrition: how to treat and to prevent? Thromb Res 2010;**126**(6):465–70.

21. van Rooden CJ, Schippers EF, Barge RM, Rosendaal FR, Guiot HF, van der Meer FJ, et al. Infectious complications of central venous catheters increase the risk of catheter-related thrombosis in hematology patients: a prospective study. J Clin Oncol 2005;**23**(12):2655–60.

22. Raad, II, Luna M, Khalil SA, Costerton JW, Lam C, Bodey GP. The relationship between the thrombotic and infectious complications of central venous catheters. JAMA 1994;**271**(13):1014–16.

23. Hanson SJ, Punzalan RC, Christensen MA, Ghanayem NS, Kuhn EM, Havens PL. Incidence and risk factors for venous thromboembolism in critically ill children with cardiac disease. Pediatr Cardiol 2012;**33**(1):103–8.

24. Alioglu B, Avci Z, Tokel K, Atac FB, Ozbek N. Thrombosis in children with cardiac pathology: analysis of acquired and inherited risk factors. Blood Coagul Fibrinolysis 2008;**19**(4):294–304.

25. Gurgey A, Ozyurek E, Gumruk F, Celiker A, Ozkutlu S, Ozer S, et al. Thrombosis in children with cardiac pathology: frequency of factor V Leiden and prothrombin G20210A mutations. Pediatr Cardiol 2003;**24**(3):244–8.

26. Lipay NV, Zmitrovich AI, Aleinikova OV. Epidemiology of venous thromboembolism in children with malignant diseases: a single-center study of the Belarusian Center for Pediatric Oncology and Hematology. Thromb Res 2011;**128**(2):130–4.

27. O'Brien SH, Klima J, Termuhlen AM, Kelleher KJ. Venous thromboembolism and adolescent and young adult oncology inpatients in US children's hospitals, 2001 to 2008. J Pediatr 2011;**159**(1):133–7.

28. Revel-Vilk S, Yacobovich J, Tamary H, Goldstein G, Nemet S, Weintraub M, et al. Risk factors for central venous catheter thrombotic complications in children and adolescents with cancer. Cancer 2010;**116**(17):4197–205.

29. Bruins B, Masterson M, Drachtman RA, Michaels LA. Deep venous thrombosis in adolescents due to anatomic causes. Pediatr Blood Cancer 2008;**51**(1):125–8.

30. Raffini L, Raybagkar D, Cahill AM, Kaye R, Blumenstein M, Manno C. May-Thurner syndrome (iliac vein compression) and thrombosis in adolescents. Pediatr Blood Cancer 2006;**47**(6):834–8.

31. Brandao LR, Williams S, Kahr WH, Ryan C, Temple M, Chan AK. Exercise-induced deep vein thrombosis of the upper extremity. 2. A case series in children. Acta Haematol 2006;**115**(3–4):221–9.

32. Chalmers E, Ganesen V, Liesner R, Maroo S, Nokes T, Saunders D, et al. Guideline on the investigation, management and prevention of venous thrombosis in children. Br J Haematol 2011;**154**(2):196–207.

33. Kearon C, Julian JA, Newman TE, Ginsberg JS. Noninvasive diagnosis of deep venous thrombosis. McMaster Diagnostic Imaging Practice Guidelines Initiative. Ann Intern Med 1998;**128**(8):663–77.

34. Manco-Johnson MJ. How I treat venous thrombosis in children. Blood 2006;**107**(1):21–9.

35. Male C, Chait P, Ginsberg JS, Hanna K, Andrew M, Halton J, et al. Comparison of venography and ultrasound for the diagnosis of asymptomatic deep vein thrombosis in the upper body in children: results of the PARKAA study. Prophylactic Antithrombin Replacement in Kids with ALL treated with Asparaginase. Thromb Haemost 2002;**87**(4):593–8.

36. Brandao LR, Williams S, Kahr WH, Ryan C, Temple M, Chan AK. Exercise-induced deep vein thrombosis of the upper extremity. 1. Literature review. Acta Haematol 2006;**115**(3–4):214–20.

37. Strouse JJ, Tamma P, Kickler TS, Takemoto CM. D-dimer for the diagnosis of venous thromboembolism in children. Am J Hematol 2009;**84**(1):62–3.

38. Sosothikul D, Seksarn P, Lusher JM. Pediatric reference values for molecular markers in hemostasis. J Pediatr Hematol/Oncol 2007;**29**(1):19–22.

39. Trame MN, Mitchell L, Krumpel A, Male C, Hempel G, Nowak-Gottl U. Population pharmacokinetics of enoxaparin in infants, children and adolescents during secondary thromboembolic prophylaxis: a cohort study. J Thromb Haemost 2010;**8**(9):1950–8.

40. Schobess R, During C, Bidlingmaier C, Heinecke A, Merkel N, Nowak-Gottl U. Long-term safety and efficacy data on childhood venous thrombosis treated with a low molecular weight heparin: an open-label pilot study of once-daily versus twice-daily enoxaparin administration. Haematologica 2006;**91**(12):1701–4.

41. Bidlingmaier C, Kenet G, Kurnik K, Mathew P, Manner D, Mitchell L, et al. Safety and efficacy of low molecular weight heparins in children: a systematic review of the literature and meta-analysis of single-arm studies. Semin Thromb Hemost 2011;**37**(7):814–25.

42. Massicotte P, Julian JA, Gent M, Shields K, Marzinotto V, Szechtman B, et al. An open-label randomized controlled trial of low molecular weight heparin compared to heparin and coumadin for the treatment of venous thromboembolic events in children: the REVIVE trial. Thromb Res 2003;**109**(2–3):85–92.

43. Bauman ME, Black KL, Massicotte MP, Bauman ML, Kuhle S, Howlett-Clyne S, et al. Accuracy of the CoaguChek XS for point-of-care international normalized ratio (INR) measurement in children requiring warfarin. Thromb Haemost 2008;**99**(6):1097–103.

44. Bajolle F, Lasne D, Elie C, Cheurfi R, Grazioli A, Traore M, et al. Home point-of-care international normalised ratio monitoring sustained by a non-selective educational program in children. Thromb Haemost 2012;**108**(4):710–18.

45. Iorio A, Guercini F, Pini M. Low-molecular-weight heparin for the long-term treatment of symptomatic venous thromboembolism: meta-analysis of the randomized comparisons with oral anticoagulants. J Thromb Haemost 2003;**1**(9):1906–13.

46. Rajgopal R, Bear M, Butcher MK, Shaughnessy SG. The effects of heparin and low molecular weight heparins on bone. Thromb Res 2008;**122**(3):293–8.

47. Deitcher SR, Kessler CM, Merli G, Rigas JR, Lyons RM, Fareed J. Secondary prevention of venous thromboembolic events in patients with active cancer: enoxaparin alone versus initial enoxaparin followed by warfarin for a 180-day period. Clin Appl Thromb Hemost 2006;**12**(4):389–96.

48. Lee AY, Levine MN, Baker RI, Bowden C, Kakkar AK, Prins M, et al. Low-molecular-weight heparin versus a coumarin for the prevention of recurrent venous thromboembolism in patients with cancer. N Engl J Med 2003;**349**(2):146–53.

49. Tousovska K, Zapletal O, Skotakova J, Bukac J, Sterba J. Treatment of deep venous thrombosis with low molecular weight heparin in pediatric cancer patients: safety and efficacy. Blood Coagul Fibrinolysis 2009;**20**(7):583–9.

50. Grace RF, Dahlberg SE, Neuberg D, Sallan SE, Connors JM, Neufeld EJ, et al. The frequency and management of asparaginase-related thrombosis in paediatric and adult patients with acute lymphoblastic leukaemia treated on Dana-Farber Cancer Institute consortium protocols. Br J Haematol 2011;**152**(4):452–9.

51. Qureshi A, Mitchell C, Richards S, Vora A, Goulden N. Asparaginase-related venous thrombosis in UKALL 2003 – re-exposure to asparaginase is feasible and safe. Br J Haematol 2010;**149**(3):410–13.

52. O'Brien SH, Smith KJ. Using thrombophilia testing to determine anticoagulation duration in pediatric thrombosis is not cost-effective. J Pediatr 2009;**155**(1):100–4.

53. Kenet G, Aronis S, Berkun Y, Bonduel M, Chan A, Goldenberg NA, et al. Impact of persistent antiphospholipid antibodies on risk of incident symptomatic thromboembolism in children: a systematic review and meta-analysis. Semin Thromb Hemost 2011;**37**(7):802–9.

54. Raffini L. Thrombolysis for intravascular thrombosis in neonates and children. Curr Opin Pediatr 2009;**21**(1):9–14.

55. Kukreja K, Vaidya S. Venous interventions in children. Tech Vasc Interv Radiol 2011;**14**(1):16–21.

56. Arthur LG, Teich S, Hogan M, Caniano DA, Smead W. Pediatric thoracic outlet syndrome: a disorder with serious vascular complications. J Pediatr Surg 2008;**43**(6):1089–94.

57. Kukreja KU, Gollamudi J, Patel MN, Johnson ND, Racadio JM. Inferior vena cava filters in children: our experience and suggested guidelines. J Pediatr Hematol/Oncol 2011;**33**(5):334–8.

58. Raffini L, Cahill AM, Hellinger J, Manno C. A prospective observational study of IVC filters in pediatric patients. Pediatr Blood Cancer 2008;**51**(4):517–20.

59. Cahn MD, Rohrer MJ, Martella MB, Cutler BS. Long-term follow-up of Greenfield inferior vena cava filter placement in children. J Vasc Surg 2001;**34**(5):820–5.

60. Chaudry G, Padua HM, Alomari AI. The use of inferior vena cava filters in young children. J Vasc Interv Radiol 2008;**19**(7):1103–6.

61. Monagle P, Adams M, Mahoney M, Ali K, Barnard D, Bernstein M, et al. Outcome of pediatric thromboembolic disease: a report from the Canadian Childhood Thrombophilia Registry. Pediatr Res 2000;**47**(6):763–6.

62. van Ommen CH, Heijboer H, Buller HR, Hirasing RA, Heijmans HS, Peters M. Venous thromboembolism in childhood: a prospective two-year registry in The Netherlands. J Pediatr 2001;**139**(5):676–81.

63. Creary S, Heiny M, Croop J, Fallon R, Vik T, Hulbert M, et al. Clinical course of postthrombotic syndrome in children with history of venous thromboembolism. Blood Coagul Fibrinolysis 2012;**23**(1):39–44.

64. Revel-Vilk S, Sharathkumar A, Massicotte P, Marzinotto V, Daneman A, Dix D, et al. Natural history of arterial and venous thrombosis in children treated with low molecular weight heparin: a longitudinal study by ultrasound. J Thromb Haemost 2004;**2**(1):42–6.

65. Manlhiot C, Menjak IB, Brandao LR, Gruenwald CE, Schwartz SM, Sivarajan VB, et al. Risk, clinical features, and outcomes of thrombosis associated with pediatric cardiac surgery. Circulation 2011;**124**(14):1511–19.

66. Estepp JH, Smeltzer M, Reiss UM. The impact of quality and duration of enoxaparin therapy on recurrent venous thrombosis in children. Pediatr Blood Cancer 2012;**59**:105–109,

67. Young G, Albisetti M, Bonduel M, Brandao L, Chan A, Friedrichs F, et al. Impact of inherited thrombophilia on venous thromboembolism in children: a systematic review and meta-analysis of observational studies. Circulation 2008;**118**(13):1373–82.

68. Kahn SR. The post-thrombotic syndrome. Hematology Am Soc Hematol Educ Program 2010;**2010**:216–20.

69. Manco-Johnson MJ. Postthrombotic syndrome in children. Acta Haematol 2006;**115**(3–4):207–13.

70. Goldenberg NA, Donadini MP, Kahn SR, Crowther M, Kenet G, Nowak-Gottl U, et al. Post-thrombotic syndrome in children: a systematic review of frequency of occurrence, validity of outcome measures, and prognostic factors. Haematologica 2010;**95**(11):1952–9.

71. Sharathkumar AA, Pipe SW. Post-thrombotic syndrome in children: a single center experience. J Pediatr Hematol/Oncol 2008;**30**(4):261–6.

72. Kuhle S, Koloshuk B, Marzinotto V, Bauman M, Massicotte P, Andrew M, et al. A cross-sectional study evaluating post-thrombotic syndrome in children. Thromb Res 2003;**111**(4–5):227–33.

73. Goldenberg NA, Knapp-Clevenger R, Manco-Johnson MJ. Elevated plasma factor VIII and D-dimer levels as predictors of poor outcomes of thrombosis in children. N Engl J Med 2004;**351**(11):1081–8.

74. Kahn SR, Hirsch A, Shrier I. Effect of postthrombotic syndrome on health-related quality of life after deep venous thrombosis. Arch Intern Med 2002;**162**(10):1144–8.

75. MacDougall DA, Feliu AL, Boccuzzi SJ, Lin J. Economic burden of deep-vein thrombosis, pulmonary embolism, and post-thrombotic syndrome. Am J Health Syst Pharm 2006;**63**(20 Suppl 6):S5–15.

76. Goldenberg NA, Brandao L, Journeycake J, Kahn S, Monagle P, Revel-Vilk S, et al. Definition of post-thrombotic syndrome following lower extremity deep venous thrombosis and standardization of outcome measurement in pediatric clinical investigations. J Thromb Haemost 2012;**10**(3):477–80.

77. Revel-Vilk S, Brandao L, Journeycake J, Goldenberg NA, Monagle P, Sharathkumar A, et al. Standardization of post-thrombotic syndrome definition and outcome assessment following upper venous system thrombosis in pediatric practice. J Thromb Haemost 2012;**10**(10):2182–5.

78. http://www.ucdenver.edu/academics/colleges/medical school/centers/HemophiliaThrombosis/research/kids dott/Pages/KidsDOTT.aspx.

79. Journeycake JM, Eshelman D, Buchanan GR. Post-thrombotic syndrome is uncommon in childhood cancer survivors. J Pediatr 2006;**148**(2):275–7.

80. Kuhle S, Spavor M, Massicotte P, Halton J, Cherrick I, Dix D, et al. Prevalence of post-thrombotic syndrome following asymptomatic thrombosis in survivors of acute lymphoblastic leukemia. J Thromb Haemost 2008;**6**(4):589–94.

81. Ruud E, Holmstrom H, Hopp E, Wesenberg F. Central line-associated venous late effects in children without prior history of thrombosis. Acta Paediatr 2006;**95**:1060–5.

82. Revel-Vilk S, Menahem M, Stoffer C, Weintraub M. Post-thrombotic syndrome after central venous catheter removal in childhood cancer survivors is associated with a history of obstruction. Pediatr Blood Cancer 2010;**55**(1):153–6.

83. Kahn SR. How I treat postthrombotic syndrome. Blood 2009;**114**:4624–31.

84. Biss TT, Kahr WH, Brandao LR, Chan AK, Thomas KE, Williams S. The use of elastic compression stockings for post-thrombotic syndrome in a child. Pediatr Blood Cancer 2009;**53**(3):462–3.

85. Pittler MH, Ernst E. Horse chestnut seed extract for chronic venous insufficiency. Cochrane Database Syst Rev 2006(1):CD003230.

86. Kahn SR, Shrier I, Shapiro S, Houweling AH, Hirsch AM, Reid RD, et al. Six-month exercise training program to treat post-thrombotic syndrome: a randomized controlled two-centre trial. CMAJ 2011;**183**(1):37–44.

87. O'Donnell MJ, McRae S, Kahn SR, Julian JA, Kearon C, Mackinnon B, et al. Evaluation of a venous-return assist device to treat severe post-thrombotic syndrome (VENOPTS). A randomized controlled trial. Thromb Haemost 2008;**99**(3):623–9.

88. Bond RT, Cohen JM, Comerota A, Kahn SR. Surgical treatment of moderate-to-severe post-thrombotic syndrome. Ann Vasc Surg 2013;**27**(2):242–58.

89. Prandoni P, Lensing AW, Prins MH, Frulla M, Marchiori A, Bernardi E, et al. Below-knee elastic compression stockings to prevent the post-thrombotic syndrome: a randomized, controlled trial. Ann Intern Med 2004;**141**(4):249–56.

Pulmonary embolism

Suzan Williams and Michael Wang

Introduction

Pulmonary embolism (PE) in the pediatric population is a relatively rare event.[1] Over the last two decades there has been an increase in the observed occurrence of PE in children (like venous thromboembolism [VTE] more generally), which has been attributed to increased recognition as well as a true increase in incidence stemming from improvements in pediatric care. Concomitant with the increased availability of relatively non-invasive methods of diagnosing PE has been a generally improved survival of previously lethal childhood diseases and an increase in use of central venous catheters (CVC).[2]

The first reported pediatric case appears to have been in 1861, when Loschner described PE in a 9-year-old boy, which followed phlebitis associated with a fracture of the tibia.[3] This case was typical of early case reports of the pre-antibiotic era, when emboli were observed to follow infection, injury to bones and muscle, or deep vein thrombosis.[4] Pediatric PE cases were later reported primarily in autopsy-proven reports. As a result, PE in children was thought to be rare and usually fatal. Autopsy-based studies from the post-antibiotic era later showed an increased prevalence of PE, with a decreased age of affected patients. In addition to infection, other risk factors were established, including congenital heart defect, cancer, and CVC. Pediatric autopsy studies have also shown that fatal, massive pulmonary thromboembolism is a rare event in infants and children. A 50-year autopsy review study reported only eight cases from a total of 17,500 autopsies.[5]

Early reports based on findings from autopsy or case series were of limited value in defining the epidemiology of thrombotic events and were consistent with the under-diagnosis of PE in children, reporting findings of PE in 0.05–4.2% of autopsies.[5–8]

Before 1970, approximately 200 cases of PE in children were reported. From 1968 to 1971, an all-Scottish hospital inpatient pediatric database identified four cases of presumed PE subsequently confirmed by autopsy among 46 cases of VTE (~9%).[9] From 1975 to 1991, 308 pediatric cases with documented deep vein thrombosis (DVT) and/or PE were published in the English and French literature.[10] Two studies from the University of Michigan Medical Center on the overall (1945 to 1954) and pediatric incidences (1955 to 1979) of autopsy-proven PE highlight the evolving profile of pediatric patients diagnosed over time.[8,11]

Epidemiology

The occurrence frequency of pediatric PE in population-based studies has been age- and gender-specific, varying from no reported cases to several per 100,000.[12–14] Studies report 8.6–57 cases of PE per 100,000 admissions in hospitalized children[15,16] and an estimated occurrence of 0.14–0.9 per 100,000 children in the community.[17,18] The variation in occurrence frequency can be explained by differences in sample size, diagnostic criteria, index of suspicion, diagnostic methods, and the inclusion of symptomatic or asymptomatic patients. Given that PE is often clinically silent and masked by symptoms of underlying diseases, even these numbers are likely an underestimate.

In a single-institution study, Buck et al. described findings of PE in 3.7% to 4.2% of autopsies.[8] Thirty-one percent of cases in which the PE was autopsy-proven were considered clinically relevant. In only 50% of the children with clinically relevant PE were there clinical signs and symptoms in retrospect associated with PE, and the diagnosis was only considered in 15% of patients.[8] The overall projected occurrence frequency

Pediatric Thrombotic Disorders, ed. Neil A. Goldenberg and Marilyn J. Manco-Johnson. Published by Cambridge University Press. © Cambridge University Press 2015.

of pediatric PE based on this study was 104 per 100,000 admissions; 25 per 100,000 admissions for clinically important cases.

Two population-based studies (Olmsted County, MN, 1966 to 1990; Germany, 2005 to 2007)[12,14] supported the age and gender dependency of the incidence rate of PE with or without associated DVT. The rates in the male and female subgroupings of age were: (1) Olmsted County study: females – 0 to 14 years: none, 15 to 19 years: 8 per 100,000/year; males – 0 to 14 years: 0.3 per 100,000/year, 15 to 19 years: 4 per 100,000/year; and (2) German Federal Statistical Office study: females – < 10 years: 0–1 per 100,000/year, 10 to 29 years: 11 per 100,000/year; males – < 10 years: 0–1 per 100,000/year, 10 to 29 years: 5–6 per 1 00,000/year).[12,14] In comparison to the incidence in children and young adults, the incidence of PE with or without DVT reaches 690–758 per 100,000/year in those over 85 years of age.[14]

More recently, data collected and published by national and international pediatric thrombosis registries have provided estimated prevalences for thrombotic events, including PE, in neonates and have increased awareness. All databases relied on voluntary submission for data collection, there was no information regarding clinical presentation, imaging, treatment, or outcome of neonatal PE, and as with autopsy studies, it is likely that the incidence of PE was under-reported. From four VTE databases containing neonatal subjects, the International Registry (n = 97), the neonatal German survey for symptomatic thromboembolism (n = 79), the Dutch VTE registry (n = 47), and the 1–800-No-Clots survey (n = 306), the percentage of cases of neonatal VTE with PE ranged from none to 3%.[17,19–21]

Prevalences of PE have subsequently been published by other groups, ranging from 8% to 16% of the total VTE number, depending on the registry.[15,17,19,22] In the first published pediatric registry (data collection: July 1990 to December 1992), the Canadian registry contained subjects aged 1 month to 18 years, with an overall VTE occurrence frequency of 5.3 per 10,000 hospital admissions.[15] Based on the positivity of ventilation–perfusion (V–Q) scans, the calculated PE occurrence was 0.86 per 10,000 admissions, significantly lower than that for hospitalized adults. In the US National Hospital Discharge Survey, which samples 8% of hospitals and 1% of discharges (data collection: ICD codes from 1979 to 2001), the estimated incidence rate of PE, which remained unchanged during the study period, was

0.9 per 100,000/year; the rate was higher between the age ranges of 0 to 1 year and 15 to 17 years (2.2 per 100,000/year and 2.0 per 100,000/year, respectively).[18] The rate of PE in black children was 2.38 (95% CI: 2.29–2.47) times higher than in white children. A large single-center-based report of PE in children disclosed an occurrence frequency of 5.7 per 10,000 admissions, representing an almost seven-fold increment compared with the previously reported Canadian pediatric PE rate.[16] Likewise, Raffini and collaborators reported the rate of VTE admissions to tertiary American children's hospitals from 2001 and 2007, showing a 70% increase of annual VTE/PE admissions from 34 to 58 cases per 10,000 admissions. As pediatric PE represented 11% of all VTE admissions included, the calculated PE rate would approximate 6.4 cases per 10,000, a similar figure to the rate reported at the tertiary Canadian center. The age distribution of children with PE, much like that for VTE more generally, shows a bimodal pattern, with an initial peak in infants < 1 year of age and a second peak during adolescence. In the Canadian registry, infants under 1 year and teenagers predominated. This bimodal higher incidence-rate distribution was subsequently confirmed by the US National Hospital Discharge Survey.[18] In infants < 1 year of age a large minority cases are actually in neonates, as shown in a Dutch report[17] which highlighted that 47% of the PE cases in infancy occurred in neonates.

Predisposing factors

In children, PE is characteristically seen in combination with underlying medical conditions. Spontaneous (i.e., unprovoked) VTE is uncommon, occurring in 0–4% of children with VTE, and truly idiopathic VTE is rare. The increase in PE rates in recent years in children, discussed above, is likely reflective of the increased number of patients placed at risk, as pediatric care has evolved. Cancer, immobility, CVC, vascular malformations, nephrotic syndrome, long-term total parenteral nutrition administration, systemic lupus erythematosus, ventriculoatrial shunts, congenital and/or acquired thrombotic tendencies, and acute DVT are all recognizable risk factors associated with PE in children.[9,10,12,15,17–21] Non-thrombotic types of PE may also occur, including tumor embolism, post-trauma-related fat embolism, septic PE, foreign bodies, and post-bone marrow transplantation cytolytic thrombi.[25–27]

Pulmonary embolism is highly associated with DVT: DVT has been identified in 72% of children presenting with PE.[16,28] Understandably, the most important predisposing factor for PE in childhood is the presence of a CVC, which is increasingly being used in pediatric care for drug administration, parenteral nutrition, and chemotherapy. Several studies have demonstrated a prevalence of CVC in 33% to 64% of children with VTE, which increases further to 89% to 94% in neonates. In adults, approximately 95% of the cases of VTE are attributed to a lower extremity DVT, whereas in children upper extremity DVT is seen in up to 20% of cases.[8,15–17,24,29] Therefore, while an upper extremity CVC may carry a lower risk of thrombosis compared to a lower extremity CVC, the use of upper extremity and jugular/subclavian CVCs placed in small caliber vessels in children remains a significant risk factor.

The presence of multiple coexisting risk factors is typical in children with PE.[8,24,30] Data from a Canadian study showed 12.4% of children with only one associated condition, 39.4% with two conditions, 35% with three conditions, and 9.6% with four conditions predisposing to thrombosis. Infection and congenital heart disease are common risk factors for PE in childhood. Oral contraceptive use is a significant risk factor for thrombosis and PE in adolescents.[31] To date, obesity does not seem to contribute greatly as a risk factor for PE in children,[16,17] but further definitive work is required on this issue. The higher risk of venous thrombosis in adult trauma patients has not been observed in children, with a PE occurrence frequency in pediatric trauma patients of 7 per 100,000.[32]

There is a risk of thromboembolism and PE in children with vascular malformations, particularly of the lower limb, and syndromes associated with these include May–Thurner, Klippel–Trenaunay, CLOVES (congenital lipomatous overgrowth, vascular malformations, and epidermal nevi), and proteus. This is especially relevant with additional concurrent thrombotic risk factors, such as surgery, pregnancy, neoplasm, or trauma.[33,34]

Data from a study in children with a hematological malignancy showed that 2.9% of the patients were diagnosed with symptomatic PE.[35] The etiology of PE in children with malignancy is multifactorial. There is the frequent use of CVC for medications and blood product administration. Furthermore, coagulation abnormalities resulting from the disease itself or the treatment, and damage to the vessel walls or alterations in a number of hemostatic proteins due to the use of particular chemotherapeutic agents such as L-asparaginase, predispose to thrombosis.[36]

In patients with nephrotic syndrome, there is an increased occurrence of PE caused by the development of a hypercoagulable state. This has been attributed to urinary losses of antithrombin and free protein S, elevated FVIII levels, elevated fibrinogen and lipoprotein(a), and hyperaggregability of platelets.[37,38] Pulmonary embolism was demonstrated in 28–40% of asymptomatic screened patients with nephrotic syndrome.[38,39]

In adults, sickle cell disease leads to a four-fold increased risk of developing PE. In a multicenter study looking at outcomes from acute chest syndrome in sickle cell disease, one-third of the deaths that occurred following presentation with acute chest syndrome were due to PE (bone marrow, fat, or thrombotic).[40] Pulmonary infarcts in sickle cell disease are often due to fat embolism from infarcted bone marrow rather than from VTE.[41,42] The risk of PE is not known in children with sickle cell disease.

Pathophysiology

Venous thromboembolism occurs when red blood cells, fibrin, platelets, and leukocytes form a mass within an intact vein. This phenomenon occurs more readily in the presence of one or more components of the Virchow triad: injury to the vessel endothelium, hemostasis, and hypercoagulability. The pathophysiological effects of PE depend on the extent to which it obstructs the pulmonary circulation, coexistent cardiopulmonary disease, and the presence of vasoactive mediators.

The consequences of pulmonary vascular occlusion can range from no or minimal effect to death of tissue (with or without clinically significant infarct) or even death. The major determinants that influence development of an infarct due to PE, and ultimately clinical severity, include vascular territory, rate of occlusion, vulnerability of the affected tissue to hypoxia, and blood oxygen content. The existence of a dual blood supply from both the pulmonary and bronchial arteries minimizes the chances of lung infarct development, especially if occurring in previously healthy patients with an intact bronchial circulation. Slowly developing obstructions are less likely to cause infarction.

Pulmonary tissue is not as sensitive to hypoxia as neuronal or myocardial cells, but coexisting cardio-pulmonary conditions (e.g., congenital heart defects with single ventricle physiology and decreased lung perfusion) can potentiate the decreased lung perfusion already caused by a thrombus. Animal studies have shown that until vascular obstruction reaches around 60% of the vascular territory, symptoms might not occur.[43] In children, unless there is coexistent cardio-pulmonary disease such as pulmonary hypertension or congenital cardiac defects, emboli obstructing < 50% of the pulmonary circulation are usually clinically silent.[44]

Hemodynamic symptoms occur from the fall in the systemic blood pressure. In cases of massive PE, the acute dilation of the right ventricle (RV) with concomitant restraining of the pericardium leads to reduced left ventricular compliance and impaired left ventricle end diastolic volume. Increased RV pressure may result in compression of the right coronary artery with cardiac ischemia[44,45] and circulatory failure.[46] A large enough obstruction may be fatal.[47] A recently published mixed prospective/retrospective cohort study of 58 consecutive children with PE showed that at presentation nearly half of the children had hypoxemia and 37% had tachycardia.[30]

Coexisting cardiopulmonary conditions (e.g., congenital heart conditions with single ventricle physiology and decreased lung perfusion) will increase the sensitivity of pulmonary tissue to hypoxia. The physiological responses to vascular obstruction are amplified by arterial hypoxemia secondary to ventilation–perfusion mismatch, right-to-left shunt, and low pressure of oxygen in the venous blood. The release of vasoactive agents (e.g., thromboxane or serotonin), can cause vasospasm of previously unobstructed vessels and ensuing pulmonary hypertension potentiating the decreased lung perfusion already caused by a thrombus.[48–50]

Decreased blood flow to areas affected by vessel blockage causes an increase in alveolar dead space (i.e., ventilated areas that are not being perfused), decreasing the lung efficiency to eliminate CO_2. Depending on the existence and/or severity of a pre-existing condition, the physiologic response of both the respiratory (hyperventilation) and circulatory systems may not support collateralization, impacting negatively on the alveolar–arterial oxygen tension gradient.[51] Additional contributors to hypoxemia include atelectasis, lung tissue infarction, patent foramen ovale, or reflex bronchoconstriction.[52]

Clinical signs

In 1878, Gerhardt gave one of the earliest descriptions of pulmonary infarction in children. He described that at first, physical signs included coarse rales followed a few days later by "dullness on percussion, increased vocal fremitus and bronchial breathing." The clinical findings of PE in children are similar to the ones encountered in adults. However, their recognition remains challenging. The diagnosis of PE based on clinical signs is difficult, because the presentation can be non-specific, young children cannot accurately describe their symptoms, underlying primary disorders or comorbid conditions may have clinical symptoms similar to those of PE, and the excellent cardiopulmonary reserve of children may minimize the hemodynamic effects of a large PE. Therefore, the diagnosis of PE may be missed completely in children, as seen in autopsy studies,[8] or delayed. The suspicion of the diagnosis by clinicians may be low.[53] Rajpurkar et al. reported that diagnoses in children were made on average 7 days (range 1–21 days) after the onset of symptoms. The most common reason for a delayed diagnosis (up to 3 weeks) was the presumptive diagnosis of pneumonia.

Classic clinical symptoms of a PE in children include shortness of breath, pleuritic chest pain, and hemoptysis.[17,54] In general, only large PEs result in such classic symptoms, whereas the presentation of smaller emboli may be subtle and mimic other diseases. In one study of adolescents diagnosed with PE, the most common presenting sign reported was pleuritic pain, seen in 84% of the patients.[31] Dyspnea (58%), cough (47%), and hemoptysis (32%) were other frequent complaints.

Presenting signs in teenagers include arterial hypoxemia, physical signs of a DVT of the lower extremity, tachypnea, and fever. Unexplained persistent tachypnea can be an important indication of pulmonary embolism in pediatric patients of all age categories.[55] Other documented signs include pulmonary hypertension, acute right heart failure, cyanosis, hypotension, dysrhythmia, pallor, syncope, cardiopulmonary arrest, or sudden death.[16,44,56,57] Rarely, PE can present with abdominal pain, resulting from diaphragmatic irritation/pleurisy or hepatic congestion.[58]

The variability of signs and symptoms illustrated in a comparison of five single-center pediatric studies is likely a result of the diversity of underlying conditions and the patients' ages.[16,24,31,59,60] From a pediatric case–control study containing mostly adolescents, shortness of breath and pleuritic pain were less likely to occur in the adolescents with proven PE in comparison to control adolescents in whom PE was judged to be highly likely on clinical evaluation but not present on imaging evaluation (69% vs. 96%, p = 0.03).[60] A similarly decreased frequency of symptoms was described in another cohort of adolescents diagnosed with PE, where dyspnea was less commonly reported in comparison to adults.[31] Asymptomatic events were highest (16%) in the report from Biss et al. (mean age, 12 years), and this cohort was comprised of 70% hospitalized patients in whom PE diagnosis was more frequently made based upon thoracic imaging obtained for other reasons, and included younger patients.[16]

Physical findings include hypoxemia, fever, DVT of the lower extremity, tachypnea, increased second heart sound, and abnormal breathing sounds. Pleurisy with friction rub may be present. Tachypnea, increased second heart sound, and abnormal breathing sounds occur less in adolescents when compared with adults.[31] If there are symptoms and signs consistent with a PE, the differential diagnosis includes pneumonia, atelectasis, intrathoracic malignancies, and trauma. Clinical suspicion plays a major role in recognition of cases.

Diagnosis of pulmonary embolism

In children, individual symptoms and signs have low sensitivity and specificity for predicting a diagnosis of PE.[60] This is quite different from the scenario for adults, where clinical prediction rules for PE have been validated. Among the most commonly used predictive rules in adults is the Wells simplified score[61] and the Geneva score,[62] which combine clinical signs and the presence of risk factors to assess the pretest probability of PE. The combination of a low clinical probability score and the negative D-dimer estimation improves the negative predictive value further and may safely exclude PE without the need for diagnostic imaging in adult patients. In children, such prediction rules have not been validated. Even when the Wells score was adapted for its use in children, it lacked discerning power between PE positive and negative children.[63]

The diagnosis of PE is difficult, and relies on clinical suspicion that takes into account the child's risk factors for PE including underlying illness, external factors such as trauma or CVC, and clinical signs and symptoms. Dyspnea, chest pain, cough, hypoxia, hemoptysis, tachycardia, and syncope raise suspicion of PE;[57,64] however, the child often cannot describe their symptoms with adequate accuracy so this additional information becomes non-specific, incomplete, or even confusing. Physical exam findings may be more sensitive but hypoxia, tachycardia, and abnormal breath sounds still lack specificity. The pairing of D-dimer and clinical probability score may not be valid to use in children. Arterial blood gases also lack sufficient sensitivity and specificity. Because of all of these factors the diagnosis of PE in children can be delayed; therefore it is the clinician's heightened awareness and acumen that integrates all of a child's risk factors and initiates the diagnostic evaluation of PE.

Electrocardiogram (ECG)

An abnormal ECG in a child with suspected PE supports the diagnosis, but an abnormal ECG is not sufficiently sensitive or specific to diagnose PE. Abnormal ECGs reflect cardiac changes secondary to the development of cor pulmonale and/or right ventricular strain; Q-wave and T-wave inversion in lead three, as well as the classical S1Q3T3 pattern, are associated with PE in adults, and these findings have not been confirmed by prospective studies in children.[30,65] A recently published mixed prospective/retrospective cohort study of 58 consecutive children with PE showed that at presentation, the classic electrocardiographic finding of S1Q3T3 was present in 12% acutely.[30] Furthermore, ECG interpretation is age dependent, and age-appropriate parameters have not been validated as a diagnostic tool for PE in children.

Chest X-ray

The chest X-ray is not particularly useful for diagnosing PE as it is often normal, but can be helpful in excluding other conditions, such as pneumothorax or pneumonia.[56,60] It may also aid in the interpretation of a V–Q scan. Non-specific signs seen in patients with PE include parenchymal infiltrates, atelectasis, and ipsilateral pleural effusion. Its lack of sensitivity and specificity has been shown in adolescents.[60] More specific signs include Westermark's sign (oligemia in parts of the lung affected by the emboli) and Hampton's hump (a peripheral wedge-shaped density with the peak directed to the hilum) but are uncommonly demonstrated.[57,66] In the prospective investigation of pulmonary embolism diagnosis (PIOPED) study, the most common abnormal finding was atelectasis and/or parenchymal areas of increased opacity.[67] However, the prevalence was not significantly different from that in patients without PE. This appears similar to a small single-institution pediatric series.[60]

Pulmonary angiography

The "gold standard" for diagnosing PE is pulmonary angiography for children and adults. Its primary advantage is that it can be diagnostic but also give potentially important hemodynamic data about the patient. The 3-month incidence of recurrent VTE after a normal pulmonary angiogram has been reported to be 1.7%, and fatal PE occurred in 0.3% of the patients.[68] The PIOPED study reported a low morbidity and mortality of the procedure, 5% and 0.5% respectively, and definitive diagnosis was obtained in up to 96% of the patients with PE;[69] a negative study may allow anticoagulation to be safely withheld.[70,71] Although low, this reported morbidity and mortality still exceeds other diagnostic modalities useful in diagnosing PE,[67] and the complexity of the images leads to less than acceptable interpreter agreement.[72] Pulmonary angiography is also an invasive and expensive procedure, and not available in every medical center. For children, it requires sedation and technical expertise, especially with neonates. Because of these limitations, pulmonary angiography is being replaced by less invasive methods,[73] and used only when these less invasive diagnostic tests give indeterminate results.[74]

Radionuclide scintigraphy (V–Q scan)

In children, perfusion scintigraphy (V–Q scan) has replaced pulmonary angiography. It is considered safe and sensitive and does not require iodinated contrast agents. In the absence of cardiac and pulmonary disease, a normal scan effectively rules out a PE. The V–Q scan has two components. Initially, the patients inhale an aerosolized radioisotope (Tc99m) that is allowed to distribute throughout the lungs (ventilation), after which images are obtained in multiple projections. Because of the inhalation technique needed for the first component of the test, younger children will likely be incapable of performing a V–Q scan. Next, [99]TC macroaggregated albumin is infused by bolus injection (perfusion), and images are obtained. These two sets of images are then compared along with the chest X-ray to detect areas where there is adequate ventilation but poor perfusion, which identifies an area with PE. A limitation of this technique is for patients with congenital heart defects whose lesions may limit the total pulmonary blood flow. In addition, lesions with right-to-left shunting may allow [99]TC macroaggregated albumin to enter and lodge in cerebral vasculature with unknown sequelae.

The V–Q scans are interpreted using criteria that have been adapted but not validated from PIOPED.[67,75] These criteria separate patients' V–Q scans into high, intermediate, and low probability. However, a high probability V–Q scan in adults has low sensitivity of 40% but a high specificity of 98%. Thus, the best diagnostic results occur when V–Q scan results are concordant with the clinical assessment. In addition, there are often patients with non-diagnostic scans, and 75% of patients with clinically suspected PE have low or intermediate probability V–Q scans, not high probability scans. Because of these data there was need for further diagnostic investigation, and the V–Q scan began losing favor to CT pulmonary angiography.

Computed tomography pulmonary angiography (CTPA)

Multidetector CTPA is becoming the diagnostic modality of choice for diagnosing PE. The clinical validity of a negative scan to rule out PE is similar to pulmonary angiography.[76] It offers additional qualities: speed, ability to evaluate for other disorders when PE is not found,[77] and discrimination to the sixth-order pulmonary artery branches.[78] It can also assess the size of the RV in patients with larger PE.[79,80] It does however require a brief time of immobility and breath-holding (1–6 seconds) and a large enough IV for rapid pump injection of iodinated contrast.

In the PIOPED II,[81] an adult study that has not been validated in children, CTPA showed a sensitivity of 83% and specificity of 95%, and was non-inferior to V–Q scanning when ruling out PE. The sensitivity increased to 95% when CT venography (CTV) was used; however, in pediatric practice, lower extremity Doppler ultrasonography would be more likely obtained as it poses no risk of ionizing radiation. As there are no prospective studies we can only speculate that the additional imaging of the lower extremity would indeed increase sensitivity. Pooled adult data revealed that the false positive rate was 9.3% and the false negative rate was 2.4% for PE detected by multidetector CTPA. With the increased sensitivity comes the question of the clinical importance of small subsegmental PE.[82] Kritsaneepaiboon *et al.* reviewed within a single institution the results of consecutive multidetector CTPA for PE in children and found a prevalence of 15%, which compares with the 23.3% from PIOPED II.[77] Finally, a meta-analysis of 23 studies looking at 4657 adult patients (some with single detector CTPA) who had a negative CTPA and received no anticoagulation found that at 3 months the subsequent rate of VTE was 1.4% and fatal PE rate was 0.51%.[83] This is comparable to conventional pulmonary angiogram.[68]

An increasing concern about the use of CT is exposure of children to iatrogenic ionizing radiation from diagnostic procedures, especially to tissues sensitive to radiation such as the thyroid gland, breast tissue and gonads, and for the concern of developing a malignancy.[84] Many studies now utilize lower-dose CT imaging algorithms. Other caveats to CTPA are the use of contrast in patients with renal insufficiency, pregnancy, and allergy to iodinated contrast.

Magnetic resonance pulmonary angiography (MRPA)

Without the use of radiation, MRPA is an alternative to CTPA in evaluating patients for PE, except for neonates and infants, where gadolinium is not approved in the USA. In PIOPED III,[85] MRPA evaluation in adults had a sensitivity of 78% and a specificity of 99%. Analogous to PIOPED II, when venography (MRV) was used sensitivity increased to 92% while preserving specificity at 96%. An important additional finding of the study was that 52% of subjects did not have a technically adequate study, suggesting that more experienced centers perform the procedure better. There are only limited data at individual institutions using MRPA in children and no outcome study based on diagnosis by MRPA is available. Despite the advantages MRPA does have limitations. Because of the length of imaging time, young children will need anesthesia, and critically ill patients may not be able to have the procedure because of limited monitoring. Children old enough to not require anesthesia may still find it difficult to hold their breath for the time necessary for a diagnostic scan. Moreover, given the technical difficulties to obtain adequate images, access to experienced centers that can reliably perform this diagnostic technique is limited.

Echocardiography

In unstable patients echocardiography can be performed at the bedside without sedation, or when more invasive procedures would not be tolerated. It is useful in these patients to determine massive PE, and the function of the RV including RV dilatation, hypokinesis, abnormal interventricular septal movement, tricuspid regurgitation, and lack of collapse of the inferior vena cava (IVC) during inspiration.[86] It can also detect thrombus in atria and around central venous lines. In neonates, echocardiography may be preferred when contrast, transport, and vessel size limit the usefulness of the other diagnostic modalities discussed above.[87] In one study, tricuspid regurgitation greater than 3 meters per second, septal flattening, and RV dilatation were each present on acute echocardiogram in 25%.[30]

Extremity imaging

Venography, akin to pulmonary angiography, is the "gold standard" for imaging the extremities for VTE. Much like pulmonary angiography, non-invasive or minimally invasive imaging is now becoming the standard.[87] In children, Doppler ultrasonography is used for diagnosis of VTE and can often define the distal and proximal end of the thrombus as well as the degree to which the vessels are occluded. Vasculature in the pelvis and central upper venous system are difficult to image with Doppler ultrasound, and modalities such as MRV and CTV may be more reliable. There is currently no widely accepted or validated treatment algorithm incorporating extremity imaging, although this may increase the sensitivity of other studies used to diagnose PE.

Treatment of pulmonary embolism

Acute PE can clinically manifest itself in ways that delay diagnosis, but once the diagnosis is achieved, it should be treated promptly as it can be rapidly life-threatening (Figure 2.1). In unstable patients where the clinical index of suspicion is high, empiric treatment may be started while awaiting diagnostic confirmation. Treatment of children with PE has been extrapolated from data from larger adult trials, pediatric single-center experiences, small pediatric studies, and expert opinion.[16,24,59,88] Pediatric clinical trials will be required if we are to treat patients based on evidence. Difficulties implementing such studies lie in the heterogeneous presentation of PE in children and the relative rarity of the condition. There are many management options for treating children with PE: anticoagulation, thrombolysis, embolectomy, and IVC filter placement.

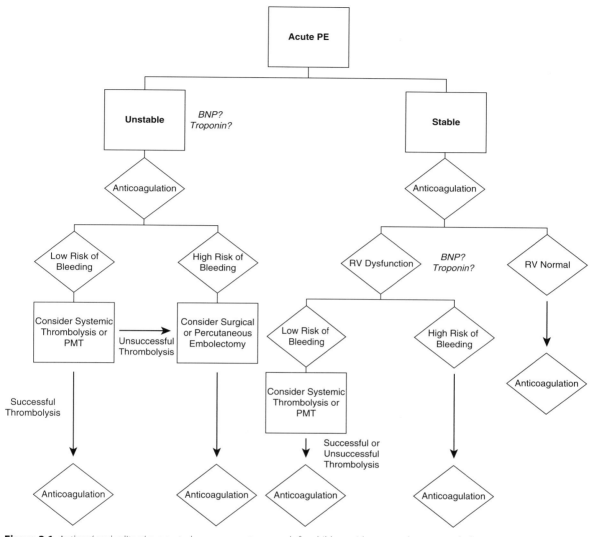

Figure 2.1 Authors' and editors' suggested management approach for children with acute pulmonary embolism.

Anticoagulation

Anticoagulation is the main therapy for treating PE in children (see Table 2.1).[89] There are increasing numbers and types of anticoagulants currently available: unfractionated heparin (UFH), low molecular weight heparin (LMWH – enoxaparin, dalteparin), vitamin K antagonists (OVKA – warfarin), oral and intravenous direct thrombin inhibitors (DTI – dabigatran, argatroban, bivalirudin), and oral and subcutaneous selective Xa inhibitors (rivaroxaban, apixaban, fondaparinux, idraparinux). For most patients with PE, anticoagulation is started with a rapid-onset anticoagulant such as UFH or LMWH for at least 5 days of therapeutic

anticoagulation, with bridging to a OVKA with a INR goal of 2.0–3.0[88] or continued use of LMWH for the subacute period. The use of LMWH for the acute period in patients with limited bleeding risk is becoming the standard. This is due to its bioavailability, longer half-life, ease of administration, infrequent but reliable monitoring, and predictable anticoagulant response. Pediatric studies show enoxaparin is equally effective as UFH when treating VTE, and may also confer a lower risk of heparin-induced thrombocytopenia (HIT).[90] Bleeding complications may occur in up to 5% of patients. There are only limited data on the efficacy and safety of DTI [91] and selective Xa inhibitors

Table 2.1 Treatment recommendations of conventional antithrombotic agents for pediatric patients with pulmonary embolism[a]

Clinical condition	Initial antithrombitic therapy		Subsequent antithrombotic therapy	Duration of therapy
	Bleeding risk[b]		Age[c]	
	Small	Significant	Infant/Young child Older child/Adolescent	
Unprovoked PE or Massive PE Provoked	LMWH[d]	UFH[e]	LMWH (VKA)[f] VKA (LMWH)	6 mo
(Risk factor resolved)	LMWH	UFH	LMWH (VKA) VKA (LMWH)	3 mo
(Risk factor persists, reversible)	LMWH	UFH	LMWH VKA	3 mo and resolution of risk factor
(Risk factor persists, potent)	LMWH	UFH	LMWH VKA	3 mo and extended/indeterminate length
Recurrent PE	LMWH	UFH	VKA (LMWH) VKA (new agent)	Indeterminate/indefinite length

PE, pulmonary embolism; LMWH, low molecular weight heparin; UFH, unfractionated heparin; VKA, vitamin K antagonist; mo, month.
[a] Table 2.1 adapted from Brandao L et al. 2011 (89).
[b] The duration of initial therapy is a minimum of 5 days (7 to 10 days in massive PE).
[c] Second-line agents within (brackets).
[d] Dose depends on age and type of LMWH used; should be adjusted to achieve an anti-FXa level of 0.5 to 1.0 U/mL.
[e] Loading dose: 75 U/kg in 10 minute IV, followed by maintenance dose: (28 U/kg/h IV [< 1 year]; 20 U/kg/h IV [> 1 year]). Dose adjusted to achieve an anti-FXa of 0.35 to 0.7 U/mL or a corresponding APTT range.
[f] Loading dose: 0.2 mg/kg on day 1 (day 5 in massive PE) followed by maintenance dose adjusted to target INR 2.0–3.0; overlap with UFH/LMWH for at least 5 days.

in children,[92] although prospective randomized control data exist for their efficacy in adults. We cannot recommend the routine use of these anticoagulants at this time in the treatment of acute pediatric PE outside of the rare occurrence of HIT, where UFH and LMWH are contraindicated. Clinical trials in children which are ongoing or completed for these new agents, will guide us in their dosing and use in acute VTE.[93,94] To serve as a reference for using anticoagulants in neonates and children, the ACCP guidelines organize the principles of anticoagulation as treatment recommendations from an expert panel of pediatric hematologists.[88] The current ACCP guidelines do not make recommendations for duration of therapy for PE, and currently, duration of therapy for pediatric patients is based upon presence or absence of a provoking factor and history of prior VTE, with a minimal course of 3 months of anticoagulation.

Thrombolysis

Today, thrombolysis is delivered locally via percutaneous catheter or systemically in patients with unstable PE, and is not for the routine treatment of PE in unselected patients.[95] Thrombolysis is used to directly facilitate a faster rate of resolution of the pulmonary artery occlusion when compared to anticoagulation by itself, thus reducing right ventricular load.[96] A more controversial group of patients are children who are hemodynamically stable but have right ventricular dysfunction and a low risk of bleeding. In this clinical scenario, it is unclear whether the benefit of thrombolysis outweighs risks of bleeding, or if stable patients who present with right ventricular dysfunction have a worse short- or long-term outcome. Arguments exist on both sides. Thrombolysis data are largely extrapolated and applied from adult studies and a limited number of smaller pediatric case studies, many of which report the use of tPA for vascular thrombosis. Gupta reported on 80 consecutive children where systemic thrombolysis for vascular thrombosis was associated with 65% complete thrombus resolution, 20% partial resolution, but 40% major and 30% minor complications (including two intracranial hemorrhages and two cerebral ischemia secondary to blood loss and hypotension).[97] Similar efficacy was obtained in a pooled analysis of systemic thrombolysis in children with fewer complications.[98] In the tissue plasminogen activator (tPA)-treated group, 69% of patients had complete resolution, 19% partial, and minor bleeding occurred in 26% and major bleeding in 17% of patients. There was 1.6% fatal bleeding. When tPA was given locally by a catheter-directed approach, the rate of complete resolution remained at 76%, partial resolution was 15%, with minor (15%) and major (6.5%) bleeding being reduced and no fatal bleeding events.[98] Meta-analysis of adult series reveal a clinical success rate of 86% and a 2.4% rate of procedural complications.[99]

The agent of choice in pediatrics is human recombinant tPA because of its low immunogenicity, in vitro clot lysis activity, and fibrin specificity. There have been no large clinical trials to determine the efficacy or safety of pharmacological thrombolysis in children. In fact, although there are ACCP recommendations concerning dosing, optimal dose and duration of tPA are unknown. Currently there are two dosing regimens that each have theoretical advantages.[89] A higher-dose regimen (0.5–0.6 mg/kg/h IV for 6 hours with an option to repeat if imaging shows incomplete resolution) has the advantage of potentially improved thrombolysis but also the potential for increased bleeding. A low-dose regimen (0.03–0.06 mg/kg/h with a maximum dose of 2 mg/h) has been shown to be efficacious in a single-institution cohort study where it was infused up to 96 hours.[100] There was less bleeding associated with this regimen. An approach combining assessment of bleeding risk with rate of clinical resolution may determine which patient may benefit most from either approach. Low-dose UFH (10 units/kg/h) is usually given with systemic or local tPA because fibrin lysis releases active clot-bound thrombin,[101] and there is an additional theoretical risk of tPA creating a procoagulant state through plasmin-mediated activation of the contact system leading to enhanced thrombin generation.[102]

A small study comparing thrombolysis versus heparin in submassive PE with RV dysfunction showed a decrease in death, recurrent VTE, RV dysfunction, and major hemorrhage at 6 months in adult patients randomized to thrombolysis.[103] In the MOPPETT trial, where adult patients were randomized to half-dose thrombolytic therapy versus heparin, a long-term reduction in the incidence of pulmonary hypertension was seen with thrombolytic therapy without excess bleeding.[104] No such trials have been reported in children.

Embolectomy

Surgical or percutaneous catheter embolectomy is considered in hemodynamically unstable patients when there is not sufficient time for anticoagulation to be effective, there is a contraindication to thrombolysis, or thrombolysis is ineffective. A direct comparison of these techniques is unavailable, and institutional experience will guide the choice. Success of both techniques for embolectomy have been reported in children.[105–107] Catheter techniques have been used with variable success for four decades, and are becoming more frequent alternatives to surgical thrombectomy.[108] Many techniques are used in clinical practice and include: aspiration thrombectomy, mechanical fragmentation thrombectomy, and rheolytic thrombectomy, with and without concomitant use of thrombolytics. Using catheter-directed thrombectomy, adult case series show major bleeding rates can be as low as 2.4% with restoration of hemodynamic stability in > 80% of patients.[108] The reported use of pharmacomechanical thrombolysis and embolectomy in PE is rare.[109] In patients with non-PE DVT, pharmacomechanical thrombolysis has been shown to be effective in a single case series of children:[110] 16 children experienced an early success rate of 94% (< 30 days) with early (< 7 days) locally recurrent DVT in 40% of cases, of which 83% were successfully treated with repeat thrombolysis. Late recurrence was 27% and there were no major bleeding complications. Physical and functional post-thrombotic syndrome at 1–2 years occurred in 13% of the cohort. Applicability of these findings to pediatric PE remains uncertain.

Vena cava filter

The IVC filters are used in patients who have proximal VTE and have a contraindication for anticoagulation, and who are > 10 kg.[111,112] They are also used in patients who continue to have recurrent or progressive thrombosis despite therapeutic anticoagulation. In both of these cases they are used to prevent PE. Retrievable IVC filters are preferable, as they can be removed when the risk for PE is reduced, or when the indication for their placement has resolved. There is limited use in pediatrics and outcome and complication data are limited. Short-term use has been associated with PE prevention and fewer complications.[16,113,114] The use of IVC filters in children is individualized, and each is placed after having discussed the risks and benefits with the patient and family. Filter retention, dislocation, thrombosis, and infection are all known complications.

Outcomes

Acute PE can be a rapidly fatal illness, even when detected and treated promptly. Data from the Canadian Childhood Thrombophilia Registry highlight this point, as four of the seven deaths reported by Monagle *et al.* occurred before treatment. Additional important sequelae from PE in children include: complications from anticoagulation, recurrence, incomplete resolution of PE, cardiac dysfunction, and pulmonary hypertension. From single-center pediatric studies, mortality ranges from 5.5% to 18%, and recurrence 5.5% to 18.5%.[16,30,59] A recent mixed retrospective–prospective inception cohort reported 9% recurrence, and no PE related-deaths.[30] These ranges highlight differing severities of PE, variability of treatment, and different follow-up times, and underscore the difficulty in examining the current pediatric data.

Complete resolution of PE is similar across a number of studies despite inhomogeneous therapies and demographics.[16,30,59] The significance of rapid or delayed resolution of PE has yet to be deciphered, but such knowledge of prognostic stratification could impact future study exploring expanded use of thrombolytics in children. Hancock *et al.* reported 58 consecutive children with acute PE.[30] In this cohort, the complete resolution rate was 82% and the partial resolution rate was 18% at 6 months, which is comparable to Biss *et al.* who reported a 78% complete resolution rate and 14% partial resolution rate.[16,30]

Chronic thromboembolic pulmonary hypertension, (CTEPH) is a serious potential long-term complication of pediatric PE. The incidence of CTEPH in adults ranges from 0.8% to 3.8%,[116,117] but no estimate can be made for children, even as they grow into adulthood. Longer-term follow-up of patients with echocardiography and pulmonary function testing may help define the magnitude of this problem, and better define a population of patients at risk for future risk-stratified (i.e., prognostically stratified) interventional trials that could inform future clinical decisions and management paradigms. Tavil *et al.* reported 3/16 patients in their series had pulmonary hypertension.[59] All had partial resolution of their PE, but nothing more can be inferred from these data. Consequences of acute ECG abnormalities and RV dysfunction secondary to PE are largely unknown. Elevated brain natriuretic peptides or troponin identifies a subgroup of adult patients with hemodynamic stability but RV dysfunction, who are at high risk for an adverse outcome.[118,119] Data on utility of such biomarkers are lacking in children. In a single-center mixed retrospective–prospective cohort study, 12% of patients presented with S1Q3T3 ECG abnormality and 25% had RV dysfunction (> 3 meters/second tricuspid regurgitation, septal flattening, and RV dilatation) by echocardiography. All ECG abnormalities resolved, and only two patients had septal flattening and RV dilation at 1 year post-event. None of these patients had a tricuspid regurgitation > 3 meters/second on follow-up.[30] It should be noted that 26% of these patients received tPA thrombolysis for occlusive iliofemoral VTE or massive PE, and nearly all children received 3 months of monitored therapeutic anticoagulation.

Conclusions and future directions

Diagnosis and management of childhood PE are highly variable. Guidelines exist that take into consideration differences between children and adults, but they are based on expert opinion which often only bridges the gap from extrapolated adult data.[88] There is an absolute paucity of high-grade evidence to guide treatment of PE in children when compared to recommendations and guidelines available and in clinical use for adults.[74,120,121] Thrombolysis in children with PE is controversial. In unstable patients with massive PE, the use of tPA has emerged in some institutions as the treatment of choice, and mirrors the use of thrombolysis in adults. However, no studies exist in children that can give clear recommendations about dose or infusion duration, and there are no meaningful outcomes data in regards to bleeding complications, CTEPH, and cardiac dysfunction. More controversial is the role of thrombolysis in submassive PE with RV dysfunction. Recent guidelines from the American Heart Association on management of massive/submassive PE, which address both adults and young patients, may help foster the design of pediatric thrombolytic trials[122] that will not merely evaluate radiologic efficacy but also (and perhaps more importantly) include more clearly clinically relevant outcomes such as CTEPH and cardiac dysfunction.

Predicting outcomes of pediatric PE is not possible with current data given the wide variability in patient demographics and treatment. This is an area in need of prospective data, which will only be achieved through multicenter trials that will help evaluate safety, patient characteristics and risk factors, standardize diagnosis and treatment, and uniformly track long-term outcomes, especially pulmonary and cardiac function.

References

1. Patocka C & Nemeth J. Pulmonary embolism in pediatrics. *J Emerg Med* **42**, 105–116 (2012).
2. Parker RI. Thrombosis in the pediatric population. *Crit Care Med* **38**, S71–75 (2010).
3. Loschner. Phlebitis venae cruralis sinistrae, peri- et myocarditis, embolis et oedema pulmonum. *Jahrb f Kinderh* **4** (1861).
4. Stevenson GF & Stevenson FL. Pulmonary embolism in childhood. *J Pediatr* **34**, 62–69 (1949).
5. Byard RW & Cutz E. Sudden and unexpected death in infancy and childhood due to pulmonary thromboembolism. An autopsy study. *Arch Pathol Lab Med* **114**, 142–144 (1990).
6. Emery JL. Pulmonary embolism in children. *Arch Dis Child* **37**, 591–595 (1962).
7. Jones RH & Sabiston DC, Jr. Pulmonary embolism in childhood. *Monogr Surg Sci* **3**, 35–51 (1966).
8. Buck JR, Connors JR, Coon WW, Weintraub WH, Wesley JR, Coran AG. Pulmonary embolism in children. *J Pediatr Surg* **16**, 385–391 (1981).
9. Jones DR & Macintyre IM. Venous thromboembolism in infancy and childhood. *Arch Dis Child* **50**, 153–155 (1975).
10. David M & Andrew M. Venous thromboembolic complications in children. *J Pediatr* **123**, 337–346 (1993).
11. Coon WW & Coller FA. Some epidemiologic considerations of thromboembolism. *Surg Gynecol Obstet* **109**, 487–501 (1959).
12. Kroger K, Moerchel C, Moysidis T, Santosa F. Incidence rate of pulmonary embolism in Germany: data from the federal statistical office. *J Thromb Thrombolysis* **29**, 349–353 (2010).
13. Oger E. Incidence of venous thromboembolism: a community-based study in Western France. EPI-GETBP Study Group. Groupe d'Etude de la Thrombose de Bretagne Occidentale. *Thromb Haemost* **83**, 657–660 (2000).
14. Silverstein MD, Heit JA, Mohr DN, *et al.* Trends in the incidence of deep vein thrombosis and pulmonary embolism: a 25-year population-based study. *Arch Intern Med* **158**, 585–593 (1998).
15. Andrew M, David M, Adams M, Ali K, Anderson R, Barnard D, Bernstein M, Brisson L, Cairney B, DeSai D, Grant R, Israels S, Jardine L, Luke B, Massicotte P, Silva Ml. Venous thromboembolic complications (VTE) in children: first analyses of the Canadian Registry of VTE. *Blood* **83**, 1251–1257 (1994).
16. Biss TT, Brandao LR, Kahr WH, Chan AK & Williams S. Clinical features and outcome of pulmonary embolism in children. *Br J Haematol* **142**, 808–818 (2008).
17. van Ommen CH, *et al.* Venous thromboembolism in childhood: a prospective two-year registry in The Netherlands. *J Pediatr* **139**, 676–681, doi: S0022-3476 (01)82380-5 [pii] 10.1067/mpd.2001.118192 (2001).
18. Stein PD, Kayali F, Olson RE. Incidence of venous thromboembolism in infants and children: data from the National Hospital Discharge Survey. *J Pediatr* **145**, 563–565 (2004).
19. Kuhle S, Massicotte P, Chan A, Adams M, Abdolell M, deVeber G, Mitchell L. Systemic thromboembolism in children. Data from the 1–800-NO-CLOTS Consultation Service. *Thromb Haemost* **92**, 722–728 (2004).
20. Nowak-Gottl U, von Kries R & Gobel U. Neonatal symptomatic thromboembolism in Germany: two year survey. *Arch Dis Child Fetal Neonatal Ed* **76**, F163–167 (1997).
21. Schmidt B & Andrew M. Neonatal thrombosis: report of a prospective Canadian and international registry. *Pediatrics* **96**, 939–943 (1995).
22. Gibson B, Chalmers EA, Bolton-Maggs P, Henderson DJ, Boshkov RL. Thromboembolism in childhood: a prospective 2-year study in the United Kingdom (interim: Feb 2001-Feb 2003). *J Thromb Haemost* **1** (2003).
23. Raffini L, Huang Y S, Witmer C, Feudtner C. Dramatic increase in venous thromboembolism in children's hospitals in the United States from 2001 to 2007. *Pediatrics* **124**, 1001–1008 (2009).
24. Rajpurkar M, Warrier I, Chitlur M, Sabo C, Frey MJ, Hollon W, Lusher J. Pulmonary embolism – experience at a single children's hospital. *Thromb Res* **119**, 699–703 (2007).
25. Kjellin IB, Boechat MI, Vinuela F, Westra SJ, Duckwiler GR. Pulmonary emboli following therapeutic embolization of cerebral arteriovenous malformations in children. *Pediatr Radiol* **30**, 279–283 (2000).
26. Farrell AG, Parikh SR, Darragh RK, Girod DA. Retrieval of "old" foreign bodies from the cardiovascular system in children. *Cathet Cardiovasc Diagn* **44**, 212–216; discussion 217 (1998).
27. Soares FA. Fatal pulmonary tumor embolism caused by chondroblastic osteosarcoma. *Arch Pathol Lab Med* **124**, 661 (2000).

28. Massicotte MP, Dix D, Monagle P, Adams M, Andrew M. Central venous catheter related thrombosis in children: analysis of the Canadian Registry of Venous Thromboembolic Complications. *J Pediatr* **133**, 770–776 (1998).

29. Sandoval JA. Sheehan MP, Stonerock CE, Shafique S, Rescorla FJ, Dalsing MC. Incidence, risk factors, and treatment patterns for deep venous thrombosis in hospitalized children: an increasing population at risk. *J Vasc Surg* **47**, 837–843 (2008).

30. Hancock HS, Wang M, Gist KM, Gibson E, Miyamoto SD, Mourani PM, Manco-Johnson MJ, Goldenberg NA. Cardiac findings and long-term thromboembolic outcomes following pulmonary embolism in children: a combined retrospective-prospective inception cohort study. *Cardiol.Young* **23**, 344–352 (2013).

31. Bernstein D, Coupey S, Schonberg SK. Pulmonary embolism in adolescents. *Am J Dis Child* **140**, 667–671 (1986).

32. McBride WJ, Gadowski GR, Keller MS, Vane DW. Pulmonary embolism in pediatric trauma patients. *J Trauma* **37**, 913–915 (1994).

33. Huiras EE, Barnes CJ, Eichenfield LF, Pelech AN, Drolet BA. Pulmonary thromboembolism associated with Klippel-Trenaunay syndrome. *Pediatrics* **116**, e596–600 (2005).

34. Alomari AI, Burrows PE, Lee EY, Hedequist DJ, Mulliken JB, Fishman SJ. CLOVES syndrome with thoracic and central phlebectasia: increased risk of pulmonary embolism. *J Thorac Cardiovasc Surg* **140**, 459–463 (2010).

35. Uderzo C, Faccini P, Rovelli A, Arosio M, Marchi PF, Riva A, Marraro G, Balduzzi A, Masera G. Pulmonary thromboembolism in childhood leukemia: 8-years' experience in a pediatric hematology center. *J Clin Oncol* **13**, 2805–2812 (1995).

36. Lee AY. Cancer and thromboembolic disease: pathogenic mechanisms. *Cancer Treat Rev* **28**, 137–140 (2002).

37. Johnson NN, Toledo A, Endom EE. Pneumothorax, pneumomediastinum, and pulmonary embolism. *Pediatr Clin North Am* **57**, 1357–1383 (2010).

38. Hoyer PF, Gonda S, Barthels M, Krohn HP, Brodehl J. Thromboembolic complications in children with nephrotic syndrome. Risk and incidence. *Acta Paediatr Scand* **75**, 804–810 (1986).

39. Huang J, Yang J, Ding J. Pulmonary embolism associated with nephrotic syndrome in children: a preliminary report of 8 cases. *Chin Med J (Engl)* **113**, 251–253 (2000).

40. Vichinsky EP, Neumayr LD, Earles AN, Williams R, Lennette ET, Dean D, Nickerson B, Orringer E, McKie V, Bellevue R, Daeschner C, Manci EA, for the National Acute Chest Syndrome Study Group. Causes and outcomes of the acute chest syndrome in sickle cell disease. National Acute Chest Syndrome Study Group. *N Engl J Med* **342**, 1855–1865 (2000).

41. Stein PD, Beemath A, Meyers FA, Skaf E, Olson RE. Deep venous thrombosis and pulmonary embolism in hospitalized patients with sickle cell disease. *Am J Med* **119**, 897, e897 (2006).

42. Oppenheimer EH & Esterly JR. Pulmonary changes in sickle cell disease. *Am Rev Respir Dis* **103**, 858–859 (1971).

43. Gibbon JH, Hopkinson M, Churchill ED. Changes in the circulation produced by gradual occlusion of the pulmonary artery. *J Clin Invest* **11**, 543–553 (1932).

44. van Ommen CH & Peters M. Acute pulmonary embolism in childhood. *Thromb Res* **118**, 13–25 (2006).

45. Tapson VF. Acute pulmonary embolism. *N Engl J Med* **358**, 1037–1052 (2008).

46. Wood KE. Major pulmonary embolism: review of a pathophysiologic approach to the golden hour of hemodynamically significant pulmonary embolism. *Chest* **121**, 877–905 (2002).

47. Schein CJ, Rifkin H, Hurwitt ES, Lebendiger A. The clinical and surgical aspects of chronic pulmonary artery thrombosis. *AMA Arch Intern Med* **101**, 592–605 (1958).

48. Goldhaber SZ & Elliott CG. Acute pulmonary embolism: part I: epidemiology, pathophysiology, and diagnosis. *Circulation* **108**, 2726–2729 (2003).

49. Smulders YM. Pathophysiology and treatment of haemodynamic instability in acute pulmonary embolism: the pivotal role of pulmonary vasoconstriction. *Cardiovasc Res* **48**, 23–33 (2000).

50. Riedel M. Acute pulmonary embolism 1: pathophysiology, clinical presentation, and diagnosis. *Heart* **85**, 229–240 (2001).

51. Elliott CG. Pulmonary physiology during pulmonary embolism. *Chest* **101**, 163S–171S (1992).

52. Benotti JR. Pulmonary angiography in the diagnosis of pulmonary embolism. *Herz* **14**, 115–125 (1989).

53. Streif W & Andrew ME. Venous thromboembolic events in pediatric patients. Diagnosis and management. *Hematol Oncol Clin North Am* **12**, 1283–1312, vii (1998).

54. Chan AK, deVeber G, Monagle P, Brooker LA, Massicotte PM. Venous thrombosis in children. *J Thromb Haemost* **1**, 1443–1455 (2003).

55. van Ommen CH, Heyboer H, Groothoff JW, Teeuw R, Aronson DC, Peters M. Persistent tachypnea in children: keep pulmonary embolism in mind. *J Pediatr Hematol/Oncol* **20**, 570–573 (1998).

56. Babyn PS, Gahunia HK, Massicotte P. Pulmonary thromboembolism in children. *Pediatr Radiol* **35**, 258–274 (2005).

57. Stein PD, Terrin ML, Hales CA, Palevsky HI, Saltzman HA, Thompson BT, Weg JG. Clinical, laboratory, roentgenographic, and electrocardiographic findings in patients with acute pulmonary embolism and no pre-existing cardiac or pulmonary disease. *Chest* **100**, 598–603 (1991).

58. Sethuraman U, Siadat M, Lepak-Hitch CA, Haritos D. Pulmonary embolism presenting as acute abdomen in a child and adult. *Am J Emerg Med* **27**, 514, e511–515, (2009).

59. Tavil B, Kuskonmaz B, Kiper N, Cetin M, Gumruk F, Gurgey A. Pulmonary thromboembolism in childhood: a single-center experience from Turkey. *Heart Lung* **38**, 56–65 (2009).

60. Victoria T, Mong A, Altes T, Jawad AF, Hernandez A, Gonzalez L, Raffini L, Dramer SS. Evaluation of pulmonary embolism in a pediatric population with high clinical suspicion. *Pediatr Radiol* **39**, 35–41 (2009).

61. Wells PS, Anderson DR, Rodger M, Ginsberg JS, Kearon C, Gent M, Turpie AGG, Bormanis J, Weitz J, Chamberlain M, Bowie D, Barnes D, Hirsh J. Derivation of a simple clinical model to categorize patients probability of pulmonary embolism: increasing the models utility with the SimpliRED D-dimer. *Thromb Haemost* **83**, 416–420 (2000).

62. Le Gal G, Righini M, Roy P-M, Sanchez O, Aujesky D, Bounameaux H, Perrier A. Prediction of pulmonary embolism in the emergency department: the revised Geneva score. *Ann Intern Med* **144**, 165–171 (2006).

63. Biss TT, Brandao LR, Kahr WH, Chan AK, Williams S. Clinical probability score and D-dimer estimation lack utility in the diagnosis of childhood pulmonary embolism. *J Thromb Haemost* **7**, 1633–1638 (2009).

64. Stein PD, Willis PW III, DeMets DL. History and physical examination in acute pulmonary embolism in patients without preexisting cardiac or pulmonary disease. *Am J Cardiol* **47**, 218–223 (1981).

65. Rodger M, Makropoulos D, Turek M, Quevillon J, Raymond F, Rasuli P, Wells PS. Diagnostic value of the electrocardiogram in suspected pulmonary embolism. *Am J Cardiol* **86**, 807–809, A810 (2000).

66. Worsley DF, Alavi A, Aronchick JM, Dhen JT, Greenspan RH, Ravin CE. Chest radiographic findings in patients with acute pulmonary embolism: observations from the PIOPED Study. *Radiology* **189**, 133–136 (1993).

67. PIOPED Investigators. Value of the ventilation/perfusion scan in acute pulmonary embolism. Results of the prospective investigation of pulmonary embolism diagnosis (PIOPED). *JAMA* **263**, 2753–2759 (1990).

68. van Beek EJ, Brouwerst EM, Song B, Stein PD, Oudkerk M. Clinical validity of a normal pulmonary angiogram in patients with suspected pulmonary embolism – a critical review. *Clin Radiol* **56**, 838–842 (2001).

69. Stein PD, Athanasoulis C, Alavi A, Greenspan RH, Hales CA, Saltzman HA, Vreim CE, Terrin ML, Weg JG. Complications and validity of pulmonary angiography in acute pulmonary embolism. *Circulation* **85**, 462–468 (1992).

70. Novelline RA. *et al.* The clinical course of patients with suspected pulmonary embolism and a negative pulmonary arteriogram. *Radiology* **126**, 561–567 (1978).

71. van Beek EJ, Reekers JA, Batchelor DA, Brandjes DP, Buller HR. Feasibility, safety and clinical utility of angiography in patients with suspected pulmonary embolism. *Eur Radiol* **6**, 415–419 (1996).

72. Stein PD, Henry JW, Gottschalk A. Reassessment of pulmonary angiography for the diagnosis of pulmonary embolism: relation of interpreter agreement to the order of the involved pulmonary arterial branch. *Radiology* **210**, 689–691 (1999).

73. Stein PD & Matta F. Acute pulmonary embolism. *Curr Probl Cardiol* **35**, 314–376 (2010).

74. Torbicki A, Perrier A, Konstantinides S, Agnelli G, Galie N, Pruszczyk P, Bengel F, Brady AJ, Ferreira D, Janssens U, Klepetko W, Mayer E, Remy-Jardin M, Bassand JP, ESC Committee for Practice Guidelines. Guidelines on the diagnosis and management of acute pulmonary embolism: the Task Force for the Diagnosis and Management of Acute Pulmonary Embolism of the European Society of Cardiology (ESC). *Eur Heart J* **29**, 2276–2315 (2008).

75. Worsley DF & Alavi A. Comprehensive analysis of the results of the PIOPED Study. Prospective Investigation of Pulmonary Embolism Diagnosis Study. *J Nucl Med* **36**, 2380–2387 (1995).

76. Quiroz R, Kucher N, Zou KH, Kipfmueller F, Costello P, Goldhaber SZ, Schoepf UJ. Clinical validity of a negative computed tomography scan in patients with suspected pulmonary embolism: a systematic review. *JAMA* **293**, 2012–2017 (2005).

77. Kritsaneepaiboon S, Lee EY, Zurakowski D, Strauss KJ, Boiselle PM. MDCT pulmonary angiography evaluation of pulmonary embolism in children. *AJR Am J Roentgenol* **192**, 1246–1252 (2009).

78. Ghaye B, Szapiro D, Mastora I, Delannoy V, Duhamel A, Remy J, Remy-Jardin M. Peripheral pulmonary arteries: how far in the lung does multi-detector row spiral CT allow analysis? *Radiology* **219**, 629–636 (2001).

79. Quiroz R, Kucher N, Schoepf UJ, Kipfmueller F, Solomon SD, Costello P, Goldhaber SZ. Right ventricular enlargement on chest computed tomography: prognostic role in acute pulmonary embolism. *Circulation* **109**, 2401–2404 (2004).

80. Schoepf UJ, Kucher N, Kipfmueller F, Quiroz R, Costello P, Goldhaber SZ. Right ventricular enlargement on chest computed tomography: a predictor of early death in acute pulmonary embolism. *Circulation* **110**, 3276–3280 (2004).

81. Stein PD, Fowler SE, Goodman LR, Gottschalk A, Hales CA, Hull RD, Leeper KV, Popovich Joh, Jr, Quinn DA, Sos TA, Sostman HD, Tapson VF, Wakefield TW, Wed JG, Woodard PK, for the PIOPED II Investigators. Multidetector computed tomography for acute pulmonary embolism. *N Engl J Med* **354**, 2317–2327 (2006).

82. Le GG, Righini M, Parent F, van SM, Couturaud F. Diagnosis and management of subsegmental pulmonary embolism. *J Thromb Haemost* **4**, 724–731 (2006).

83. Moores LK, Jackson WL, Jr., Shorr AF, Jackson JL. Meta-analysis: outcomes in patients with suspected pulmonary embolism managed with computed tomographic pulmonary angiography. *Ann Intern Med* **141**, 866–874 (2004).

84. Macdougall RD, Strauss KJ, Lee EY. Managing radiation dose from thoracic multidetector computed tomography in pediatric patients: background, current issues, and recommendations. *Radiol Clin North Am* **51**, 743–760 (2013).

85. Stein PD, Fowler SE, Goodman LR, Gottschalk A, Hales CA, Hull RD, Leeper KV, Popovich Joh, Jr, Quinn DA, Sos TA, Sostman HD, Tapson VF, Wakefield TW, Wed JG, Woodard PK, for the PIOPED II Investigators. Gadolinium-enhanced magnetic resonance angiography for pulmonary embolism: a multicenter prospective study (PIOPED III). *Ann Intern Med* **152**, 434–433 (2010).

86. Goldhaber SZ. Echocardiography in the management of pulmonary embolism. *Ann Intern Med* **136**, 691–700 (2002).

87. Goldenberg NA & Bernard TJ. Venous thromboembolism in children. *Hematol Oncol Clin North Am* **24**, 151–166 (2010).

88. Monagle P, Chan AKC, Goldenberg NA, Ichord RN, Journeycake JM, Nowak-Gottl U, Vesely SK. Antithrombotic therapy in neonates and children: Antithrombotic Therapy and Prevention of Thrombosis, 9th edn: American College of Chest Physicians Evidence-Based Clinical Practice Guidelines. *Chest* **141**, e737S–801S (2012).

89. Brandao LR, Labarque V, Diab Y, Williams S, Manson DE. Pulmonary embolism in children. *Semin Thromb Hemost* **37**, 772–785 (2011).

90. Warkentin TE, Levine MN, Hirsh J, Horsewood P, Roberts RS, Gent M, Kelton JG. Heparin-induced thrombocytopenia in patients treated with low-molecular-weight heparin or unfractionated heparin. *N Engl J Med* **332**, 1330–1335 (1995).

91. Young G, Boshkov LK, Sullivan JE, Raffini LJ, Cox DS, Boyle DA, Kallender H, Tarka EA, Soffer J, Hursting MJ. Argatroban therapy in pediatric patients requiring nonheparin anticoagulation: an open-label, safety, efficacy, and pharmacokinetic study. *Pediatr Blood Cancer* **56**, 1103–1109 (2011).

92. Young G, Yee DL, O'Brien SH, Khanna R, Barbour A, Nugent DJ. FondaKIDS: a prospective pharmacokinetic and safety study of fondaparinux in children between 1 and 18 years of age. *Pediatr Blood Cancer* **57**, 1049–1054 (2011).

93. Yee DL, O'Brien SH, Young G. Pharmacokinetics and pharmacodynamics of anticoagulants in paediatric patients. *Clin Pharmacokinet*, doi:10.1007/s40262-013-0094-1 [doi] (2013).

94. Young G. New anticoagulants in children: a review of recent studies and a look to the future. *Thromb Res* **127**, 70–74 (2011).

95. Wan S, Quinlan DJ, Agnelli G & Eikelboom JW. Thrombolysis compared with heparin for the initial treatment of pulmonary embolism: a meta-analysis of the randomized controlled trials. *Circulation* **110**, 744–749 (2004).

96. Agnelli G & Becattini C. Acute pulmonary embolism. *N Engl J Med* **363**, 266–274 (2010).

97. Gupta AA, Leaker M, Andrew M, Massicotte P, Liu L, Benson LN, McCrindle BW. Safety and outcomes of thrombolysis with tissue plasminogen activator for treatment of intravascular thrombosis in children. *J Pediatr* **139**, 682–688 (2001).

98. Albisetti M. Thrombolytic therapy in children. *Thromb Res* **118**, 95–105 (2006).

99. Kuo WT, Gould MK, Louie JD, Rosenberg JK, Sze DY, Hofmann LV. Catheter-directed therapy for the treatment of massive pulmonary embolism: systematic review and meta-analysis of modern techniques. *J Vasc Interv Radiol* **20**, 1431–1440 (2009).

100. Wang M, Hays T, Balasa V, Bagatell R, Gruppo R, Grabowski EF, Valentino LA, Tsao-Wu G, Manco-Johnson MJ; Pediatric Coagulation Consortium. Low-dose tissue plasminogen activator thrombolysis in children. *J Pediatr Hematol/Oncol* **25**, 379–386 (2003).

101. Weitz JI, Hudoba M, Massel D, Maraganore J, Hirsh J. Clot-bound thrombin is protected from inhibition by heparin-antithrombin III but is susceptible to

inactivation by antithrombin III-independent inhibitors. *J Clin Invest* **86**, 385–391 (1990).

102. Hoffmeister HM, Szabo S, Helber U, Seipel L. The thrombolytic paradox. *Thromb Res* **103**(Suppl 1), S51–55 (2001).

103. Fasullo S, Scalzo S, Maringhini G, Ganci F, Cannizzaro S, Basile I, Cangemi D, Terrazzino G, Parrinello G, Sarullo FM, Baglini R, Paterna S, Di Pasquale P. Six-month echocardiographic study in patients with submassive pulmonary embolism and right ventricle dysfunction: comparison of thrombolysis with heparin. *Am J Med Sci* **341**, 33–39 (2011).

104. Sharifi M, Bay C, Skrocki L, Rahimi F, Mehdipour M. Moderate pulmonary embolism treated with thrombolysis (from the "MOPETT" Trial). *Am J Cardiol* **111**, 273–277 (2013).

105. Eini ZM, Houri S, Cohen I, Sion R, Tamir A, Sasson L, Mandelberg A. Massive pulmonary emboli in children: does fiber-optic-guided embolectomy have a role? Review of the literature and report of two cases. *Chest* **143**, 544–549 (2013).

106. Jean N, Labombarda F, De La Gastine G, Raisky O, Boudjemline Y. Successful pulmonary embolectomy in a 4-year-old girl with antithrombin III deficiency. *Pediatr Cardiol* **31**, 711–713 (2010).

107. Sur JP, Garg RK, Jolly N. Rheolytic percutaneous thrombectomy for acute pulmonary embolism in a pediatric patient. *Catheter Cardiovasc Interv* **70**, 450–453 (2007).

108. Todoran TM & Sobieszczyk P. Catheter-based therapies for massive pulmonary embolism. *Prog Cardiovasc Dis* **52**, 429–437 (2010).

109. Manco-Johnson MJ, Wang M, Goldenberg NA, Soep J, Gibson E, Knoll CM, Mourani PM. Treatment, survival, and thromboembolic outcomes of thrombotic storm in children. *J Pediatr* **161**, 682–688, e681 (2012).

110. Goldenberg NA, Branchford B, Wang M, Ray C, Jr, Durham JD, Manco-Johnson MJ. Percutaneous mechanical and pharmacomechanical thrombolysis for occlusive deep vein thrombosis of the proximal limb in adolescent subjects: findings from an institution-based prospective inception cohort study of pediatric venous thromboembolism. *J Vasc Interv Radiol* **22**, 121–132 (2011).

111. Chaudry G, Padua HM, Alomari AI. The use of inferior vena cava filters in young children. *J Vasc Interv Radiol* **19**, 1103–1106 (2008).

112. Reed RA, Teitelbaum GP, Stanley P, Mazer MJ, Tonkin IL, Rollins NK. The use of inferior vena cava filters in pediatric patients for pulmonary embolus prophylaxis. *Cardiovasc Intervent Radiol* **19**, 401–405 (1996).

113. Kai R, Imamura H, Kumazaki S, Kamiyoshi Y, Koshikawa M, Hanaoka T, Kogashi K, Koyama J,

Tsutsui H, Yazaki Y, Kinoshita O, Ikeda U. Temporary inferior vena cava filter for deep vein thrombosis and acute pulmonary thromboembolism: effectiveness and indication. *Heart Vessels* **21**, 221–225 (2006).

114. Kukreja KU, Gollamudi J, Patel MN, Johnson ND, Racadio JM. Inferior vena cava filters in children: our experience and suggested guidelines. *J Pediatr Hematol/Oncol* **33**, 334–338 (2011).

115. Monagle P, Adams M, Mahoney M, Ali K, Barnard D, Bernstein M, Brisson L, David M, Desai S, Scully MF, Halton J, Israels S, Jardine L, Leaker M, McCusker P, Silva M, Wu J, Anderson R, Andrew M, Massicotte MP. Outcome of pediatric thromboembolic disease: a report from the Canadian Childhood Thrombophilia Registry. *Pediatr Res* **47**, 763–766 (2000).

116. Becattini C, Agnelli G, Pesavento R, Silingardi M, Poggio R, Taliani MR, Ageno W. Incidence of chronic thromboembolic pulmonary hypertension after a first episode of pulmonary embolism. *Chest* **130**, 172–175 (2006).

117. Pengo V, Lensing AW, Prins MH, Marchiori A, Davidson BL, Tiozzo F, Albanese P, Biasiolo A, Pegoraro C, Iliceto S, Prandoni P; Thromboembolic Pulmonary Hypertension Study Group. Incidence of chronic thromboembolic pulmonary hypertension after pulmonary embolism. *N Engl J Med* **350**, 2257–2264 (2004).

118. Binder L, Pieske B, Olschewski M, Geibel A, Klostermann B, Reiner C, Konstantinides S. N-terminal pro-brain natriuretic peptide or troponin testing followed by echocardiography for risk stratification of acute pulmonary embolism. *Circulation* **112**, 1573–1579 (2005).

119. Becattini C, Vedovati MC & Agnelli G. Prognostic value of troponins in acute pulmonary embolism: a meta-analysis. *Circulation* **116**, 427–433 (2007).

120. Goldhaber SZ. Advanced treatment strategies for acute pulmonary embolism, including thrombolysis and embolectomy. *J Thromb Haemost* **7**(Suppl 1), 322–327 (2009).

121. Kearon C, Akl EA, Comerota AJ, Prandoni P, Bounameaux H, Goldhaber SZ, Nelson ME, Wells PS, Gould MK, Dentali F, Crowther M, Kahn SR; American College of Chest Physicians. Antithrombotic therapy for VTE disease. Antithrombotic Therapy and Prevention of Thrombosis, 9th edn: American College of Chest Physicians Evidence-Based Clinical Practice Guidelines. *Chest* **141**, e419S–494S (2012).

122. Jaff MR, McMurtry MS, Archer SL, Cushman M, Goldenberg N, Goldhaber SZ, Jenkins JS, Kline JA, Michaels AD, Thistlethwaite P, Vedantham S, White

RJ, Zierler BK; American Heart Association Council on Cardiopulmonary, Critical Care, Perioperative and Resuscitation; American Heart Association Council on Peripheral Vascular Disease; American Heart Association Council on Arteriosclerosis, Thrombosis and Vascular Biology. Management of massive and submassive pulmonary embolism, iliofemoral deep vein thrombosis, and chronic thromboembolic pulmonary hypertension: a scientific statement from the American Heart Association. *Circulation* **123**, 1788–1830 (2011).

Cerebral sinovenous thrombosis in children and neonates

Mahendranath Moharir and Gili Kenet

Introduction

Cerebral venous sinus (sinovenous) thrombosis (CSVT) is a serious and rare disorder, whose etiology and pathophysiology has not yet been completely clarified. Unlike in adults with CSVT, management in children and neonates remains controversial. Nonetheless, mortality and morbidity associated with neurologic sequelae among survivors are significant.

Stroke and cerebrovascular diseases are increasingly recognized and diagnosed in pediatric patients, including neonates, due to mounting awareness and advances in neuroimaging techniques. Stroke is defined as the sudden occlusion or rupture of cerebral arteries or veins resulting in brain injury. Stroke due to vascular occlusion is broadly divided into *arterial ischemic stroke* (AIS) and *cerebral sinovenous thrombosis* (CSVT). In AIS, brain injury occurs due to arterial occlusion secondary to thromboembolism resulting in cerebral infarction. In CSVT, brain dysfunction occurs due to thrombotic occlusion of cerebral veins and/or dural venous sinuses resulting in venous congestion and intracranial venous hypertension, which may or may not be associated with "venous infarction."

Although there is overlap in the conditions predisposing to neonatal AIS and CSVT, the clinical and radiographic features, management, and outcomes are distinct. The condition of CSVT is under-recognized in neonates due to the subtle and non-specific presentation, resulting in delayed or missed diagnosis. While randomized controlled trials (RCTs) have established the usefulness of anticoagulant therapy for adults with CSVT, pediatric data are limited to multicenter (childhood CSVT) and single-center (neonatal CSVT) cohort studies. Important developmental differences in the hemostatic, sinovenous, and neurologic systems in children and neonates prevent the direct extrapolation of adult treatment data to pediatrics. Current knowledge, though limited due to sample size or single-center enrolment, addresses the epidemiology, symptoms, neuroimaging diagnostic findings, treatment practices, and outcome of pediatric and neonatal CSVT, and will be summarized in this chapter.

Epidemiology

An accurate incidence of CSVT remains largely unknown and is currently estimated between 0.34 and 0.67/100,000 children annually, with neonates comprising 27–50% of all cases in childhood [1–6]. In the Canadian Pediatric Ischemic Stroke Registry, the annual incidence of pediatric CSVT (neonates included) was approximately 0.67 cases per 100,000 per year and a large proportion of these patients were newborns [1]. The German Pediatric Thrombophila Registry estimated an incidence of 0.35 cases per 100,000 per year for childhood CSVT and 2.6 per 100,000 per year for neonatal CSVT [2].

Interestingly, a more recent Dutch study has provided, for the first time, data documenting a 7-year rise in the incidence of neonatal CSVT from 1.2 to 12 per 100,000 term newborns per year, from 2000 to 2007 [3]. This rising incidence could be attributed to higher awareness, improvement in diagnostic neuroimaging, and increasing survival of neonates with previously lethal conditions like extreme prematurity, complex congenital heart disease, and multiorgan dysfunction that places them at risk for CSVT. In the last few years, neonatal CSVT has been more systematically reported by larger cohort studies [1,3–10]. Most of these studies have documented CSVT more frequently in male as compared to female newborns; CSVT has also been reported to occur in utero [11,12].

Pediatric Thrombotic Disorders, ed. Neil A. Goldenberg and Marilyn J. Manco-Johnson. Published by Cambridge University Press. © Cambridge University Press 2015.

Anatomic and pathophysiologic considerations

The intracranial venous system consisting of the dural venous sinuses and cerebral veins are traditionally categorized into the superficial and deep cerebral venous systems (Figure 3.1). In the superficial venous system, cortical veins drain into the superior sagittal sinus, which drains into the torcular and then predominantly into the dominant right transverse (lateral) sinus, and right internal jugular vein. The deep system includes the inferior sagittal sinus, the basal vein of Rosenthal, and two paired internal cerebral veins that empty into the vein of Galen and straight sinus and then into the torcular and the smaller-caliber left transverse (lateral) sinus and left internal jugular vein [13]. The flow in the dural venous system occurs typically in a rostro-caudal direction. Although the internal jugular veins are the major common exit for cerebral venous drainage, extra-jugular pathways such as vertebral venous plexus are also apparently active [14]. The vertebral venous plexus has connections with transverse sinus–jugular system that are poorly understood. The internal jugular veins appear to drain blood primarily in the supine position whereas the vertebral venous plexus drainage occurs mainly in the upright position in humans [15].

The cerebral sinovenous system lacks valves and is a low pressure–slow velocity circuit. The dural lining of the venous sinuses is rigid and the walls are therefore non-collapsible. This results in a passive drainage of blood flow to the heart [16]. The flow in the sinuses is gravity- and respiration-dependent and can be bidirectional depending upon the venous pressure gradient [17]. Reduction in systemic blood pressure can lead to stasis or reversal of sinovenous blood flow. Cerebrospinal fluid (CSF) is absorbed via arachnoid granulations into the venous blood mainly within the superior saggital and transverse sinuses.

The most frequently involved sites of CSVT are the superior saggital sinus (90% of all cases in most studies), the transverse sinuses of the superficial venous system, and the straight sinus of the deep system [20]. Neonatal CSVT frequently involves multiple sites (about 70–80% of neonates in the Toronto study) [6,8]. The superficial sinovenous system, including the superior saggital sinus and right transverse sinus, is involved in the majority of neonates (over 50–60%); and the deep system and left transverse sinus in the remainder.

The physiology of the immature sinovenous system probably differs from that of older children and adults. In neonates, the presence of factors that are poorly understood but potentially important in maturational changes include: prematurity; persistence/involution of embryonic venous collaterals; venous pressure gradients and their effect on cerebral

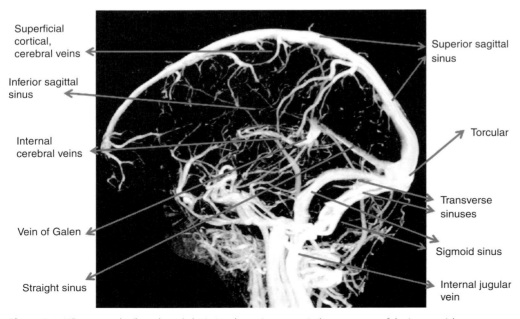

Superficial cortical, cerebral veins

Inferior sagittal sinus

Internal cerebral veins

Vein of Galen

Straight sinus

Superior sagittal sinus

Torcular

Transverse sinuses

Sigmoid sinus

Internal jugular vein

Figure 3.1 MR venography (lateral view) depicting the major anatomical components of the intracranial venous system.

perfusion pressure and CSF pressure; immaturity of arachnoid villi in CSF absorption; development of venous collaterals in the wake of obstruction; and obstruction of the posterior portion of the superior saggital sinus with compression by the mobile bony plates of the skull in supine position [22]. This emphasizes the consideration to develop and study animal models of neonatal CSVT in the future (see also below).

The severity and duration of clinical symptoms associated with CSVT are dependent upon anatomic involvement, how acutely a clot develops, and the extent and number of occluded venous channels. If collateral venous circulation develops adequately and rapidly, significant venous obstruction can be potentially tolerated without decompensation. The brain tolerates venous thrombi poorly in certain sites such as the torcular or the dominant transverse–jugular system since these are the final exit points for cerebral venous drainage. This understanding of the above pathophysiologic mechanisms predominantly comes from adult literature, which is extrapolated to childhood and neonatal CSVT.

In CSVT, the mechanisms underlying venous infarction are initiated by the obstruction of venous drainage resulting in retrograde venous congestion in the absence of collateral venous drainage [23]. The venous congestion and intracranial venous hypertension result in increased tissue and capillary hydrostatic pressure with consequent extravasation of fluid into the interstitium, producing focal or sometimes diffuse cerebral edema. Hemorrhage results from diapedesis of red blood cells through the leaky capillaries. This explains the high rate of spontaneous hemorrhage within areas of venous infarction in CSVT. Hemorrhage has been reported at all levels of varying severity: intraparenchymal, intraventricular (IVH), subdural, and subarachnoid. In a study of IVH in term neonates, about one-third was found to have had CSVT [24]. The cerebral edema and congestion may be transient if venous flow is re-established, or may be associated with permanent tissue infarction if the increased regional tissue pressure ultimately exceeds the arterial perfusion pressure. Eventually the delivery of arterial blood glucose and oxygen are compromised and ischemic injury with "venous" infarction results [23,25]. Cytotoxic edema preceding the onset of vasogenic edema has been documented early in acute CSVT, signifying the presence of neuronal injury early in venous infarction [26]. Once the

initial thrombus has formed, the ensuing obstruction and venous stasis can promote propagation of the initial thrombus. Relief of venous obstruction, even if delayed, can ease the circulatory congestion in CSVT completely with potentially improved clinical outcome. Occlusion of the superior saggital sinus or the dominant transverse sinus impairs the function of arachnoid granulations, which inteferes with the absorption of CSF. This further increases the extent of cerebral swelling and occasionally results in communicating hydrocephalus [23].

To date, no animal models of CSVT have been developed to the best of our knowledge. Very likely, differences would be expected between the mature and immature brain in its ability to tolerate and react to venous obstruction. In this regard, there are some elementary data to suggest that venous congestion could interfere with the myelin maturation process in the white matter of human newborns [27].

Etiology and risk factors

Cerebral sinovenous thrombosis is a multifactorial disease. The etiology and pathophysiology of CSVT in the pediatric population are still poorly understood, and the role of thrombophilic risk factors remains to be elucidated [1–5,33,34]. CSVT can result from local or regional structural or inflammatory abnormalities exerting mechanical effects on the sinovenous system, or systemic comorbid conditions. Among children with CSVT, either chronic or acute health disorders are frequently reported. Trauma, infections (especially sinusitis, mastoiditis, and other conditions affecting the head and neck area), collagen vascular disorders, hemoglobinopathies, metabolic disorders, and inflammatory bowel disease have been suggested as potential risk factors for CSVT occurrence in small cohort studies and case series [35–42]. Several case–control studies have dealt with the role of prothrombotic risk factors in the pathphysiology of CSVT [1–2,33,34,43–49]. In a recent meta-analysis of pediatric case–control studies, thrombophilia increased the risk of stroke or CSVT in patients aged 0–18 years old, especially when combined thrombophilic traits were diagnosed [49]. A statistically significant association with first event occurrence was demonstrated for each thrombophilia trait evaluated, with no difference found between arterial ischemic stroke and CSVT.

Neonates are vulnerable to CSVT due to many physiological and pathological factors. Physiological factors may include: the maternal hypercoagulable state of pregnancy [50]; moulding of the infants skull bones [51] and instrumentation during labor causing mechanical damage to underlying dural sinuses; a relatively high hematocrit; venous flow that is dependent on head positioning [52]; and lower than adult levels of natural coagulation inhibitors such as protein C, protein S, and antithrombin [53]. Compression of the posterior superior saggital sinus by the occipital bone due to dependent head position has been invoked as another potential mechanism predisposing to stasis and probable increase in the risk of thrombus formation [22]. Pathological disorders in the pre- or perinatal period have been reported in approximately 50% of neonates with CSVT and include maternal infections, gestational diabetes, premature rupture of membranes, abruptio placentae, and birth asphyxia [1–3,8]. Other neonatal disorders associated with CSVT include dehydration, bacterial sepsis, meningitis, and congenital heart disease [1,54,55]. Prothrombotic abnormalities have been reported in 15–50% of neonates with CSVT [1,2,8,49,56–61]. In another report, low carnitine levels were found in two neonates with CSVT in association with hypoxic ischemic encephalopathy [62]. Overall, neonatal CSVT can result from local or regional structural or inflammatory abnormalities exerting mechanical effects on the sinovenous system, or systemic comorbid conditions.

In the normal term neonate, there is a delicate balance of procoagulant and anticoagulant or fibrinolytic processes. Particularly in the setting of a clinical provoking factor (e.g., endothelial damage, venous stasis), thrombosis can develop once a relative excess of procoagulant factors or a relative deficiency of the anticoagulant or fibrinolytic mechanisms evolves, a condition often referred to as a "hypercoagulable state."

Despite the reporting of several prothrombotic abnormalities in CSVT, their role in the pathogenesis of CSVT and neonatal CSVT is not fully established. The main issue with the thrombophilia laboratory work-up with regard to the native anticoagulants is "how low" below the accepted normal values (for age) should be considered "pathologically low"? Another problem is the fact that laboratories across different centers have differing levels of normal ranges and variable methods of testing. There is a need to develop universally acceptable and reproducible methods of testing for prothrombotic risk factors as thrombophila testing does have some added value, mostly with

regard to therapy considerations. Genetic thrombophilia, and especially presence of prothrombin G20210A mutation, significantly increase the risk of recurrent thromboembolism in CSVT patients older than 2 years of age, paticularly when acquired hypercoagulability aggravates the underlying constitutional prothrombotic state [34]. Nonetheless, lack of systematic studies currently precludes application of this information to neonates with neonatal CSVT.

Clinical features of CSVT

It is apparent that the clinical manifestations of CSVT are non-specific and may be subtle. Clinical scenarios occur at all ages, and the clinician should consider this diagnosis in a wide range of acute neurological presentations in childhood. These include seizures, coma, altered consciousness, focal deficits, stroke, headache, and increased intracranial pressure [1–2,6]. Particularly in non-neonates, massive/extensive CSVT may include presentation with diffuse signs or altered level of consciousness. Common illnesses (e.g., ear infections, meningitis, anaemia, diabetes, and head injury) may lead to CSVT evolution, particularly when thrombogenesis has been precipitated by various clinical settings such as sepsis, dehydration, renal failure, trauma, cancer, and hematological disorders [28]. Although presentation with pseudotumour cerebri has been well documented, there are few data on the prevalence of CSVT in otherwise unexplained hydrocephalus or in convulsive and non-convulsive seizures and status epilepticus. It has been suggested that toddlers frequently present with seizures and focal signs, mainly hemiparesis, whereas in older children, seizures are less common and the presentation is typically with headache and changes in mental status [29].

Neonatal CSVT can occur either in isolation or more commonly as part of a coexisting intracranial or systemic disorder. When CSVT presents with signs/symptoms in neonates, seizures and encephalopathy are the chief clinical manifestations. The clinical features are typically diffuse and often overlap with manifestations of other comorbid neurological problems such as perinatal brain insults and intracranial infection. It may not be possible in individual cases to differentiate symptoms caused by neonatal CSVT from those caused by the coexisting neurological disease. Seizures are the predominant presenting feature in neonates, documented recently in 70% of 104 neonates with CSVT [8]. Despite focal venous infarction in many cases, clinical focal neurologic deficits are rare in neonates. The second most common manifestation of neonatal CSVT is encephalopathy, ranging from irritability and lethargy to frank coma. Raised intracranial pressure (due to retrograde venous congestion) – manifested by a tense, bulging, non-pulsatile fontanelle, split sutures, and dilated scalp veins – has been reported in severe neonatal CSVT [30]. Constitutional symptoms such as vomiting and poor feeding are other features. Rare manifestations of neonatal CSVT include head tremor [31] and palpebral ecchymosis [32]. Coexistent systemic (below neck) thrombosis is not uncommon in neonates with CSVT due to the existence of a hypercoagulable state and/or regional stasis. Concurrent systemic venous thrombosis was observed in 20% of Canadian neonates with CSVT [6,8]. Thus, neonates with CSVT should be potentially considered for screening for systemic thrombosis, and physical examination should at least be vigilant in this regard.

Imaging studies and diagnosis of CSVT

A number of radiographic modalities are available to evaluate the cerebral venous system and dural sinuses. However, systematic studies comparing diagnostic modalities against a gold standard are lacking, especially in neonates. Knowledge of the normal variations in the venous anatomy, as well as variations due to the imaging techniques in neonates, and correctly applying newly available techniques are clearly important.

Cranial ultrasound (for neonatal CSVT)

Because of their open fontanelles, cranial ultrasound (US) is helpful for diagnosing centrally located venous infarcts or hemorrhages in neonates. It is regularly used in neonatal intensive care units (NICUs) across most centers. The major advantage of US is that it is a bedside non-invasive procedure without radiation exposure. Doppler US can define absent or, less reliably, reduced flow in the sinovenous channels, mainly the superior saggital sinus. Assessment of the transverse sinuses and deep system is more limited [63]. Power Doppler, which measures the amplitude or strength of the Doppler signal instead of the velocity and direction of flow, is a measure of the number of flowing red cells, and in limited work to date has been reported to be better than conventional color Doppler in evaluation of CSVT [64]. As overall US is highly operator-dependent, it has clear limitations and treatment decisions cannot be based upon cranial ultrasound alone. Further research in ultrasound techniques for CSVT diagnosis is desirable.

Computed tomography (CT) and venography (CTV)

The main advantages of CT include ease of availability, short procedure time, and capacity to detect acute hemorrhage. In the Toronto study, just over 50% of neonates had their CSVT diagnosed by CT/CTV [6]. Signs indicative of CSVT on a non-contrast CT are the "filled triangle" or "dense triangle" sign or the "cord sign," reflecting the increased density of an intraluminal thrombus in sinovenous channels [23]. On contrast-enhanced CT, "empty triangle" or "empty delta" sign refers to a non-contrast enhancing thrombus surrounded by the dural walls of the sinus, which enhance with contrast. Although the same radiographic signs have been found in neonates, unenhanced CT has limitations, since it may miss CSVT in 20–40% of pediatric patients and underestimate both the extent of sinus involvement and the presence and extent of venous infarction [1,65]. The CT can also yield false positive results in neonates, in whom the increased hematocrit, presence of fetal hemoglobin, and decreased density of unmyelinated brain can combine to produce a high-density triangle in the torcular area on a non-contrast CT that can simulate the dense triangle sign [65–67]. In addition, unless thinly sliced coronal CT images are obtained, it can be difficult to differentiate subdural hemorrhage along the edges of tentorium cerebelli from intraluminal thrombus in the transverse or sigmoid sinus. Using CT venography with a multislice technique has been reported to be better than routine CT and a good alternative to MR venography (MRV) in adults [68]. There are no similar head-to-head comparison studies yet in children and newborns. However, the radiation dose with multislice CT might be concerning in newborns and increasing awareness of radiation hazard in the long term is precluding its routine use [69]. With recent advances in CT technology, optimizing the yield of CTV with even lower doses of radiation are expected in the future.

Magnetic resonance imaging (MRI) and venography (MRV)

The MRI technique is at present the preferred diagnostic modality in general because of its capability to demonstrate flow, thrombus, edema, infarction, and concurrent abnormalities [70]. However, few studies have addressed the role of MRI in neonatal CSVT [71]. In the Toronto study, nearly 50% of neonates had MRI to diagnose CSVT [6,8]. On conventional MR images, acute thrombus within a cerebral vein or dural sinus is isointense on T1-weighted images and hypointense on T2-weighted images. In the subacute stage, thrombus is hyperintense on T1- as well as T2-weighted images. Slow flow, turbulent flow, angled flow, or flow-related enhancement may cause an increased signal that can imitate intraluminal thrombus. The two-dimensional time-of-flight (TOF) MRV has flow gaps in the transverse sinus especially in the non-dominant transverse sinus, which can mimic thrombosis. In neonates, two-dimensional TOF–MRV has limitations [72], as moulding of the skull in the occipital region often partially compresses the posterior portion of the superior saggital sinus resulting in loss of signal on TOF–MRV. Subdural blood adjacent to the tentorium and the torcular can be falsely interpreted as transverse sinus thrombosis on MRI or CT. However, subtentorial subdural hemorrhage and thrombosis in the torcular or transverse sinuses may coexist in the same patient and further complicate the issue. Three-dimensional gadolinium-enhanced MRV techniques are being increasingly used in adults, but there are no pediatric or neonatal studies yet. Notably, unmyelinated brain presents challenges to T2-weighted imaging of venous infarcts. Sedation issues and the availability of urgent/emergent time slots for MRI are also problematic. For the direct imaging of thrombosis within veins or sinuses, CTV with multislice CT is comparable to gadolinium-enhanced MRV in most stages of evolution of CSVT, and both of these techniques are more accurate than TOF–MRV. There is limited experience with diffusion-weighted imaging (DWI) in neonates with CSVT; however, it has shed light on the presence of cytotoxic and vasogenic edema during venous infarction in adults with CSVT and the potential reversibility of such changes [73]. The use of DWI has been reported to be of value in the diagnosis of acute CSVT as well as a potential predictor for recanalization [74]. In acute CSVT, restricted DWI can be seen in the actual clot itself in the affected venous sinus and its presence potentially predicts incomplete recanalization in neonates as well [75].

Other modalities

Conventional catheter cerebral angiography is now rarely used for CSVT diagnosis by itself due to its invasive nature. Classic angiographic findings are similar to those in adults and include partial or complete lack of filling of cerebral veins or sinuses, enlarged collateral veins, delayed venous emptying, reversal of normal venous flow direction, abnormal cortical veins (broken or corkscrew-like), and regional or global delayed venous flow.

Indirect radiologic evidence of CSVT: Venous infarction with/without hemorrhage

Between 50–90% of neonates and children with CSVT have parenchymal lesions loosely referred to as venous infarcts [1,5,76]. In neonates, the majority of these are hemorrhagic. Diffusion restriction may or may not be seen in venous infarcts depending on the degree of venous congestion and reduced arterial inflow with resultant true ischemia. With thrombosis of the superficial system, infarcts are usually located in the cortex and white matter and may be bilateral (Figure 3.2). Typically, superior saggital sinus thrombosis gives rise to uni- or bilateral high parasagittal venous infarcts. With thrombosis of the deep system, infarcts (typically hemorrhagic) are usually located in one or both thalami or the cerebellum. In term neonates with IVH or thalamic hemorrhage, sinovenous thrombosis involving the deep system is the underlying cause in up to one-third and should be sought [4] (Figure 3.3). In the Toronto study, venous infarction was documented in about 60% of neonates [6,8]. Of these, about half were frankly hemorrhagic infarcts and the remaining half were deep white matter petechial hemorrhagic venous infarcts. The topographic distribution of brain lesions associated with CSVT correlates well the expected known drainage territories of the dural venous sinuses in newborns [76]. Kersbergen and colleagues have shown differences in the location of ischemic lesions related to CSVT between preterm and term newborns; white matter involvement was more common in preterm infants while thalamic involvement was more common in term babies [77].

Approximately 65% of neonates with CSVT have brain parenchymal lesions, frequently detected in the frontal and parietal lobes [21].

Recanalization rate

In adults, maximum recanalization occurs by 4–6 months after diagnosis, and almost none thereafter [78]. Neonates clearly recanalize faster and more completely than older children, with the maximal rate of

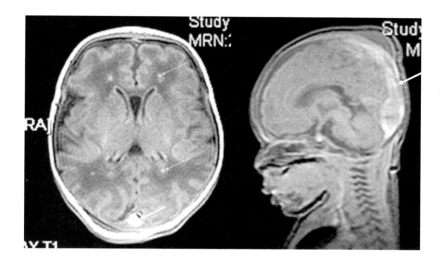

Figure 3.2 Axial (left) and sagittal (right) T1-weighted MRI of a 9-day-old male neonate with *E. coli* sepsis, showing increased signal in the superior sagittal sinus and torcular (thick arrows) and bilateral small areas of increased signal suggestive of petechial hemorrhagic venous infarction in the deep white matter (thin arrows).

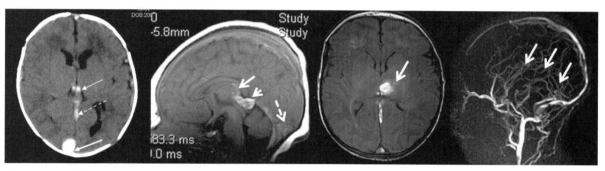

Figure 3.3 Far left panel is an axial non-contrast CT scan of a 5-day-old male neonate with hyperdense signal in the superior torcular (thick arrow), the vein of Galen (broken arrow), and both internal cerebral veins (thin arrow), suggestive of acute thrombosis. The second panel is a sagittal T1-weighted MRI scan of the brain showing bright signal in the internal cerebral veins (long arrow), vein of Galen (short arrow), and torcular (dashed arrow), suggestive of thrombus. The third panel is an axial T1-weighted MRI of the brain showing a hemorrhagic venous infarct in the left thalamus. The panel on the far right is an MR venogram showing absence (arrows) of blood flow in the internal cerebral vein, vein of Galen, and straight sinus.

recanalization in the first 3 months after diagnosis. About 50% of all neonates were fully recanalized by 6 weeks to 3 months after diagnosis; the rate increased to 65% by 6 months and to 75% by 1 year [6,8]. In older children, non-recanalization is considered a poor prognostic sign and has been associated with higher risk of recurrent venous thromboembolism [34].

Management of CSVT

Treatment of CSVT should consist of a three-pronged approach. Firstly, efforts should be concentrated on mitigating underlying risk factor(s), as amenable. Secondly, neuroprotective measures should be adopted in all newborns with CSVT. Thirdly, judicious consideration should be given to target the thrombotic process by way of specific antithrombotic agents. Two

pediatric stroke treatment guidelines have discussed the above three steps to some extent, mainly based on expert and consensus-based parameters [79 (ACCP Guidelines, Chest journal), 80 (AHA Guidelines, Stroke journal)]. Most recently, specific treatment guidelines for CSVT in general, including both adult and pediatric CSVT, have discussed these three targets in the neonatal population as well [81,82].

Management of underlying risk factors

As the majority of patients seem to have an associated risk factor at the time of CSVT, the benefit of identifying the potentially treatable or modifiable risk factor causing or provoking or aggravating CSVT cannot be underestimated. As far as prothrombotic risk factors (thrombophila states) are concerned, although many centers do undertake a systematic search, the cost-effectiveness and yield of this line of investigations, especially in neonates, remains to be established (AHA class II, level of evidence B). Please see also discussion of hypercoagulable states/thrombophilias, above.

Neuroprotection

Neuroprotective measures are expected to be beneficial in limiting the extent of brain injury in CSVT in young patients. Simple measures like maintenance of normal temperature, blood pressure, blood volume, blood sugar, and treatment of seizures, has been shown in adult studies to prevent worsening of existing brain injury, and is recommended in children and neonates (AHA class I, level of evidence C). Seizures, which are a frequent feature of CSVT (particularly in neonates), should be treated aggressively, as seizures can increase infarct volume and ultimately increase the area of brain injury. There are, however, insufficient data to routinely recommend prophylactic anticonvulsants in children and neonates with CSVT. There could be potentially some benefit in monitoring neonates with CSVT by continuous EEG monitoring; however, systematic studies are required to address this issue (AHA class IIb, level of evidence C). Neonatal CSVT is accompanied by venous congestion, cerebral edema, and intracranial venous hypertension. Although adults and children with CSVT may sometimes be treated with specific agents to manage elevated intracranial pressure (such as mannitol, acetazolamide, and controlled hyperventilation), there are no data to support the use of these measures in newborns. Moreover, the patent anterior fontanelle in newborns might serve as a protective feature against raised intracranial pressure. Overall, the role of supportive neuroprotective measures in pediatric CSVT, especially in neonates, requires further systematic investigation.

Antithrombotic therapy

Currently available treatment for CSVT in general includes anticoagulant therapy and thrombolytic therapy. Antiplatelet agents, such as aspirin, traditionally have not been used in CSVT treatment in adults and hence has not been considered during CSVT treatment in children and newborns. As a result, most of the pediatric treatment data address the role of anticoagulation as opposed to antiplatelet therapy in CSVT. The AHA 2008, ACCP 2008, and AHA 2011 guidelines address the evidence regarding both anticoagulant and

thrombolytic therapies in childhood and neonatal CSVT. Currently there are no high-quality evidence-based recommendations for antithrombotic therapy in pediatric CSVT due to the lack of randomized controlled trials. The aim of antithrombotic therapy after CSVT is maintenance of patency and mitigation of thrombus growth in the acute treatment period and avoidance of a new thrombosis in the subsequent phase of secondary prophylaxis. To the extent that attenuating the hypercoagulable state may also optimize intrinsic fibrinolytic potential (e.g., down-regulating thrombin production may decrease activation of thrombin activatable fibrinolysis inhibitor), anticoagulation may perhaps also act to hasten recanalization, although the clinical correlation of this mechanistic hypothesis remains unclear. Although not treating CSVT may significantly increase the risk of thrombus propagation that is associated with new venous infarctions and worse clinical outcomes, safety issues (i.e., presence or risk of clinically significant bleeding) should simultaneously be considered. In the context of present guidelines and in the absence of RCT-based evidence, factors influencing treatment decision include the extent and location of the thrombus, CSVT propagation, intracranial hemorrhage, the reversibility or irreversibility of risk factors for the CSVT, and the capacity to monitor anticoagulant therapy.

The Canadian registry was the first large study to address the use of anticoagulation in pediatric CSVT. One-third of 69 neonates in that cohort received anticoagulant therapy without significant hemorrhagic complications [1]. Following that study and given prior adult [83,84] and early pediatric data [85,86], there has been an increasing tendency to treat infants and children with CSVT with anticoagulation. A large prospective cohort study addressing the safety of protocol-based anticoagulants for a variety of childhood thrombotic events [86], including 146 children (33% were neonates, 15% had CSVT) treated with therapeutic doses of low molecular weight heparin, yielded 5% major bleeds in neonates and children. Another recent study documented the safety of low molecular weight heparin in preterm neonates with systemic thrombosis [87]. Data from adult CSVT trials have also shown that even patients presenting with hemorrhagic infarction benefited from heparin therapy [83,84].

Two recent studies have provided data on safety of anticoagulation specifically in newborns with CSVT, even in the presence of coexisting intracranial hemorrhage (ICH) [3,8]. In the study from Toronto [8],

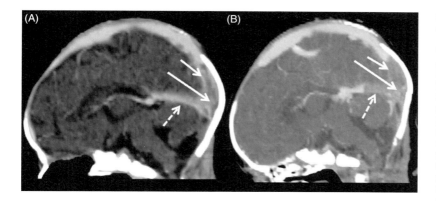

Figure 3.4 Panel A is a midline sagittal contrast-enhanced CT venogram of a newborn with CSVT showing thrombus in the posterior superior sagittal sinus (short arrow) and torcular (long arrow), as well as bilateral transverse sinuses (not seen in this image). Note the patent straight sinus (dashed arrow). This child was not anticoagulated, based on the attending physician's preference. Panel B is the follow-up CT venogram of the same newborn revealing propagation of the thrombus in the superior sagittal sinus (short arrow; note the increased bulk of the thrombus), torcular (long arrow; note the increased bulk of the thrombus), and straight sinus (dashed arrow; note the previously patent sinus is now occluded with new clot, which extended retrograde from the clot in the torcular).

53/104 newborns with CSVT received anticoagulation. Major hemorrhagic complications (all non-fatal) were seen in 5.6% of all treated newborns. Among 56 infants with radiographically confirmed significant ICH at presentation, 14 were treated with anticoagulation without any worsening of ICH. The same study demonstrated 35% thrombus propagation (Figure 3.4) in those not treated, vs. 2% in those treated, with anticoagulation. Moreover, clinically silent propagation of CSVT resulted in new venous infarction in 40% of all neonates. This clearly shows that untreated CSVT is not benign in neonates; it can result in worsening of thrombosis, which increases the risk of subclinical parenchymal brain injury. Thus, it appears essential to monitor those neonates not receiving anticoagulation for thrombus propagation with imaging, and if propagation is documented, institution of anticoagulation should be strongly considered.

Despite emerging observational data supporting the safety of anticoagulant therapy in pediatric CSVT, many centers are still not treating newborns, and treatment appears to be geographically based [5,7]. In addition, use of anticoagulation is likely linked with clinical severity at CSVT presentation and with underlying disease. Presence of ICH at diagnosis essentially reflects the severity of brain injury due to CSVT and therefore strengthens the notion supporting the need to consider anticoagulant therapy even in newborns with CSVT in the presence of ICH.

In the absence of RCT evidence, the presence of significant inherited thrombophilia and/or lack of transient risk factors (namely: idiopathic CSVT) in non-neonatal children typically warrants a prolonged course of anticoagulant therapy. Notably, prospective follow-up of the European pediatric CSVT cohort reflected the use of secondary anticoagulant prophylaxis in subsequent high-risk situations. This was especially true in children with thrombophilia and lack of thrombus recanalization following acute-phase therapy [34].

With regard to thrombolytic therapy, neither the AHA nor ACCP pediatric guidelines endorse the use the thrombolytic therapy for childhood and neonatal CSVT. Thrombolysis is generally limited to severe cases with high risk of mortality, or patients who experience clinical deterioration despite adequate anticoagulant therapy [88]. There are some case reports documenting the successful thrombolytic treatment of CSVT in neonates or children [89–92]. Major hemorrhagic complications have also been reported with this treatment [92].

Outcomes

A mortality rate of 4% has recently been reported for childhood CSVT, whereas mortality from neonatal CSVT has been difficult to gauge based on existing data, and ranges from 2.5% to 19% [3,6]. Wasay *et al.* [96] reported a higher mortality rate from CSVT in neonates as compared to older children, which was further associated with coma and seizures at presentation.

The neurological outcome following neonatal CSVT would be anticipated to be better than older infants or children due to theoretically enhanced brain plasticity. However, as with any neurologic insult occurring in the neonatal period, detection of the clinical sequelae could be understandably delayed, since the young brain may not exhibit many of the neurologic deficits that can be evident at older ages [93]. Indeed, initial CSVT studies indicated that neonates have a more favorable outcome as compared to older children [94]. Nevertheless, in the majority of studies, the authors did not adequately distinguish outcomes between children and neonates. The mean age of follow-up varied across the studies, and disabilities were variably classified [95]. With more recent accrual of data, it seems that neonates have a worse outcome than children [3,5–8,101]. To date, there has been substantial heterogeneity in reporting of neurodevelopment outcome in neonates and children with CSVT, mainly due to lack of standardized assessment protocols. Neurologic deficits including epilepsy, motor impairments, and a range of cognitive impairments were reported for 40% to 80% of all neonates on follow-up. Long-term epilepsy, including infantile spasms [55], is estimated to occur in approximately 20% [3,8] of neonatal CSVT patients, although some studies quote a much higher figure of up to 40% [5]. Data are now available from recent cohort studies regarding the neurological outcome from childhood CSVT as well [6,101]. In general, the frequency of adverse neurological outcome (including a range of moderate to severe neurological deficits consisting of sensorimotor, visual, cognitive, hearing, and behavioral problems) ranges from 10–20% in children [6,101]. Presence of comorbid neurological conditions, prolonged follow-up period, and presence of ICH at diagnosis were predictors of poorer outcome [6,8]. Interestingly, radiological recanalization beyond the acute period does not seem to have any effect on the clinical outcome, yet it appears that the *rate* of recanalization in the acute period might influence prognosis [6], and thrombus propagation does potentially adversely affect it.

Other predictors of poor neurologic outcome in pediatric CSVT include coagulation abnormalities, multiple sinus thrombosis, seizures at presentation, and venous infarction [97,98]. Notably, childhood CSVT prognosis was found to be better when compared to arterial ischemic stroke [99,100]; nearly 50% of CSVT patients do not have infarcts and may suffer fewer motor deficits or no permanent damage [102].

Recurrent CSVT or other systemic thromboses have been reported in 6–13% of children with CSVT [1,34], and not reported in neonatal cohorts followed so far. The multicenter European study has documented a recurrent venous thromboembolism risk of 6% in 396 children with CSVT, half of these being cerebral [34]. Significantly, none of the recurrences were documented in children experiencing CSVT under the age of 2 years.

Conclusions

Cerebral sinovenous thrombosis is increasingly encountered in children and neonates and should remain in the differential diagnosis of neurological symptoms, especially in the setting of complicated delivery or acute illnesses. Neuroimaging of sinovenous channels must be specifically undertaken or the diagnosis will be missed. The etiology of CSVT is multifactorial and the role of thrombophilic risk factors has not yet been fully established. Although anticoagulation appears to provide benefit when administered and managed via experienced clinicians, it is not uniformly applied within and across centers, especially in neonates. Infants not receiving anticoagulation for CSVT should be closely monitored for thrombosis propagation. Although mortality is low, there is risk of adverse long-term neurological sequelae, particularly in neonates. Further cooperative cohort studies are needed to define the natural history (including long-term outcomes and risk strata) in childhood and neonatal CSVT. In addition, multicenter randomized controlled trials must be conducted in order to provide key evidence for the standard of care in childhood and neonatal CSVT.

References

1. deVeber G, Andrew M, Adams M, et al. Canadian Pediatric Ischemic Stroke Study Group. Cerebral sinovenous thrombosis in children. New Eng J Med 2001; **345**: 417–23.

2. Heller C, Heinecke A, Junker C, et al. Childhood Stroke Study Group. Cerebral venous thrombosis in children: a multifactorial origin. Circulation 2003; **108**: 1362–7.

3. Berfelo FJ, Kersbergen KJ, van Ommen CH, et al. Neonatal cerebral sinovenous thrombosis from symptom to outcome. Stroke 2010; **41**: 1382–8.

4. Wu YW, Miller SP, Chin K, Collins AE, Lomeli SC, Chuang NA, Barkovich AJ, Ferriero DM. Multiple risk factors in neonatal sinovenous thrombosis. Neurology 2002; **59**: 438–40.

5. Fitzgerald KC, Williams LS, Garg BP, Carvalho KS, Golomb MR. Cerebral sinovenous thrombosis in the neonate. Arch Neurol 2006; **63**: 405–9.

6. Moharir MD, Shroff M, Stephens D, et al. Anticoagulants in pediatric cerebral sinovenous

thrombosis: a safety and outcome study. Ann Neurol 2010; **67**: 590–9.

7. Jordan LC, Rafay MF, Smith SE, et al; International Pediatric Stroke Study Group. Antithrombotic treatment in neonatal cerebral sinovenous thrombosis: results of the International Pediatric Stroke Study. J Pediatr 2010; **156**: 704–10.

8. Moharir M, Shroff M, Pontigon A, et al. A prospective outcome study of neonatal cerebral sinovenous thrombosis. J Child Neurol 2011; **26**: 1137–44.

9. Kersbergen K, Groenendaal F, Benders M, de Vries L. Neonatal cerebral sinovenous thrombosis: neuroimaging and long-term follow-up. J Child Neurol 2011; **26**: 1111–20.

10. Pergami P, Abraham L. Impact of anticoagulation on the short-term outcome in a population of neonates with cerebral sinovenous thrombosis: a retrospective study. J Child Neurol 2011; **26**: 844–50.

11. Laurichesse Delmas H, Winer N, Gallot D, et al. Prenatal diagnosis of thrombosis of the dural sinuses: report of six cases, review of the literature and suggested management. Ultrasound Obstet Gynecol 2008; **32**: 188–98.

12. Legendre D, Picone O, Levaillant JM, et al. Prenatal diagnosis of spontaneous dural sinus thrombosis. Prenat Diagn 2009; **29**: 808–13.

13. Woodhall B. Variations of the cranial venous sinuses in the region of the torcular herophili. Arch Surg 1936; **33**: 297–314.

14. Schreiber SJ, Lurtzing F, Gotze R, et al. Extrajugular pathways of human cerebral venous drainage assessed by duplex ultrasound. J Appl Physiol 2003; **94**: 1802–5.

15. Valdueza JM, von Munster T, Hoffman O, et al. Postural dependency of cerebral venous outflow. Lancet 2000; **355**: 200–1.

16. Capra N, Anderson K. Anatomy of the cerebral venous system. In Knapp JP and Schmidek HH, editors. *The Cerebral Venous System and its Disorders*. Orlando, FL: Grune and Stratton, Inc.; 1984: pp 1–36.

17. Kudo L, Terae S, Ishii A, et al. Physiologic change in flow velocity and direction of dural venous sinuses with respiration: MR venography and flow analysis. Am J Neuroradiol 2004; **25**: 551–7.

18. Lasjaunias P, Burrows P, Planet C. Developmental venous anomalies (DVA): The so-called venous angioma. Neurosurg Rev 1986; **9**: 233–42.

19. Lai PH, Chen PC, Pan HB, Yang CF. Venous infarction from a venous angioma occurring after thrombosis of a drainage vein. AJR Am J Roengenol 1999; **172**: 1698–99.

20. Sarwar M, McCormic WF. Intracerebral venous angioma. Case report and review. Arch Neurol 1978; **35**: 323–5.

21. San Millan Ruiz D, Delavelle J, Yilmaz H, Gailloud P, Piovan E, Bertramello A, Pizzini F, Rufenacht DA. Parenchymal abnormalities associated with developmental venous anomalies. Neuroradiology 2007; **49**: 987–5.

22. Tan M, deVeber G, Shroff M, et al. Sagittal sinus compression is associated with neonatal cerebral sinovenous thrombosis. Pediatrics 2011; **128**: e429–35.

23. Bousser MG, Russell RR. *Cerebral Venous Thrombosis*. Toronto: WB Saunders Company Ltd, 1997.

24. Wu YW, Hamrick SE, Miller SP, et al. Intraventricular hemorrhage in term neonates caused by sinovenous thrombosis. Ann Neurol 2003; **54**: 123–6.

25. Ungersbock K, Heimann A, Kempski O. Cerebral blood flow alterations in a rat model of cerebral sinus thrombosis. Stroke 1993; **24**: 563–9.

26. Forbes KP, Pipe JG, Heiserman JE. Evidence for cytotoxic edema in the pathogenesis of cerebral venous infarction. Am J Neuroradiol 2001; **22**: 450–5.

27. Porto L, Kieslich M, Yan B, et al. Accelerated myelination associated with venous congestion. Eur Radiol 2006; **16**: 922–6.

28. Barron TF, Gusnard DA, Zimmerman RA, Clancy RR. Cerebral venous thrombosis in neonates and children. Pediatr Neurol 1992; **8**: 112–16.

29. Carvalho KS, Bodensteiner JB, Connolly PJ, Garg BP. Cerebral venous thrombosis in children. J Child Neurol 2001; **16**: 574–80.

30. Hartmann A, Wappenschmidt J, Solymosi L. Clinical findings and differential diagnosis of cerebral vein thrombosis. In Einhaupl K, editor. *Cerebral Sinus Thrombosis. Experimental and Clinical Aspects*. New York: Plenum Press; 1987: pp. 171–86.

31. Sagrera FX, Raspall TF, Sala CP, et al. Cephalic trembling as a result of neonatal cerebral venous thrombosis. Ann Espanol Pediatr 1996; **45**: 431–3.

32. Fumagalli M, Ramenghi LA, Mosca F. Palpebral ecchymosis and cerebral venous thrombosis in a near term infant. Arch Dis Childhood Fetal Neonatal Ed 2004; **89**: F530.

33. Kenet G, Waldman D, Lubetsky A, Kornbrut N, et al. Paediatric cerebral sinus vein thrombosis. A multi-center, case-controlled study. Thromb Haemost 2004; **92**: 713–18.

34. Kenet G, Kirkham F, Neiderstadt T, et al; the European Thromboses Study Group. Risk factors for recurrent venous thromboembolism in the European collaborative database on cerebral venous thrombosis: a multicentre cohort study. Lancet Neurol 2007; **6**: 595–603.

35. Stiefel D, Eich G, Sacher P. Posttraumatic dural sinus thrombosis in children. Eur J Pediatr Surg 2000; **10**: 41–4.

36. Matsushige T, Nakaoka M, Kiya K. Cerebral sinovenous thrombosis after closed head injury. J Trauma 2009; **66**: 1599–604.

37. Krishnan A, Karnad DR, Limaye U. Cerebral venous and dural sinus thrombosis in severe falciparum malaria. J Infect 2004; **48**: 86–90.

38. Prasad R, Singh R, Joshi B. Lateral sinus thrombosis in neurocysticercosis. Trop Doct 2005; **35**: 182–3.

39. Standridge S, de los Reyes E. Inflammatory bowel disease and cerebrovascular arterial and venous thromboembolic events in 4 pediatric patients: a case series and review of the literature. J Child Neurol 2008; **23**: 59–66.

40. Uziel Y, Laxer RM, Blaser S. Cerebral vein thrombosis in childhood systemic lupus erythematosus. J Pediatr 1995; **126**: 722–7.

41. Yoshimura S, Ago T, Kitazono T. Cerebral sinus thrombosis in a patient with Cushing's syndrome. J Neurol Neurosurg Psychiatr 2005; **76**: 1182–3.

42. Siegert CE, Smelt AH, de Bruin TW. Superior sagittal sinus thrombosis and thyrotoxicosis. Possible association in two cases. Stroke 1995; **26**: 496–7.

43. Bonduel M, Sciuccati G, Hepner M. Factor V Leiden and prothrombin gene G20210A mutation in children with cerebral thromboembolism. Am J Hematol 2003; **73**: 81–6.

44. Cakmak S, Derex L, Berruyer M. Cerebral venous thrombosis: clinical outcome and systematic screening of prothrombotic factors. Neurology 2003; **60**: 1175–8.

45. Johnson MC, Parkerson N, Ward S. Pediatric sinovenous thrombosis. J Pediatr Hematol/Oncol 2003; **25**: 312–5.

46. Vorstman E, Keeling D, Leonard J. Sagittal sinus thrombosis in a teenager: homocystinuria associated with reversible antithrombin deficiency. Dev Med Child Neurol 2002; **44**: 498.

47. Martinelli I, Battaglioli T, Pedotti P. Hyperhomocysteinemia in cerebral vein thrombosis. Blood 2003; **102**: 1363–6.

48. Cantu C, Alonso E, Jara A. Hyperhomocysteinemia, low folate and vitamin B12 concentrations, and methylene tetrahydrofolate reductase mutation in cerebral venous thrombosis. Stroke 2004; **35**: 1790–4.

49. Kenet G, Lütkhoff LK, Albisetti M, et al. Impact of thrombophilia on risk of arterial ischemic stroke or cerebral sinovenous thrombosis in neonates and children: a systematic review and meta-analysis of observational studies. Circulation 2010; **121**: 1838–47.

50. Ballem P. Acquired thrombophilia in pregnancy. Semin Thromb Hemost 1998; **24 (Suppl 1)**: 41–7.

51. Newton TH, Gooding CA. Compression of superior sagittal sinus by neonatal calvarial molding. Neuroradiology 1975; **115**: 635–639.

52. Cowan F, Thoresen M. Changes in superior sagittal sinus blood velocities due to postural alterations and pressure on the head of the newborn infant. Pediatrics 1985; **75**: 1038–47.

53. Andrew M, Paes B, Johnston M. Development of the hemostatic system in the neonate and young infant. Am J Pediatr Hematol/Oncol 1990; **12**: 95–104.

54. Farstad H, Gaustad P, Kristiansen P, et al. Cerebral venous thrombosis and Escherichia coli infection in neonates. Acta Paediatr 2003; **92**: 254–7.

55. Soman TB, Moharir M, deVeber G, Weiss S. Infantile spasms as an adverse outcome of neonatal cortical sinovenous thrombosis. J Child Neurol 2006; **21**: 126–31.

56. deVeber G, Monagle P, Chan A, et al. Prothrombotic disorders in infants and children with cerebral thromboembolism. Arch Neurol 1998; **55**: 1539–43.

57. Ramenghi LA, Gill BJ, Tanner SF, et al. Cerebral venous thrombosis, intraventricular haemorrhage and white matter lesions in a preterm newborn with factor V (Leiden) mutation. Neuropediatrics 2002; **33**: 97–9.

58. Baumeister FA, Auberger K, Schneider K. Thrombosis of the deep cerebral veins with excessive bilateral infarction in a premature infant with the thrombogenic 4G/4G genotype of plasminogen activator inhibitor-1. Eur J Pediatr 2000; **159**: 239–42.

59. Friese S, Muller-Hansen I, Schoning M, et al. Isolated internal cerebral venous thrombosis in a neonate with increased lipoprotein (a) level: diagnostic and therapeutic considerations. Neuropediatrics 2003; **34**: 36–9.

60. Tardy-Poncet B, Rayet I, Damon G, et al. Protein C concentrates in a neonate with a cerebral venous thrombosis due to heterozygous type 1 protein C deficiency. Thromb Haemost 2001; **85**: 1118–9.

61. Burneo JG, Elias SB, Barkley GL. Cerebral venous thrombosis due to protein S deficiency in pregnancy. Lancet 2002; **359**: 892.

62. Ezgu FS, Atalay Y, Hasanolu A, et al. Intracranial venous thrombosis after hypoxic-ischemic brain insult in two newborns: could low serum carnitine levels have contributed? Nutr Neurosci 2004; **7**: 63–5.

63. Bezinque SL, Slovis TL, Touchette AS. Characterization of superior sagittal sinus blood flow velocity using colour flow Doppler in neonates and infants. Pediatr Radiol 1995; **25**: 175–9.

64. Tsao PN, Lee WT, Peng SF, et al. Power Doppler ultrasound imaging in neonatal cerebral venous sinus thrombosis. Pediatr Neurol 1999; **21**: 652–5.

65. Davies RP, Slavotinek JP. Incidence of the empty delta sign in computed tomography in the paediatric age group. Austral Radiol 1994; **38**: 17–9.

66. Hamburger C, Villringer A, Bauer M. Delta (empty triangle) sign in patients without thrombosis of the

superior sagittal sinus. In: Einhaupl K, Kempski O, Baethmann A, editors. *Cerebral Sinus Thrombosis: Experimental and Clinical Aspects.* New York: Plenum Press; 1990: pp 211–7.

67. Kriss VM. Hyperdense posterior falx in the neonate. Pediatr Radiol 1998; **28**: 817–9.

68. Ozsvath RR, Casey SO, Lustrin ES, et al. Cerebral venography: comparison of CT and MR projection venography. Am J Roentgenol 1997; **169**: 1699–707.

69. Brenner D, Elliston C, Hall E. Estimated risks of radiation-induced fatal cancer from pediatric CT. Am J Roentgenol 2001; **176**: 289–96.

70. Medlock MD, Olivero WC, Hanigan WC, et al. Children with cerebral venous thrombosis diagnosed with magnetic resonance imaging and magnetic resonance angiography. Neurosurgery 1992; **31**: 870–6.

71. Puig J, Pedraza S, Mendez J, Trujillo A. Neonatal cerebral venous thrombosis: diagnosis by magnetic resonance angiography. Radiologia 2006; **48**: 169–71.

72. Widjaja E, Shroff M, Blaser S. 2D time-of-flight MR venography in neonates: anatomy and pitfalls. Am J Neuroradiol 2006; **27**: 1913–8.

73. Ducreux D, Oppenheim C, Vandamme X, et al. Diffusion-weighted imaging patterns of brain damage associated with cerebral venous thrombosis. Am J Neuroradiol 2001; **22**: 261–8.

74. Favrole P, Guichard J-P, Crassard I, et al. Diffusion weighted imaging of intravascular clots in cerebral venous thrombosis. Stroke 2004; **35**: 99–105.

75. Moharir M, Shroff M, deVeber G. Diffusion weighted imaging of venous clots in childhood cerebral sinovenous thrombosis: An aid to diagnosis and a potential predictor of recanalization outcome. Ann Neurol 2006; **60**: S157 [Abstract].

76. Teksam M, Moharir M, deVeber G, Shroff M. Frequency and topographic distribution of brain lesions in pediatric cerebral venous thrombosis. Am J Neuroradiol 2008; **29**: 1961–5.

77. Kersbergen K, Groenendaal F, Benders M, et al. The spectrum of associated brain lesions in cerebral sinovenous thrombosis: relation to gestational age and outcome. Arch Dis Child Fetal Neonatal Ed 2011; **96**: F404–9.

78. Baumgartner RW, Studer A, Arnold M, Georgiadis, D. Recanalization of cerebral venous thrombosis. J Neurol Neurosurg Psych 2003; **74**: 459–61.

79. Monagle P, Chalmers E, Chan A, et al. Antithrombotic therapy in neonates and children: American College of Chest Physicians Evidence-Based Clinical Practice Guidelines (8th Edition). Chest 2008; **133(6 Suppl)**: 887S-968S.

80. Roach ES, Golomb MR, Adams R, et al. Management of stroke in infants and children: a scientific statement from a Special Writing Group of the American Heart Association Stroke Council and the Council on Cardiovascular Disease in the Young. Stroke 2008; **39**: 2644–91.

81. Saposnik G, Barrinagarrementaria, Brown RD, et al. Diagnosis and Management of Cerebral Venous Thrombosis: A Statement for Healthcare Professionals From the American Heart Association/American Stroke Association. Stroke 2011; **42**: 1158–92.

82. Nwosu ME, Williams LS, Edwards-Brown M, et al. Neonatal sinovenous thrombosis: presentation and association with imaging. Pediatr Neurol 2008; **39**: 155–61.

83. Einhaupl KM, Villringer A, Meister W, et al. Heparin treatment in sinus venous thrombosis. Lancet 1991; **338**: 597–600.

84. de Bruijn SF, Stam J. Randomized, placebo-controlled trial of anticoagulant treatment with low molecular weight heparin for cerebral sinus thrombosis. Stroke 1999; **30**: 484–8.

85. deVeber G, Chan A, Monagle P, et al. Anticoagulation therapy in pediatric patients with sinovenous thrombosis: a cohort study. Arch Neurol 1998; **55**: 1533–7

86. Dix D, Andrew M, Marzinotto V, et al. The use of low molecular weight heparin in pediatric patients: a prospective cohort study. J Pediatr 2000; **136**: 439–95.

87. Michaels LA, Gurian M, Hegyi T, Drachtman RA. Low molecular weight heparin in the treatment of venous and arterial thromboses in the premature infant. Pediatrics 2004; **114**: 703–7.

88. Ciccone A, Canhao P, Falcao F. Thrombolysis for cerebral vein and dural sinus thrombosis. Cochrane Database Syst Rev. 2004; **1**: CD003693.

89. Higashida RT, Helmer E, Halbach VV, Hieshima GB. Direct thrombolytic therapy for superior sagittal sinus thrombosis. Am J Neuroradiol 1989; **10**: S4–6.

90. Griesemer DA, Theodorou AA, Berg RA, Spera TD. Local fibrinolysis in cerebral venous thrombosis. Pediatr Neurol 1994; **10**: 78–80.

91. Tsai FY, Wang AM, Matovich VB, et al. MR staging of acute dural sinus thrombosis: correlation with venous pressure measurements and implications for treatment and prognosis. Am J Neuroradiol 1995; **16**: 1021–9.

92. Horowitz M, Purdy P, Unwin H, et al. Treatment of dural sinus thrombosis using selective catheterization and urokinase. Ann Neurol 1995; **38**: 58–67.

93. Bouza H, Rutherford M, Acolet D, et al. Evolution of early hemiplegic signs in full term infants with unilateral brain lesions in the neonatal period: a prospective study. Neuropediatrics 1994; **25**: 201–7.

94. deVeber GA, MacGregor D, Curtis R, Mayank S. Neurologic outcome in survivors of childhood arterial

ischemic stroke and sinovenous thrombosis. J Child Neurol 2000; **15**: 316–24.

95. Sebire G, Tabarki B, Saunders DE, et al. Cerebral venous sinus thrombosis in children: risk factors, presentation, diagnosis and outcome. Brain 2005; **128**: 477–89.

96. Wasay M, Dai AI, Ansari M, Shaikh Z, Roach ES. Cerebral venous sinus thrombosis in children: a multicenter cohort from the United States. J Child Neurol 2008; **23**: 26–31.

97. Johnson MC, Parkerson N, Ward S, de Alarcon PA. Pediatric sinovenous thrombosis. J Pediatr Hematol/Oncol 2003; **25**: 312–5.

98. Jacobs K, Moulin T, Bogousslavsky J, Woimant F, Dehaene I, Tatu L. The stroke syndrome of cortical vein thrombosis. Neurology 1996; **47**: 376–82.

99. De Schryver EL, Blom I, Braun KP, Kappelle LJ, Rinkel GJ, Peters AC, et al. Long-term prognosis of cerebral venous sinus thrombosis in childhood. Dev Med Child Neurol 2004; **46**: 514–9.

100. de Bruijn SF, de Haan RJ, Stam J, for the Cerebral Venous Sinus Thrombosis Study. Clinical features and prognostic factors of cerebral venous sinus thrombosis in a prospective series of 59 patients. J Neurol Neurosurg Psychiatr 2001; **70**: 105–8.

101. Grunt S, Wingeier K, Wehrli E, et al; Swiss Neuropaediatric Stroke Registry. Cerebral sinus venous thrombosis in Swiss children. Dev Med Child Neurol 2010; **52**(12): 1145–50.

102. Huisman TA, Holzmann D, Martin E, Willi UV. Cerebral venous thrombosis in childhood. Eur Radiol 2001; **11**: 1760–5.

Gastrointestinal and visceral thromboembolism

Courtney A. Lyle and Christoph Male

Introduction

Although thrombosis of the gastrointestinal and visceral vasculature, including hepatic vein and inferior vena cava thrombosis (Budd–Chiari syndrome) and splanchnic vein thrombosis (portal, splenic, or mesenteric vein thrombosis) is a rare phenomenon in childhood, it is associated with considerable morbidity and mortality. The overall incidence is unknown in children, but portal vein thrombosis (PVT) and Budd–Chiari syndrome are the most frequently reported. In general, the natural history of these thrombotic disorders is not well described in the pediatric literature; thus risk factors, diagnostic strategies, and therapeutic interventions are often extrapolated from the adult literature to supplement the experience reported in children.

An anatomical understanding of the abdominal venous vasculature is critical in identifying risk factors and recognizing signs and symptoms of gastrointestinal VTE. The portal vein originates behind the pancreas in the right upper quadrant of the abdomen and is formed by the confluence of the splenic and superior mesenteric veins (Figure 4.1). The inferior mesenteric vein drains directly into the splenic vein. The portal vein typically ascends behind the common bile duct and hepatic artery and divides into the right and left portal branches at the porta hepatis, delivering nearly two-thirds of the blood flow to the liver. In neonates, the umbilical vein traverses the portal vein to connect with the ductus venosus, which enables blood to bypass the liver to flow directly to the inferior vena cava (Figure 4.2) [1,2]. A thrombus may form anywhere along the portal vein as well as along any associated tributaries and/or branches. Veno-occlusion may be described as either partial or complete obstruction of the vessel. Nearly two-thirds of PVT are isolated to the portal vein, while 28% of PVT are found to involve the splenic vein and 15% involve the superior mesenteric vein [3]. Patients may also have isolated splenic or isolated mesenteric vein thrombosis.

Hepatic venous outflow occurs primarily via three major hepatic veins that drain into the inferior vena cava just below the level of the diaphragm. Hepatic vein thrombosis may range from single-vessel involvement to severe obstruction that extends either to the right atrium or to the portal venous system [4]. The accepted nomenclature of hepatic vein thrombosis is Budd–Chiari syndrome, defined as obstruction of hepatic venous outflow at any level [5]. Thus, obstruction may occur at the level of the small hepatic veins, large hepatic veins, or at the inferior vena cava up to the level of the right atrium (obstruction as a result of cardiac disease and hepatic veno-occlusive disease/sinusoidal obstruction syndrome are excluded from this definition) [5].

Although gastrointestinal thrombosis is frequently reported as idiopathic, it is likely that similar mechanisms contribute to the development of gastrointestinal thrombosis as for the formation of VTE in other areas, namely Virchow's triad, consisting of endothelial damage, venous stasis, and hypercoagulability [3,6].

Portal venous thrombosis

Introduction

Thrombosis of the portal vein accounts for approximately 6% of all venous thromboembolism in the pediatric population and is the most common form of splanchnic venous thrombosis [7,8]. Children of all ages may be diagnosed with PVT. The mean age at presentation is 6 years and there does not appear to be any predilection for either sex [6].

Risk factors

Risk factors that contribute to direct injury of the portal vein include umbilical venous catheters (UVC),

---

Pediatric Thrombotic Disorders, ed. Neil A. Goldenberg and Marilyn J. Manco-Johnson. Published by Cambridge University Press. © Cambridge University Press 2015.

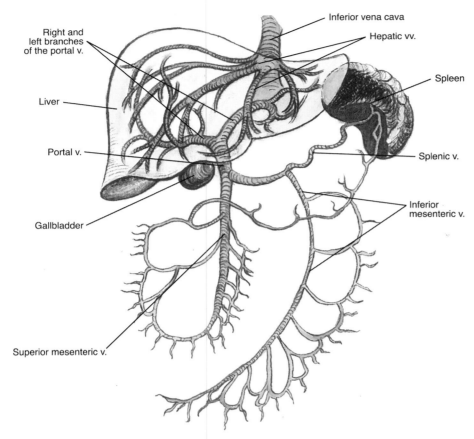

Figure 4.1 Mesenteric and portal vein system. (A black and white version of this figure will appear in some formats. For the color version of this figure, please refer to the plate section.)

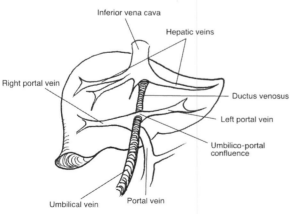

Figure 4.2 Umbilical vein.

infection (omphalitis and peritonitis), splenectomy, liver transplant, trauma, malignancy, and chemotherapeutic agents [2,3,6,9–13]. The most common risk factor causing direct injury to the portal vein occurs during catheterization of the umbilical vein. Although there is considerable heterogeneity in studies reporting incidence of PVT following umbilical vein catheterization, it has been reported as high as 43% in neonates who have had a UVC, and ranges from 0–43% in published literature [1,2,14]. The criteria for thrombosis evaluation in the neonatal period may influence the incidence rates of PVT, as global evaluation of all children with a UVC may identify cases that will resolve spontaneously, while imaging only in the presence of associated symptoms may miss those cases that present with delayed portal hypertension that occur beyond the neonatal period [2,9,15].

There are several factors associated with UVC placement that increase the risk of PVT. The left portal vein may be inadvertently cannulated during umbilical vein catheterization attempts, as a result of the proximity of the portal vein to the ductus venous. This cannulation can result in direct trauma to the vein itself, while the catheter material may also be thrombogenic [1,2]. Kim *et al.* also identified prolonged catheterization (longer than 6 days) as an additional factor that increases the risk of PVT [2]. In addition, patients requiring a UVC are typically critically ill as a result of sepsis/infection, hypoxia, and congenital malformations, which all can contribute to the overall risk of VTE formation.

Infection is also considered a major risk factor for PVT in neonates and during childhood that may cause direct injury to the portal vein. Omphalitis and peritonitis can cause local damage to the portal vein and its branches in addition to a systemic inflammatory response that may result in endothelial damage [1,3]. In a single-site cohort study (including both children and adults), Webb *et al.* reported that 39% of cases were associated with either umbilical sepsis or an intra-abdominal infection.

Surgical procedures, trauma, malignancy, and congenital vascular malformations also can be associated with direct trauma to the portal vein and increase the risk of thrombosis. Although rare, PVT has been reported following splenectomy in children [11,12]. The overall risk of VTE is increased following splenectomy as a result of venous stasis and thrombocytosis, and the risk of PVT is likely related to endothelial damage of portal vein tributaries (splenic vein) during surgery [11]. Liver transplant is associated with complex portal vein anastomoses, which can result in stasis and endothelial damage [13]. Trauma, either accidental or surgical, may result in injury to the portal vein, while malignancy such as hepatoblastoma or hepatocellular carcinoma (tumors at the porta hepatis) may cause direct damage to the portal vein or obstruction of the portal vein. [3] Treatment of malignancy may also further exacerbate the overall risk of PVT as a result of chemotherapy-induced endothelial damage [16]. Although cirrhosis is a common cause for PVT in adults, it is infrequently encountered in children [17]. Patients with congenital malformations of the vascular system involving the portal vein and/or its branches or tributaries, including stenosis, atresia, and agenesis, are also at higher risk of developing PVT [18].

Additional systemic risk factors that may contribute to an increased risk of thrombosis include sepsis, dehydration, and inherited or acquired thrombophilias. Although the role of thrombophilias in the pathogenesis of PVT is not completely understood and is frequently debated, several studies do suggest that thrombophilia is a risk factor for PVT in children. Pietrobattista *et al.* reported in a case–control study comparing children with PVT to healthy controls, that 32% of children with PVT had at least one inherited factor (factor V Leiden or prothrombin G20210A mutation, or deficiencies of protein C or protein S) compared to only 4% in the control population [19]. El-Karaksy and colleagues presented similar findings in a separate case–control study, noting that 62.5% of children with PVT had evidence of inherited thrombophilia (including factor V Leiden mutation or deficiencies of protein C, protein S, or antithrombin) [20]. Antiphospholipid antibodies have also been reported in children with PVT [21–23]. Conversely, however, Seixas and colleagues reported no difference in protein C and protein S levels in a small case–control study comparing children with PVT with healthy controls, and FVL was infrequently identified [21,24]. Elevated factor VIII levels have been reported in both children and adults with PVT; however, there is insufficient evidence to determine the overall causal association [25]. Myeloproliferative disorders, often with a JAK2 mutation, and paroxysmal nocturnal hemoglobinuria are frequently identified in adults with PVT [17,26]. While larger collaborative studies would be beneficial to further characterize the risk of PVT associated with thrombophilia, a comprehensive evaluation for hypercoagulable conditions, consistent with evaluation of other forms of VTE, could be considered if other risk factors or etiologies are not apparent.

Clinical presentation

The presenting signs and symptoms of PVT vary greatly and are dependent on the timing of diagnosis, associated conditions, and extent of venous involvement. Portal venous thrombosis in its initial phases may be asymptomatic or associated with vague symptoms such as transient abdominal pain that is not severe enough to warrant an extensive evaluation, and thus may often be overlooked in the early phase. Some cases may, in fact, resolve spontaneously before diagnosis ever occurs. If, however, the thrombus extends beyond the portal vein into the superior mesenteric vein or involves the proximal mesenteric venous arches, initial symptoms may be more severe and prompt a more extensive evaluation (see mesenteric venous thrombosis section below). Patients with septic pylephlebitis will also present with a more significant constellation of symptoms in the acute period, including fever, chills, and a painful liver [17]. These patients often have liver abscesses and a *Bacteroides* species detected in a blood culture.

Chronic PVT is most notably associated with the presence of a portal cavernoma. Within days to weeks following an acute PVT, collateral vessels begin to form around the obstructed portal venous segment to improve venous return to the hepatic system, resulting in a hepatopetal network of collaterals [17]. Despite the compensatory network of collateral flow, portal hypertension typically results in associated variceal formation and splenic enlargement leading to both upper gastrointestinal bleeding and hypersplenism. In addition, chronic PVT is associated with growth retardation, ascites, coagulation disorders, and portal biliopathy [10,27–29].

Upper gastrointestinal bleeding manifesting as hematemesis is the most frequently recognized symptom of PVT, which is also the most common cause of severe upper gastrointestinal bleeding in children [30]. Although varices have been noted as early as 1 month following an acute episode of PVT, upper gastrointestinal bleeding is often encountered many months to years following the initial event. Despite medical interventions, nearly three-quarters of children will suffer at least one episode of upper gastrointestinal bleeding and nearly a quarter of children will suffer from two or more occurrences [10,30]. In children who were diagnosed with PVT prior to an initial episode of upper gastrointestinal bleeding, the mean time to first episode of upper gastrointestinal bleeding is 4 years, and the frequency and severity of upper gastrointestinal bleeding may increase during adolescence [6].

Children may have concomitant splenomegaly with upper gastrointestinal bleeding, or may have isolated splenomegaly identified on physical exam. Splenomegaly is the second most common clinical manifestation (following upper gastrointestinal bleeding) at time of initial presentation in children and ultimately develops in the majority of patients [6,19,31]. The associated hypersplenism may result in leukopenia or thrombocytopenia [3].

Chronic abnormalities in venous flow secondary to the obstructed portal venous segment may also result in portal biliopathy [29]. Abnormalities of the intra- and extrahepatic bile ducts may occur secondary to compression from collateral vessels or altered venous return, resulting in biliary strictures, biliary stones, or displacement of the bile ducts. Associated symptoms range from being asymptomatic to severe abdominal pain, jaundice, pruritus, and fever. Clinically significant portal biliopathy occurs in approximately 3–6% of children affected by PVT [10,32].

Children with chronic PVT are also at risk of significant growth delays. Sarin and colleagues reported that more than 50% of children with PVT suffered from growth retardation [28]. Delayed growth has also been reported as the initial presenting sign of PVT [27]. The etiology for this, however, is unclear and may be multifactorial. A chronic anemia secondary to upper gastrointestinal bleeding or hypersplenism may contribute to decreased growth velocity, while diminished hepatic flow could also interfere with hepatrophic hormone signaling [33]. In addition, Mehrotra *et al.* proposed that a resistance to growth hormone may also contribute to the delay in growth [34].

Diagnosis

The modality used most frequently to diagnose PVT in both the acute and the chronic stages is ultrasonography with Doppler. Ultrasound findings consistent with PVT include echogenic material in the portal vein, dilatation of vessels proximal to the identified thrombus, and either decreased flow through the portal vein with partial obstruction or absence of flow with complete occlusion [35]. Visualization of new vessels providing venous flow around the obstructed segment, termed cavernous transformation, helps to establish the chronicity of the thrombus. Cavernous transformation has been identified as early as 5 weeks following an initial thrombotic event, but may take as long as 12 months before changes are visualized on ultrasound [36]. Ultrasound is a preferred modality as it is non-invasive, relatively quick, inexpensive, and sedation is not required even in young infants. Ultrasonography is however limited by the technician's expertise and can be non-diagnostic in patients who are obese, have a fatty liver, or have significant bowel gas.

Computed tomography (CT) or magnetic resonance imaging (MRI) may be used to confirm a diagnosis if initial ultrasound is not optimal, there is suspicion that additional vasculature is affected such as the mesenteric veins, or there is suspicion of abscess formation or bowel ischemia. Ultrasound findings consistent with PVT include an intraluminal soft tissue density in the portal vein with reduced/absent flow on Doppler, often associated with enlarged and sharply defined collateral vessels [37]. A major benefit of CT is that it is not limited by the technician's expertise. Disadvantages include the need for IV contrast, exposure to radiation, and greater expense of this exam.

With MRI, a thrombus visualized within approximately 5 weeks of formation will appear as a bright signal on T1- and T2-weighted images, while more chronic PVT will typically appear hyperintense on T2-weighted images [36]. While MRI provides additional information with regards to tributary veins as well as possible signs of bowel infarct, it is a much more expensive study than ultrasound, requires sedation in the young infant, and is optimized by the use of intravenous contrast (gadolinium).

Laboratory examination

In children with acute PVT or chronic PVT without associated portal biliopathy, liver transaminases usually remain within normal limits or just beyond the upper limit of normal [30]. Children with significant portal hypertension or portal biliopathy may have hyperbilirubinemia, elevated transaminases, and hepatic dysfunction. Children frequently do show laboratory abnormalities associated with hypersplenism, including thrombocytopenia, anemia, and neutropenia [27]. Anemia may also be further exacerbated by associated upper gastrointestinal bleeding. Portal venous thrombosis that occurs in the context of disseminated intravascular coagulation (DIC) may be associated with abnormalities of the prothrombin time (PT), partial thromboplastin time (PTT), and fibrinogen level, as well as thrombocytopenia. As discussed previously (section on risk factors), PVT is frequently associated with hypercoagulability, thus testing may reveal deficiencies of protein C, protein S, or antithrombin, the presence of antiphospholipid antibodies (lupus anticoagulant, anticardiolipin antibodies, and anti β_2 glycoprotein antibodies), or an elevated factor VIII level.

Treatment

In the treatment of PVT, one must consider acute interventions to prevent thrombus progression and promote vessel recanalization, determine prevention strategies to minimize long-term complications, and implement therapeutic interventions to treat associated morbidities.

When PVT is identified in the acute setting, anticoagulation should be considered to limit thrombus progression and attenuate overall hypercoagulability [38]. Although there is a paucity of data both in adults and children, it appears that early anticoagulation may prevent progression and recurrent thrombosis and decrease the overall risk of intestinal ischemia [39–41]. The optimal duration of therapy is also unknown, but is extrapolated from outcomes research for DVT in other locations, such that therapy may be discontinued after 3 months if the inciting risk factor has resolved, and to continue therapy for at least 6 months in the absence of any identifiable risk factor [39]. Initial therapy may commence with either unfractionated heparin (UFH) or low molecular weight heparin (LMWH) and may be transitioned to a vitamin K antagonist (VKA) if there is no evidence of liver disease or thrombocytopenia. It is recognized that anticoagulation for PVT is associated with additional challenges, including the risk of bleeding secondary to varices and thrombocytopenia associated with splenomegaly; however, initial treatment may lessen the risk of developing portal hypertension and its associated complications [39]. Additional measures that may be considered acutely include the removal of an umbilical venous catheter if feasible in a neonate and emergency surgical thrombectomy if a patient is suffering from intestinal ischemia as a result of the PVT. While thrombolysis has been reported as a therapeutic intervention for children with PVT, there is insufficient evidence to confirm benefits of this approach [42].

More frequently, children are diagnosed with chronic PVT as a result of complications secondary to portal hypertension. In the chronic phase, the use of anticoagulation is generally not recommended as there is likely limited benefit from anticoagulation and there is also an increased risk of bleeding associated with portal hypertension [38,39]. Strategies in the chronic phase are directed toward preventing the development of portal hypertension and associated sequelae and determining optimal intervention strategies for complications of portal hypertension.

Historically, the management of extrahepatic portal hypertension has been primarily non-surgical, including the use of endoscopic procedures such as sclerotherapy and endoscopic variceal band ligation (EVBL) to mitigate the presence of varices [43]. More recently, however, the meso-Rex bypass procedure, a mesenteric–left portal vein bypass, has been increasingly used to both prevent and treat the associated complications of extrahepatic portal venous obstruction [38,44]. By restoring mesenteric blood flow, there is improved blood flow to the liver and it is possible to control or lessen the effects of portal hypertension. Retrospective cohort studies suggest that children may suffer fewer (or no) episodes of variceal bleeding, have improved linear growth, and improved splenomegaly and hypersplenism, while a prospective series reports improved cognitive ability following a mesenteric–left portal vein bypass [44–46]. Thus, indications to consider the meso-Rex bypass procedure include growth impairment, neurocognitive impairment related to encephalopathy, hypersplenism with thrombocytopenia, portal biliopathy, and hepatopulmonary syndrome [38].

While expert opinion also suggests the meso-Rex bypass should be considered for children with grade II or III varices and used for secondary prophylaxis in children, there is no consensus regarding the optimal strategy in an asymptomatic patient with extrahepatic portal vein obstruction [38]. Additional considerations for primary prophylaxis in an asymptomatic patient to prevent a first-episode of variceal bleeding is the use of either a non-selective beta-blocker or endoscopic therapy; however, there are limited data and there is no consensus regarding the optimal approach to prophylaxis [38].

Prognosis

Despite the significant morbidity associated with PVT, the mortality rate in children is estimated to be quite low. In a retrospective review of 82 children with PVT with a mean follow-up duration of 15 years, there were no deaths observed, and in a slightly smaller cohort study, with a mean follow-up period of 5.5 years, 1/55 children with PVT died [10,31].

Splenic vein thrombosis

Introduction

Isolated splenic vein thrombosis (SPVT) is a rare occurrence in childhood. Although there are case reports documenting isolated SPVT, there were no cases of SPVT in two childhood VTE cohort studies [8,47]. Splenic vein thrombosis may also occur in association with mesenteric vein thrombosis or PVT.

Risk factors

The primary risk factors for isolated SPVT appear to be related to local factors contributing to venous stasis and endothelial damage. The local inflammation associated with both acute and chronic pancreatitis may cause damage to the nearby vessels, namely the splenic vessels that lie along the tail of the pancreas [48]. This may cause a disturbance in the venous flow and create a nidus for coagulation activation and, subsequently, thrombus formation. Splenic vein

thrombosis following splenectomy has been reported in children [49]. Not only does post-splenectomy thrombocytosis increase the risk of VTE, but local damage and stasis in the remaining splenic vein may also augment thrombus formation. Umbilical venous catheter placement has also been identified as a risk factor for SPVT, likely as a result of local vessel damage [50]. In addition, SPVT may occur in the context of other splanchnic thromboses; thus, risk factors such as inherited/acquired thrombophilias and myeloproliferative disorders must also be considered.

Clinical presentation

The extent of vessel involvement and rapidity of disease progression may affect the severity of presentation. If SPVT is diagnosed in the acute setting, presenting symptoms are often associated with the underlying condition, such as pancreatitis or a post-surgical state. In the chronic setting, nearly 50% of patients will have splenomegaly and patients may present with variceal-associated hematemesis [50,51]. With efferent splenic flow obstructed, collateral vessels form to relieve splenic congestion and may result in gastric, esophageal, or colonic varices [51].

Diagnosis

Thrombosis of the splenic vein may be visualized with ultrasound with Doppler, CT, or MRI techniques. Visualization of the splenic vein, however, can be difficult with ultrasound. If collateral vessels and/or splenomegaly are visualized, further diagnostic imaging should be completed to evaluate the patency of vessels.

Treatment

There are no specific guidelines informing pediatric treatment strategies for SPVT. In the ACCP adult guidelines, anticoagulation is recommended over no anticoagulation in the setting of symptomatic splanchnic VTE (including splenic vein), and recommendations are given against anticoagulation if the thrombosis is an incidental finding [39]. In the presence of severe variceal hemorrhage, splenectomy may be considered [50,52].

Mesenteric venous thrombosis

Introduction

Although mesenteric venous thrombosis (MVT) is infrequently encountered in pediatrics, it is an important consideration for an acute abdomen and intestinal ischemia. While MVT may occur in the context of thrombosis of other splanchnic veins as well as with mesenteric artery thrombosis, it is also recognized as a separate diagnostic entity [53].

Risk factors

Risk factors for MVT are similar to those described for PVT (see PVT risk factors above). Inherited and acquired thrombophilias are frequently associated with both pediatric and adult MVT. In a case–control study of 12 adult patients with MVT and 431 controls, factor V Leiden, prothrombin G20210A, and MTHFR mutations were each associated with increased odds of MVT [54]. Pediatric case reports have indicated associations of MVT with a homozygous MTHFR mutation and protein S deficiency [55,56]; it can also present in the setting of moderate/severe protein C deficiency (homozygous/compound heterozygous mutations) with and without superimposed heterozygous factor V Leiden (Goldenberg NA and Manco-Johnson MJ, personal communication; January 2014). Furthermore, MVT has also been reported in pediatric patients with inflammatory bowel disease and nephrotic syndrome [56,57]. Other local inflammatory conditions to consider include pancreatitis or the presence of an intra-abdominal abscess, and inflammation or trauma secondary to abdominal surgery [53].

Clinical presentation

Presenting signs and symptoms of MVT depend on the extent of venous involvement and whether or not collateral vessels have formed to relieve venous congestion. Symptoms consistent with an acute presentation include abdominal pain, often described as colicky pain located in the mid-abdomen, distension, vomiting, diarrhea, and if ischemia and necrosis are present, rebound tenderness will be noted [53,56,58–60]. Notably, the physical examination can range from normal to a surgical abdomen in the acute period. In the subacute or chronic phase, abdominal pain is common, but a surgical abdomen is unlikely. Hematemesis or upper gastrointestinal bleeding may occur if the occlusion has extended into the portal or splenic vein and varices have developed. Hematochezia, melena, and occult blood may also be noted at diagnosis of MVT [53,60]. While portal hypertension may occur if the portal or splenic vein are affected, the primary concern in MVT is intestinal ischemia and hemorrhagic infarct as a result of insufficient venous drainage [53].

Diagnosis

There are several imaging modalities that may assist a clinician in diagnosing MVT and determining the severity of the condition. An abdominal X-ray may be notable for non-specific bowel gas patterns or demonstrate pneumatosis intestinalis in severe cases, but will not provide visualization of the mesenteric thrombosis. Ultrasound is a relatively quick and inexpensive technique that may demonstrate thrombus in the mesenteric vein; however, the location of the mesenteric veins often precludes visualization with this modality. The CT is typically the modality of choice to establish a diagnosis of MVT. Thrombus may be visualized with CT, and this technique will also demonstrate the degree of infarcted or ischemic bowel, the presence of pneumatosis intestinalis or portal venous gas, and the presence of collateral vessels [61,62]. Magnetic resonance imaging also has good sensitivity/specificity in diagnosing MVT, but is less often utilized [63].

Laboratory evaluation

While a patient presenting with severe abdominal pain will likely warrant a comprehensive evaluation, the laboratory evaluation is typically non-diagnostic for MVT [59]. Evidence of inflammation or infection or the presence of a thrombophilia trait may suggest an etiology for MVT.

Treatment

As recommended by the adult ACCP guidelines for splanchnic vein thrombosis, anticoagulation should be initiated after diagnosis in a symptomatic patient [39]. While there are no randomized controlled clinical trials (RCT) to determine optimal therapy, it is suggested that acute anticoagulation is associated with improved survival and decreased rates of recurrence [64]. Subacute therapy is considered with either LMWH or VKA; however, the optimal duration of therapy is unknown [39]. Thrombolysis has also been reported as a successful intervention acutely; however, there is insufficient evidence to offer guidance regarding this approach [65]. In a patient without evidence of bowel ischemia, pharmacologic management may be sufficient, but in the presence of bowel ischemia or infarct, a patient will likely require emergency surgery [53].

If MVT is diagnosed incidentally or in the chronic phase, anticoagulation is usually not recommended unless a prothrombotic state is present and the patient is at risk of recurrence [39]. Therapy in this phase is directed toward prevention and treatment of any associated varices or portal hypertension.

Prognosis

The natural history of MVT in children is unknown, but in children who present acutely with extensive veno-occlusion and intestinal ischemia, immediate intervention is indicated as the risk of death is considerable [59].

Hepatic vein thrombosis (Budd–Chiari syndrome)

Introduction

Although thrombosis of the hepatic veins is rare in childhood, it has been reported to account for up to 8% of VTE cases in a cohort study of children and adolescents [47]. Thrombosis of the hepatic veins, or Budd–Chiari syndrome (BCS), results in obstruction of the hepatic venous outflow tract and leads to venous stasis and congestion in the liver. This further causes increased hepatic sinusoidal pressure leading to liver injury and ultimately irreversible liver damage if not alleviated through the development of a collateral venous system or a therapeutic intervention to restore hepatic venous outflow.

Risk factors

Risk factors for BCS, consistent with other forms of VTE, may be understood in the context of Virchow's triad, including acquired/inherited thrombophilias resulting in hypercoagulability, congenital or acquired IVC webs which may result in venous stasis, and local or systemic processes that result in endothelial damage [66–70]. While prothrombotic conditions are identified in the majority of adult cases of BCS (most frequently myeloproliferative disorders with JAK2 mutations), the overall prevalence in children with BCS is still unknown as there are a limited number of pediatric studies with a comprehensive thrombophilia evaluation [26]. In a small study of 16 children with BCS, 25% had an identified prothrombotic trait [71]. Reported cases of thrombophilia associated with BCS in children include the presence of a factor V Leiden or prothrombin G20210A mutation, the

presence of antiphospholipid antibodies, and paroxysmal nocturnal hemoglobinuria [71–74]. Protein C, protein S, and antithrombin deficiencies have also been associated with BCS; however, it is difficult to distinguish acquired from inherited deficiencies in the context of hepatic synthetic dysfunction [71,75]. In addition, inflammatory bowel disease, infection, and TPN have been reported in children with BCS, likely associated with activation of the coagulation pathway and/or endothelial damage [70,76].

Clinical presentation

The presenting signs/symptoms of BCS in children can vary significantly depending on the severity of the venous obstruction and rapidity of disease progression [5]. In cases of limited vessel involvement, children may be asymptomatic, while children with significant occlusion and limited hepatic venous outflow may present with fulminant hepatic dysfunction and encephalopathy, especially if progression is rapid and additional collateral vessels are not yet present [72]. The most frequent presenting signs/symptoms in children include abdominal distension secondary to ascites and hepatomegaly [71,77]. Additional findings may include prominent superficial abdominal veins, jaundice, splenomegaly, and portal hypertension [71,72,77,78]. As BCS is a rare diagnosis in children, a high level of suspicion is warranted in children presenting with ascites, hepatomegaly, and abdominal pain in order to diagnose the condition promptly.

Diagnosis

A diagnosis of BCS can often be made using non-invasive ultrasonography with Doppler. The sensitivity of this examination is approximately 85% [79]. Findings on ultrasound may include the absence of a flow signal in the intrahepatic veins or reversed or turbulent venous flow, the presence of collateral vessels supporting venous flow, and subcapsular hepatic venous collaterals [75,80]. If the obstruction extends into the portal venous system, splenoportal flow may also be reduced [72]. Ultrasound may also identify hepatomegaly and ascites [72]. Limitations of ultrasonography include reduced resolution in obesity and dependence on the expertise of the technician. In addition, ultrasonography may be limited in identifying thrombosis of the small hepatic veins.

Magnetic resonance imaging or CT should be utilized if ultrasound is inconclusive or if the extent of disease is not ascertained. These modalities can aid in the diagnosis and treatment planning by offering better visualization of the venous anatomy and identifying any abnormalities of the liver anatomy. Limitations include their costs, use of contrast media, radiation exposure with CT, and the need for sedation with MRI in a small child.

If the diagnosis is not easily ascertained with the available imaging techniques, a liver biopsy may be warranted. A liver biopsy may be useful in differentiating BCS affecting the small hepatic veins from sinusoidal obstruction syndrome [75,81].

Laboratory evaluation

The degree of laboratory abnormalities will depend on the severity of the disease [5]. In many cases, liver transaminases may be normal to only slightly abnormal unless severe hepatic venous obstruction is present [77]. As the disease state progresses, bilirubin and ammonia levels may increase and coagulopathies may develop secondary to decreased hepatic synthetic function [78]. Thrombophilias may be uncovered with a thorough hypercoagulability investigation. In certain cases, evaluation for infection or possible inflammatory diseases is also warranted.

Treatment

Therapeutic considerations for BCS include treatment of existing symptoms such as ascites and portal hypertension, anticoagulation, re-establishing hepatic flow with either an interventional radiologic (IR) approach (angioplasty, stenting, transjugular intrahepatic portosystemic shunt [TIPS]) or surgical shunt, and intervening in the event of irreversible liver damage with liver transplantation [5]. While there is a paucity of data in both the adult and pediatric literature to inform optimal therapeutic strategies, the ACCP and the European Group for the Study of Hepatic Vascular Diseases have established guidelines to assist the clinician in complex treatment decisions [5,39]. Often, however, treatment is guided by institutional experience [67].

Anticoagulation should be considered during the acute period to limit thrombus progression and attenuate hypercoagulability [5,39]. Although coagulopathies may also present acutely, this finding is not an absolute contraindication to acute anticoagulation [39]. Early treatment of veno-occlusion may improve flow and hepatic function; however, the treating clinician must weigh risks and benefits of anticoagulation. The ideal therapeutic agent is also unknown. Heparin

is often preferred in the setting of clinical instability or if there is considerable risk of bleeding as the half-life is short in comparison to LMWH. In a stable patient, however, LMWH may be considered as a first-line agent for anticoagulation. For subacute therapy, LMWH is preferred over VKA in the setting of hepatic dysfunction. There is insufficient evidence to determine the optimal duration of anticoagulation. An approach extrapolated from treatment of DVT is to anticoagulate for 3–6 months for a first BCS episode if there is a reversible risk factor, continue for 6–12 months in the setting of idiopathic BCS, and indefinite therapy in the setting of irreversible risk factors [39,82]. Subacute therapy with antiplatelet agents has also been reported following an IR approach in a small retrospective cohort study (6 children) and in a pediatric case report [71,78]. Although the authors report that this intervention has been successful, there are insufficient data by which to determine the overall risks and benefits of this approach. In a patient with incidentally detected BCS, anticoagulation may not be warranted unless a potent hypercoagulable state or ongoing coagulation activation is disclosed [39].

Thrombolysis may be considered acutely and has been reported in the pediatric literature with favorable outcomes; however, there is insufficient evidence to recognize the true risk or benefit from this intervention [68,83]. A percutaneous IR approach is conducted to restore venous drainage from the liver. The type of approach offered (angioplasty, stenting, and TIPS) depends on the site and extent of vessel occlusion, and size of the patient [71,83,84]. While an intervention in children may be more technically difficult owing to the small caliber of the veins than in adults, successful IR approaches have been reported in young patients [71,78,85]. Historically, portosystemic shunts were conducted more routinely to decompress the liver, but have been decreasing in frequency secondary to the success of IR approaches and increasing acceptance and availability of liver transplantation [5,86]. A liver transplant should be considered in a patient with encephalopathy, irreversible liver damage, or who has failed pharmacologic or interventional treatment [5,72].

The guidelines proposed by Janssen et al., although not pediatric-specific, suggest initiating anticoagulation acutely and initiating treatment for any underlying cause, as well as any concomitant symptoms including ascites and portal hypertension [5]. For patients who fail medical management, consideration should first be given to intervention with angioplasty and stenting with possible thrombolysis. In patients who are not an IR candidate, TIPS, or surgical portosystemic shunting should be considered. If this approach is unsuccessful or the condition rapidly progresses, liver transplantation should be offered [5]. The treatment of BCS is quite complex and associated with significant risks; thus, it is optimal to treat a patient in a center with experienced personnel who can also coordinate services with gastro-enterology, hematology, surgery, radiology, and a liver transplant service.

Prognosis

Despite medical and surgical interventions, the morbidity of symptomatic BCS is still considerable and overall survival is approximately 80% [5,71]. Further longitudinal studies are indicated to determine the natural course of asymptomatic BCS.

Conclusion

Budd–Chiari syndrome and SPVT comprise a rare and heterogeneous group of VTE. Clinical severity depends on the extent of veno-occlusion and the duration of time in which the occlusion occurred. Severity may range from an asymptomatic case identified incidentally to an acute presentation of fulminant liver failure or intestinal ischemia. Prompt diagnosis is required in order to offer early interventions such as anticoagulation, surgical, and percutaneous interventions aimed at improving outcomes, in addition to treatments targeting underlying diseases and associated signs/symptoms. Management is thus ideally undertaken at a center with expertise in the management of rare pediatric VTE in addition to pediatric gastrointestinal disorders.

References

1. Williams S, Chan AK. Neonatal portal vein thrombosis: Diagnosis and management. Semin Fetal Neonatal Med. Netherlands: Elsevier Ltd, 2011, **vol 16**, pp. 329–339.

2. Kim JH, Lee YS, Kim SH, Lee SK, Lim MK, Kim HS. Does umbilical vein catheterization lead to portal venous thrombosis? Prospective US evaluation in 100 neonates. Radiology 2001;**219**:645–650.

3. Orloff MJ, Orloff MS, Rambotti M. Treatment of bleeding esophagogastric varices due to extrahepatic portal hypertension: Results of portal-systemic shunts during 35 years; J Pediatr Surg 1994;**29**:142–151; discussion 151–154.

4. Mahmoud AE, Mendoza A, Meshikhes AN, Olliff S, West R, Neuberger J, Buckels J, Wilde J, Elias E. Clinical spectrum, investigations and treatment of Budd-Chiari syndrome. QJM 1996;**89**:37–43.

5. Janssen HL, Garcia-Pagan JC, Elias E, Mentha G, Hadengue A, Valla DC. Budd-Chiari syndrome: A review by an expert panel. J Hepatol 2003;**38**;364–371.

6. Webb LJ, Sherlock S. The aetiology, presentation and natural history of extra-hepatic portal venous obstruction. Q J Med 1979;**48**:627–639.

7. Raffini L, Huang YS, Witmer C, Feudtner C. Dramatic increase in venous thromboembolism in children's hospitals in the United States from 2001 to 2007. Pediatrics 2009;**124**:1001–1008.

8. van Ommen CH, Heijboer H, Buller HR, Hirasing RA, Heijmans HS, Peters M. Venous thromboembolism in childhood: A prospective two-year registry in the Netherlands. J Pediatr 2001;**139**:676–681.

9. Morag I, Epelman M, Daneman A, Moineddin R, Parvez B, Shechter T, Hellmann J. Portal vein thrombosis in the neonate: Risk factors, course, and outcome. J Pediatr 2006;**148**:735–739.

10. Maksoud-Filho JG, Goncalves ME, Cardoso SR, Gibelli NE, Tannuri U. Long-term follow-up of children with extrahepatic portal vein obstruction: Impact of an endoscopic sclerotherapy program on bleeding episodes, hepatic function, hypersplenism, and mortality. J Pediatr Surg 2009;**44**:1877–1883.

11. Skarsgard E, Doski J, Jaksic T, Wesson D, Shandling B, Ein S, Babyn P, Heiss K, Hu X. Thrombosis of the portal venous system after splenectomy for pediatric hematologic disease. J Pediatr Surg 1993;**28**:1109–1112.

12. Brink JS, Brown AK, Palmer BA, Moir C, Rodeberg DR. Portal vein thrombosis after laparoscopy-assisted splenectomy and cholecystectomy. J Pediatr Surg 2003;**38**:644–647.

13. Alvarez F. Portal vein complications after pediatric liver transplantation. Curr Gastroenterol Rep 2012;**14**:270–274.

14. Yadav S, Dutta AK, Sarin SK. Do umbilical vein catheterization and sepsis lead to portal vein thrombosis? A prospective, clinical, and sonographic evaluation. J Pediatr Gastroenterol Nutr 1993;**17**:392–396.

15. Morag I, Shah PS, Epelman M, Daneman A, Strauss T, Moore AM. Childhood outcomes of neonates diagnosed with portal vein thrombosis. J Paediatr Child Health 2011;**47**:356–360.

16. Brisse H, Orbach D, Lassau N, Servois V, Doz F, Debray D, Helfre S, Hartmann O, Neuenschwander S. Portal vein thrombosis during antineoplastic chemotherapy in children: Report of five cases and review of the literature. Eur J Cancer 2004;**40**:2659–2666.

17. Primignani M. Portal vein thrombosis, revisited. Dig Liver Dis. Netherlands, 2009 Editrice Gastroenterologica Italiana S.R.L.: Elsevier Ltd, 2010, **vol 42**, pp. 163–170.

18. Sarin SK, Sollano JD, Chawla YK, Amarapurkar D, Hamid S, Hashizume M, Jafri W, Kumar A, Kudo M, Lesmana LA, Sharma BC, Shiha G, Janaka de Silva H. Consensus on extra-hepatic portal vein obstruction. Liver Int 2006;**26**:512–519.

19. Pietrobattista A, Luciani M, Abraldes JG, Candusso M, Pancotti S, Soldati M, Monti L, Torre G, Nobili V. Extrahepatic portal vein thrombosis in children and adolescents: Influence of genetic thrombophilic disorders. World J Gastroenterol 2010;**16**:6123–6127.

20. El-Karaksy H, El-Koofy N, El-Hawary M, Mostafa A, Aziz M, El-Shabrawi M, Mohsen NA, Kotb M, El-Raziky M, El-Sonoon MA, A-Kader H. Prevalence of factor v Leiden mutation and other hereditary thrombophilic factors in Egyptian children with portal vein thrombosis: Results of a single-center case-control study. Ann Hematol 2004;**83**:712–715.

21. Seixas CA, Hessel G, Siqueira LH, Machado TF, Gallizoni AM, Annichino-Bizzacchi JM. Study of hemostasis in pediatric patients with portal vein thrombosis. Haematologica 1998;**83**:955–956.

22. Pati HP, Srivastava A, Sahni P. Extra hepatic portal vein thrombosis in a child associated with lupus anticoagulant. J Trop Pediatr 2003;**49**:191–192.

23. Ferri PM, Rodrigues Ferreira A, Fagundes ED, Xavier SG, Dias Ribeiro D, Fernandes AP, Borges KB, Liu SM, de Melo Mdo C, Roquete ML, Penna FJ. Evaluation of the presence of hereditary and acquired thrombophilias in Brazilian children and adolescents with diagnoses of portal vein thrombosis. J Pediatr Gastroenterol Nutr 2012;**55**:599–604.

24. Seixas CA, Hessel G, Ribeiro CC, Arruda VR, Annichino-Bizzacchi JM. Factor v Leiden is not common in children with portal vein thrombosis. Thromb Haemost 1997;**77**:258–261.

25. Kurekci AE, Gokce H, Akar N. Factor VIII levels in children with thrombosis. Pediatr Int 2003;**45**:159–162.

26. Primignani M, Barosi G, Bergamaschi G, Gianelli U, Fabris F, Reati R, Dell'Era A, Bucciarelli P, Mannucci PM. Role of the jak2 mutation in the diagnosis of chronic myeloproliferative disorders in splanchnic vein thrombosis. Hepatology 2006;**44**:1528–1534.

27. Gurakan F, Eren M, Kocak N, Yuce A, Ozen H, Temizel IN, Demir H. Extrahepatic portal vein thrombosis in children: Etiology and long-term follow-up. J Clin Gastroenterol 2004;**38**:368–372.

28. Sarin SK, Bansal A, Sasan S, Nigam A. Portal-vein obstruction in children leads to growth retardation. Hepatology 1992;**15**:229–233.

29. Khuroo MS, Yattoo GN, Zargar SA, Javid G, Dar MY, Khan BA, Boda MI. Biliary abnormalities associated with extrahepatic portal venous obstruction. Hepatology 1993;**17**:807–813.

30. Alvarez F, Bernard O, Brunelle F, Hadchouel P, Odievre M, Alagille D. Portal obstruction in children. I. Clinical investigation and hemorrhage risk. J Pediatr 1983;**103**:696–702.

31. Ferri PM, Ferreira AR, Fagundes ED, Liu SM, Roquete ML, Penna FJ. Portal vein thrombosis in children and adolescents: 20 years experience of a pediatric hepatology reference center. Arq Gastroenterol 2012;**49**:69–76.

32. Gauthier-Villars M, Franchi S, Gauthier F, Fabre M, Pariente D, Bernard O. Cholestasis in children with portal vein obstruction. J Pediatr 2005;**146**:568–573.

33. Sarin SK, Agarwal SR. Extrahepatic portal vein obstruction. Semin Liver Dis 2002;**22**:43–58.

34. Mehrotra RN, Bhatia V, Dabadghao P, Yachha SK. Extrahepatic portal vein obstruction in children: Anthropometry, growth hormone, and insulin-like growth factor I. J Pediatr Gastroenterol Nutr 1997;**25**:520–523.

35. Schwerk WB. Portal vein thrombosis: Real-time sonographic demonstration and follow-up. Gastrointest Radiol 1986;**11**:312–318.

36. Cohen J, Edelman RR, Chopra S. Portal vein thrombosis: A review. Am J Med 1992;**92**:173–182.

37. Mathieu D, Vasile N, Grenier P. Portal thrombosis: Dynamic CT features and course. Radiology 1985;**154**:737–741.

38. Shneider BL, Bosch J, de Franchis R, Emre SH, Groszmann RJ, Ling SC, Lorenz JM, Squires RH, Superina RA, Thompson AE, Mazariegos GV. Portal hypertension in children: Expert pediatric opinion on the report of the Baveno v consensus workshop on methodology of diagnosis and therapy in portal hypertension. Pediatr Transplant 2012;**16**:426–437.

39. Kearon C, Akl EA, Comerota AJ, Prandoni P, Bounameaux H, Goldhaber SZ, Nelson ME, Wells PS, Gould MK, Dentali F, Crowther M, Kahn SR. Antithrombotic therapy for VTE disease: Antithrombotic therapy and prevention of thrombosis, 9th edn: American College of Chest Physicians Evidence-Based Clinical Practice Guidelines. Chest 2012;**141**:e419S–494S.

40. Condat B, Pessione F, Hillaire S, Denninger MH, Guillin MC, Poliquin M, Hadengue A, Erlinger S, Valla D. Current outcome of portal vein thrombosis in adults: Risk and benefit of anticoagulant therapy. Gastroenterology 2001;**120**:490–497.

41. Plessier A, Darwish-Murad S, Hernandez-Guerra M, Consigny Y, Fabris F, Trebicka J, Heller J, Morard I,

Lasser L, Langlet P, Denninger MH, Vidaud D, Condat B, Hadengue A, Primignani M, Garcia-Pagan JC, Janssen HL, Valla D. Acute portal vein thrombosis unrelated to cirrhosis: A prospective multicenter follow-up study. Hepatology 2010;**51**:210–218.

42. Rehan VK, Cronin CM, Bowman JM. Neonatal portal vein thrombosis successfully treated by regional streptokinase infusion. Eur J Pediatr 1994;**153**:456–459.

43. Zargar SA, Yattoo GN, Javid G, Khan BA, Shah AH, Shah NA, Gulzar GM, Singh J, Shafi HM. Fifteen-year follow up of endoscopic injection sclerotherapy in children with extrahepatic portal venous obstruction. J Gastroenterol Hepatol 2004;**19**:139–145.

44. Sharif K, McKiernan P, de Ville de Goyet J. Mesoportal bypass for extrahepatic portal vein obstruction in children: Close to a cure for most! J Pediatr Surg 2010;**45**:272–276.

45. Mack CL, Zelko FA, Lokar J, Superina R, Alonso EM, Blei AT, Whitington PF. Surgically restoring portal blood flow to the liver in children with primary extrahepatic portal vein thrombosis improves fluid neurocognitive ability. Pediatrics 2006;**117**:e405–412.

46. Stringer MD. Improved body mass index after mesenterico-portal bypass. Pediatr Surg Int 2007;**23**:539–543.

47. Wright JM, Watts RG. Venous thromboembolism in pediatric patients: Epidemiologic data from a pediatric tertiary care center in Alabama. J Pediatr Hematol/Oncol 2011;**33**:261–264.

48. Koklu S, Koksal A, Yolcu OF, Bayram G, Sakaogullari Z, Arda K, Sahin B. Isolated splenic vein thrombosis: An unusual cause and review of the literature. Can J Gastroenterol 2004;**18**:173–174.

49. Lederman HM, Fieldston E. Splenic and portal vein thrombosis following laparoscopic splenectomy in a pediatric patient with chronic myeloid leukemia. Sao Paulo Med J 2006;**124**:275–277.

50. Vos LJ, Potocky V, Broker FH, de Vries JA, Postma L, Edens E. Splenic vein thrombosis with oesophageal varices: A late complication of umbilical vein catheterization. Ann Surg 1974;**180**:152–156.

51. Butler JR, Eckert GJ, Zyromski NJ, Leonardi MJ, Lillemoe KD, Howard TJ. Natural history of pancreatitis-induced splenic vein thrombosis: A systematic review and meta-analysis of its incidence and rate of gastrointestinal bleeding. HPB (Oxford) 2011;**13**:839–845.

52. Bradley EL, 3rd. The natural history of splenic vein thrombosis due to chronic pancreatitis: Indications for surgery. Int J Pancreatol 1987;**2**:87–92.

53. Kumar S, Sarr MG, Kamath PS. Mesenteric venous thrombosis. N Engl J Med 2001;**345**:1683–1688.

54. Amitrano L, Brancaccio V, Guardascione MA, Margaglione M, Iannaccone L, Dandrea G, Ames PR, Marmo R, Mosca S, Balzano A. High prevalence of thrombophilic genotypes in patients with acute mesenteric vein thrombosis. Am J Gastroenterol 2001;**96**:146–149.

55. Hayakawa T, Morimoto A, Nozaki Y, Kashii Y, Aihara T, Maeda K, Momoi MY. Mesenteric venous thrombosis in a child with type 2 protein s deficiency. J Pediatr Hematol/Oncol 2011;**33**:141–143.

56. Ulinski T, Guigonis V, Baudet-Bonneville V, Auber F, Garcette K, Bensman A. Mesenteric thrombosis causing short bowel syndrome in nephrotic syndrome. Pediatr Nephrol 2003;**18**:1295–1297.

57. Ross AS, Gasparaitis A, Hurst R, Hanauer SB, Rubin DT. Superior mesenteric vein thrombosis after colectomy in a patient with Crohn's disease. Nat Clin Pract Gastroenterol Hepatol 2005;**2**:281–285; quiz 281.

58. Gertsch P, Matthews J, Lerut J, Luder P, Blumgart LH. Acute thrombosis of the splanchnic veins. Arch Surg 1993;**128**:341–345.

59. Oguzkurt P, Senocak ME, Ciftci AO, Tanyel FC, Buyukpamukcu N. Mesenteric vascular occlusion resulting in intestinal necrosis in children. J Pediatr Surg 2000;**35**:1161–1164.

60. Boley SJ, Kaleya RN, Brandt LJ. Mesenteric venous thrombosis. Surg Clin North Am 1992;**72**:183–201.

61. Vogelzang RL, Gore RM, Anschuetz SL, Blei AT. Thrombosis of the splanchnic veins: CT diagnosis. AJR Am J Roentgenol 1988;**150**:93–96.

62. Kim JY, Ha HK, Byun JY, Lee JM, Yong BK, Kim IC, Lee JY, Park WS, Shinn KS. Intestinal infarction secondary to mesenteric venous thrombosis: CT-pathologic correlation. J Comput Assist Tomogr 1993;**17**:382–385.

63. Haddad MC, Clark DC, Sharif HS, al Shahed M, Aideyan O, Sammak BM. MR, CT, and ultrasonography of splanchnic venous thrombosis. Gastrointest Radiol 1992;**17**:34–40.

64. Abdu RA, Zakhour BJ, Dallis DJ. Mesenteric venous thrombosis – 1911 to 1984. Surgery 1987;**101**:383–388.

65. Robin P, Gruel Y, Lang M, Lagarrigue F, Scotto JM. Complete thrombolysis of mesenteric vein occlusion with recombinant tissue-type plasminogen activator. Lancet 1988;**1**:1391.

66. Mohanty D, Shetty S, Ghosh K, Pawar A, Abraham P. Hereditary thrombophilia as a cause of Budd-Chiari syndrome: A study from Western India. Hepatology 2001;**34**:666–670.

67. Menon KV, Shah V, Kamath PS. The Budd-Chiari syndrome. N Engl J Med 2004;**350**:578–585.

68. Alioglu B, Avci Z, Aytekin C, Mercan S, Ozcay F, Kurekci E, Ozbek N. Budd-Chiari syndrome in a child due to a membranous web of the inferior vena cava resolved by systemic and local recombinant tissue plasminogen activator treatment. Blood Coagul Fibrinolysis 2006;**17**:209–212.

69. Odell JA, Rode H, Millar AJ, Hoffman HD. Surgical repair in children with the Budd-Chiari syndrome. J Thorac Cardiovasc Surg 1995;**110**:916–923.

70. Nylund CM, Goudie A, Garza JM, Crouch G, Denson LA. Venous thrombotic events in hospitalized children and adolescents with inflammatory bowel disease. J Pediatr Gastroenterol Nutr 2012;**128**(19):2023–2027.

71. Nagral A, Hasija RP, Marar S, Nabi F. Budd-Chiari syndrome in children: Experience with therapeutic radiological intervention. J Pediatr Gastroenterol Nutr 2010;**50**:74–78.

72. Gomes AC, Rubino G, Pinto C, Cipriano A, Furtado E, Goncalves I. Budd-Chiari syndrome in children and outcome after liver transplant. Pediatr Transplant 2012;**16**:E338–341.

73. Sipahi T, Duru F, Yarah N, Akar N. Compound heterozygosity for factor v Leiden and prothrombin G20210a mutations in a child with Budd-Chiari syndrome. Eur J Pediatr 2001;**160**:198.

74. Wyatt HA, Mowat AP, Layton M. Paroxysmal nocturnal haemoglobinuria and Budd-Chiari syndrome. Arch Dis Child 1995;**72**:241–242.

75. Plessier A, Valla DC. Budd-Chiari syndrome. Semin Liver Dis 2008;**28**:259–269.

76. McClead RE, Birken G, Wheller JJ, Hansen NB, Bickers RG, Menke JA. Budd-Chiari syndrome in a premature infant receiving total parenteral nutrition. J Pediatr Gastroenterol Nutr 1986;**5**:655–658.

77. Gentil-Kocher S, Bernard O, Brunelle F, Hadchouel M, Maillard JN, Valayer J, Hay JM, Alagille D. Budd-Chiari syndrome in children: Report of 22 cases. J Pediatr 1988;**113**:30–38.

78. Chaudhuri M, Jayaranganath M, Chandra VS. Percutaneous recanalization of an occluded hepatic vein in a difficult subset of pediatric Budd-Chiari syndrome. Pediatr Cardiol 2012;**33**:806–810.

79. Bolondi L, Gaiani S, Li Bassi S, Zironi G, Bonino F, Brunetto M, Barbara L. Diagnosis of Budd-Chiari syndrome by pulsed Doppler ultrasound. Gastroenterology 1991;**100**:1324–1331.

80. Chawla Y, Kumar S, Dhiman RK, Suri S, Dilawari JB. Duplex doppler sonography in patients with Budd-Chiari syndrome. J Gastroenterol Hepatol 1999;**14**:904–907.

81. Valla DC. Budd-Chiari syndrome and veno-occlusive disease/sinusoidal obstruction syndrome. Gut 2008;**57**:1469–1478.

82. Monagle P, Chan AK, Goldenberg NA, Ichord RN, Journeycake JM, Nowak-Gottl U, Vesely SK. Antithrombotic therapy in neonates and children: Antithrombotic therapy and prevention of thrombosis, 9th edn: American College of Chest Physicians Evidence-Based Clinical Practice Guidelines. Chest 2012;**141**:e737S–801S.

83. Cauchi JA, Oliff S, Baumann U, Mirza D, Kelly DA, Hewitson J, Rode H, McCulloch M, Spearman W, Millar AJ. The Budd-Chiari syndrome in children: The spectrum of management. J Pediatr Surg 2006;**41**:1919–1923.

84. Rerksuppaphol S, Hardikar W, Smith AL, Wilkinson JL, Goh TH, Angus P, Jones R. Successful stenting for Budd-Chiari syndrome after pediatric liver transplantation: A case series and review of the literature. Pediatr Surg Int 2004;**20**:87–90.

85. Carnevale FC, Caldas JG, Maksoud JG. Transjugular intrahepatic portosystemic shunt in a child with Budd-Chiari syndrome: Technical modification and extended follow-up. Cardiovasc Intervent Radiol 2002;**25**:224–226.

86. Botha JF, Campos BD, Grant WJ, Horslen SP, Sudan DL, Shaw BW, Jr., Langnas AN. Portosystemic shunts in children: A 15-year experience. J Am Coll Surg 2004;**199**:179–185.

Renal and adrenal vein thromboses

Robert Francis Sidonio, Jr. and Leonardo R. Brandao

Introduction

Historical perspective

Renal vein thrombosis (RVT) poses a diagnostic and management challenge to pediatric hematologists, nephrologists, radiologists and neonatologists [1,2]. Such challenges are exemplified by one of the first descriptions of RVT in the literature in 1837 in which Pierre Rayer described the association between RVT and infancy. Three years later he described the association between nephrotic syndrome and RVT [3].

These first descriptions are fitting as the vast majority of cases occur in the neonatal period while the rare cases that do occur outside this period are typically associated with either primary or secondary renal disease or local vascular compression. Many of the first descriptions of RVT were reported in the European literature from the 1840s to the 1920s [3,4]. Subsequently, from the 1920s to the 1960s, the descriptions of RVT were noted mostly in the setting of its discovery at the time of surgery in a decompensating neonate followed by nephrectomy or at autopsy [5–7]. Although described nearly 190 years ago, the exact etiology of RVT remains still largely unknown but is likely related to the underlying disease, host characteristics and local and systemic risk factors. These factors include a reduced renal perfusion in the perinatal period, local inflammation and/or vascular obstruction, and coagulation-related issues either related to developmental hemostasis (i.e., the physiologic reduction of natural anticoagulants early in life) or to an inherited/acquired thrombophilia trait. In fact, thrombophilia was not recognized as a potential association until the 1990s, when most of the currently recognized inherited traits were characterized and initially thought to be the etiology of many pediatric thrombotic events.

The diagnosis and management recommendations in pediatric RVT, with/without adjacent adrenal vein thrombosis, are largely based on a few international registries and retrospective single-institution studies. In terms of imaging studies, while inferior venocavography and selective renal venography were initially considered the gold standard methods, they are currently rarely performed and have largely been replaced by ultrasound due to its excellent sensitivity and minimal side effects.

Even though RVT has been long recognized in children, systemic anticoagulation and/or thrombolytic therapy have been considered only in the last few decades, but not without controversy [1,2,8,9]. The aim of acute treatment is to prevent long-term poor renal outcomes ranging from mild renal insufficiency and chronic hypertension to atrophy and renal failure as well as to prevent direct extension in the inferior vena cava. While mortality is rare, prevention of significant morbidity remains the greatest challenge. Current treatment recommendations focus on thrombus burden, reserving thrombolysis for bilateral involvement of the renal veins and anticoagulation for unilateral involvement of the renal vein with extension into the IVC. A continuing challenge is a lack of an evidence-based risk-stratified algorithm to guide acute management of RVT. Predictors of poor renal outcome have not been fully validated but potential risk factors include severely decreased renal perfusion, subcapsular fluid collections, renal length and patchy renal cortex echogenicity.

This chapter describes the current knowledge of RVT as well as delineating areas in need of additional research. Throughout most of the text, we use the term "RVT" to indicate RVT with/without adjacent adrenal vein thrombosis. Near the conclusion of the chapter, we also briefly discuss isolated adrenal vein thrombosis, for which the available literature in pediatrics is quite limited.

Pediatric Thrombotic Disorders, ed. Neil A. Goldenberg and Marilyn J. Manco-Johnson. Published by Cambridge University Press. © Cambridge University Press 2015.

Epidemiology

Prevalence estimates of thrombosis in children are often difficult to determine since there is a paucity of large registries or prospective studies in pediatric thrombosis and prevalence differs by registry. A Dutch registry estimated the overall incidence of thrombosis in children at 0.14 per 10,000 [10]. Neonates comprised 20% of all cases of thrombosis in children, second only to the rate (27%) in teenagers [11]. The annual rate of VTE in neonates (< 28 days of life) grew 70% over a 6-year period ending in 2007 to 75 cases per 10,000 admissions, higher than the overall annual rate of VTE in children at 58 cases per 10,000 admissions [11]. Renal vein thrombosis remains the most common non-catheter related thrombotic event in the neonatal period and is also seen in the non-neonates, usually associated with nephrotic syndrome or following renal transplant (cadaveric conveying a greater risk than live-related donor transplant). Based on a single-institution study, a reasonable overall estimate of RVT in children is 0.17 cases per 1,000 admissions [12], while a Canadian registry estimated the prevalence of neonatal RVT at 0.5 per 1,000 neonatal intensive care admissions [13]. In general, RVT comprises 10–20% of all venous thrombotic events in the newborn period [13,14]; less is known about the incidence of RVT outside of the neonatal period. Renal vein thrombosis outside the first week of life is rarer and nearly always associated with an inherited thrombophilia or an acute or chronic medical disorder, predominantly primary renal disease (i.e., nephrotic syndrome). Although data are lacking on the true prevalence of RVT associated with nephrotic syndrome in children, it is likely similar to adults, estimated at 22–28% [15,16]. Renal vein thrombosis is the second most common cause, following acute and chronic rejection, for renal graft failure [17]. Thrombosis of the transplanted kidney graft occurs mostly in transplant recipients age 0–5, likely related to small vessel size, and is the cause of 12.8% of total pediatric renal transplant graft failures [17]. Investigations of the role of antiphospholipid antibodies or inherited thrombophilia in graft failure have not been conclusive.

Pathophysiology

Since most RVTs occur in neonates we will focus on pathophysiology during the perinatal period. While 89% of all neonatal thromboses are associated with an indwelling vascular catheter, RVT is the most common non-catheter-related thrombosis in the neonatal period [13]. The exact pathophysiology is still not fully elucidated but likely it is multifactorial.

In neonates it is likely that RVTs originate intra-renally due to the following factors: (1) low renal perfusion pressure, (2) elevated renal vascular resistance and (3) a double intracapillary network (see Figure 5.1). When these physiologic factors are coupled with hypovolemia and acidosis, the result appears to be a "fertile soil" for stasis and subsequent thrombosis. Because of the unique neonatal renal physiology, the vast majority of renal vein thromboses begin within the small intra-renal veins, specifically the arcuate or interlobular veins. Less commonly, RVT may originate from the IVC moving inward to the renal veins [18].

There is likely an interaction between acquired and underlying risk factors leading to a thrombotic event. Approximately 80% of affected neonates had at least one risk factor [14]. Overall, risk factors can be sub-categorized into three groups: (1) disease-related, (2) host-related and (3) treatment-related (see Table 5.1).

The most common disease-related risk factors for neonatal RVT are associated with altered blood rheology and include dehydration, perinatal asphyxia, sepsis/DIC and maternal diabetes. Acquired antiphospholipid antibodies are emerging as a potential independent risk factor in neonates and children with VTE [19]. It is presumed that most of the cases identified were likely related to passively transferred antibodies from the mother but this assumption has not been verified. In a German case–control study, anticardiolipin antibodies were identified in 5% of children with RVT but not seen as significant in multivariate analysis. Since evaluation for antiphospholipid antibodies (typically anticardiolipin and beta-2-glycoprotein 1 antibodies) is not routinely performed, true prevalence is not known.

Other disease-related risk factors include primary renal disease, specifically nephrotic syndrome and maternally transferred antiphospholipid antibodies. Membranous nephritis seems to be particularly associated with RVT, accounting for 37% of all cases of nephrotic syndrome and RVT. Nephrotic syndrome leads to anticoagulant protein wasting, most importantly antithrombin and protein S, increased fibrinogen production, enhanced platelet activation and aggregation, all of which creates an ideal environment for thrombosis development [15,16]. Beyond the neonatal period, in addition to primary renal disease,

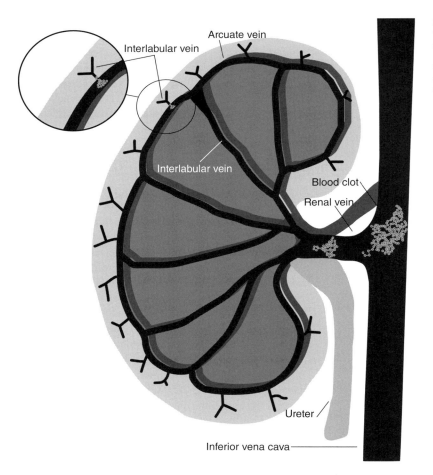

Figure 5.1 Most cases of RVT originate in the interlobular and arcuate veins and less commonly in the IVC, extending into the renal vein. (A black and white version of this figure will appear in some formats. For the color version of this figure, please refer to the plate section.)

RVT remains a significant cause of graft loss [20]. Prevalence of RVT following renal transplantation may be as high as 6% with recent evidence showing that surgical changes and use of aspirin has reduced the prevalence of RVT to < 2% [20].

Since RVT occurs predominantly in the neonatal period, a reasonable assumption would be a physiologic or anatomic predisposition. Regarding the coagulation system, one theory suggests that physiologic decreases in natural anticoagulants and fibrinolytic factors causes a vulnerability in the capacity of the hemostatic system to limit thrombus propagation, predisposing newborn infants to thrombotic events during episodes of excess thrombin generation [21,22]. Most natural anticoagulants such as protein S, protein C, antithrombin and tissue factor pathway inhibitor are approximately 50% that of adult levels at term gestation. Physiologic deficiencies in coagulation, regulatory and fibrinolytic proteins would support the predominance of RVT in the perinatal period.

Other prothrombotic factors at term include increased hematocrit and viscosity, increased concentration and larger molecular weight multimers of the von Willebrand factor and elevated soluble tissue factor. In contrast, only 28.7% of RVT occurs in preterm infants, and those RVT events are usually delayed beyond 1 week and related to other conditions related to prematurity. As most healthy infants do not develop RVT, physiologic differences at birth may contribute to, but not necessarily be causal for, RVT.

Inherited or host-related risk factors leading to RVT include inherited thrombophilia that predispose to DVT and PE in older children and adults. Studies to date have not shown an association of inherited thrombophilia and RVT and there are no prospective studies further investigating this association. Evidence discussed here is largely derived from case reports and small case series, which may overestimate their significance. Hereditary prothrombotic states likely play a large role in the development

Table 5.1 Pediatric Causes of Renal Vein Thrombosis

Treatment-related
- Renal transplant
- Indwelling intravascular catheter

Disease-related
- Nephrotic syndrome
- Antiphospholipid antibodies
- Systemic lupus erythematosus
- Cancer (Wilms tumor, neuroblastoma, etc.)
- Infant of a diabetic mother
- Sepsis/DIC/Infection
- Perinatal asphyxia

Host-related
- Inferior vena cava anomaly
- Protein S deficiency
- Protein C deficiency
- Antithrombin deficiency
- Activated protein C resistance (factor V Leiden mutation)
- Prothrombin 20210 gene mutation
- Elevated homocysteine
- Elevated lipoprotein(a)
- Elevated factor VIII activity
- Dehydration/Hemorrhage
- Complex cardiac disease

of neonatal RVT. The literature indicates that up to 53–85% of neonates with RVT had at least one of the following inherited or acquired thrombophilias: (1) factor V Leiden mutation, (2) prothrombin G20210A mutation, (3) elevated homocysteine level, (4) elevated anticardiolipin antibody titers, (5) elevated lipoprotein(a), (6) protein C/S deficiency and (7) homozygous methyltetrahydrofolate reductase (MTHFR) C677T polymorphism. Heller *et al.* reported in a case–control study of abdominal venous thrombosis that 45.2% of the cases of RVT had at least one inherited thrombophilia compared to 7% in an age- and sex-matched control group [23].

Factor V Leiden mutation (FVL) is the most common prothrombotic risk factor associated with thrombosis in children. In general, FVL has been shown to be associated with first VTE onset in children with an OR of 3.56 (95% confidence interval [CI]: 2.57–4.93) [24]. Since neonatal RVT is one of the first VTEs seen in children occurring as early as during the last trimester to the first week of life, one can assume that this association also holds for RVT. When combined with other abdominal venous thrombotic events (portal vein thrombosis and hepatic vascular occlusion), FVL demonstrated a significant association with an OR of 5.2 (95% CI: 1.77–15.3) [23]. In a German

case–control study, FVL was associated with RVT in multivariate analysis with an OR of 9.4 (95% CI: 3.3–26.6) [25]. Factor V Leiden mutation was identified in 14% to 37% of cases of RVT [23,25,26].

Prothrombin (PT) 20210 gene mutation is also rather common and associated with thrombosis in children. Overall, PT 20210 gene mutation was associated with first VTE onset in children with an OR of 2.63 (95% CI: 1.61–4.29) [24]. In a German case–control study, PT 20210 mutation was not associated with RVT (OR of 4.3, 95% CI: 0.8–24.2) [25]. The PT 202010 gene mutation was identified in 1–8.5% of cases of RVT [23,25,26].

Protein C and protein S are important anticoagulants imparting negative feedback once excessive thrombin is generated. Both natural anticoagulants are significantly lower in infants compared to adults possibly conveying a hypercoagulable state, particularly when combined with acquired underlying conditions that cause increased thrombin generation. Protein C deficiency is associated with first VTE onset in children with an OR of 7.75 (95% CI: 4.48–13.38) while protein S deficiency is associated with a lower OR of 3.76 (95% CI: 1.76–8.04) [24]. However, the strength of these data can be questioned as these reports do not describe whether repeat testing was performed to confirm a persistent deficiency compared to an acute consumption during the thrombotic phenomena. In a German case–control study, protein C deficiency was seen in 5% of cases of RVT in children while protein S deficiency was not identified in either the cases or controls [25]. A deficiency of either protein C or protein S was identified in 18% (5 of 28) of children with RVTs in a Canadian retrospective cohort study [26].

Antithrombin (AT) deficiency is a rare diagnosis and has been associated with VTE, particularly abdominal thrombosis. AT deficiency has been associated with first VTE in children with an OR of 8.73 (95% CI: 3.12–24.42) [24]. AT deficiency has been reported in 3.2–5% of cases of RVT [23,25,26]. In a German case–control study, AT deficiency was seen in 5% of cases of RVT in children but not determined as significant in multivariate analysis. Again it is not clear whether persistence of AT deficiency was determined in the reported cases.

Less commonly evaluated potential risk factors for RVT include elevated lipoprotein(a) and elevated FVIII activity. The former has been associated with first episode VTE in children with an OR of 4.5 (95%

CI: 3.19–6.35) while the latter has not been rigorously evaluated in this setting. Elevated lipoprotein(a) was seen in 28.8% of children with RVT in a German case–control study and was associated with RVT with a significant OR of 7.6 (95% CI: 2.4–23.8) [25]. Since lipoprotein(a) has not been widely (or broadly) evaluated in reported cases or series, the true prevalence is not known and results from small series may overestimate the true prevalence. Persistence of elevated FVIII activity (> 150 IU/dl) correlates with a poorer thrombotic composite outcome as measured by death, post-thrombotic syndrome or recurrent VTE. This has not been rigorously investigated in the setting of RVT and is not included in a recent systematic review of inherited thrombophilia in children [24,27].

Well-known risk factors that are treatment-related include renal transplant and RVT occurring in the setting of an indwelling intravascular catheter. Overall prevalence of RVT following renal transplant is estimated at 1–2% [20].

Clinical Presentation

The classic RVT triad of thrombocytopenia, abdominal mass and macroscopic hematuria has been well described (see Figure 5.2). Based on a large case series and retrospective review of neonatal RVT, 50–56.2% had macroscopic hematuria, 41–45.4% had a palpable abdominal mass and 29–47.5% had thrombocytopenia [14,28]. Most cases of neonatal RVT have at least one sign, but only 13–22% will have all three at presentation [29,30]. Such findings become extremely relevant, as the differential of a neonate or young child with a palpable flank mass includes but is not limited to Wilms tumor, hydronephrosis, neuroblastoma and multicystic kidney disease. All of these conditions are usually easily discriminated from RVT with Doppler and imaging ultrasound. Since renal failure and hypertension were not consistently evaluated in the largest case review, prevalence estimates are based on smaller studies, which described presentations of 14–56% with renal insufficiency/failure, 17.6% with hypertension and 7% with dehydration [14,26]. Renal insufficiency/failure and hypertension are more common when the presentation of RVT is bilateral, and have been reported in 41% and 70% of cases, respectively [14,26].

Renal vein thrombosis largely is unilateral, left-sided, and more common in males, usually presenting in the first days of life in term infants, and a few days later in preterm infants. In the largest review available to date, which compiled English-language case series

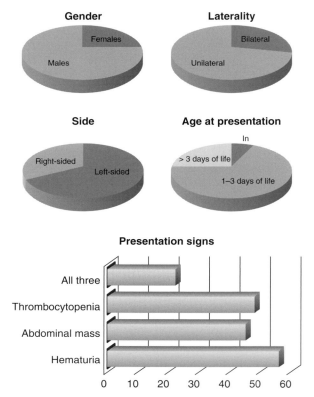

Figure 5.2 Clinical presentation of RVT in the neonatal period: 67% are males, 72% are unilateral, 67% left-sided, occurring on day of life 1–3 in 67% of cases. The classic triad of neonatal RVT is seen in 22% of cases, with 48% having thrombocytopenia, 56% hematuria and 45% a palpable mass.

over a 15-year period, 67.2% of cases were males [28], with similar gender predominance in a Canadian registry study (65%) [14]. A simple proposed explanation is that males are more likely to have congenital renal abnormalities thus potentially predisposing males to RVTs [29]. Moreover, there are renal perfusion differences that may also contribute to this gender discrepancy [14], but the exact etiology is still not fully understood.

Male gender and left-sided predominance in RVT have been reported in adults [31]. Left-sided predominance was confirmed in neonatal RVT in 2004, based on the Canadian registry, and is likely the result of the left renal vein coarsing under the aorta, making it susceptible to thrombosis in the setting of decreased renal perfusion [14]. In addition to male predominance in RVT, the majority of RVT cases are unilateral (70.3–72%) with a predilection for the left side (63.6–67%) [14,28].

Based on the largest review of RVTs, the vast majority of infants affected were term (71.3%) [28]. The median age of RVT presentation was 2 days, with 43% presenting on the first day of life and 67.1% presenting within the first 3 days of life [14,28]. An additional 25.6% present after 3 days of life and 7.3% present in utero [14,28]. It is rare for RVT to present outside the first 30 days of life unless it is associated with primary renal disease [28]. Renal vein thrombosis has been called a perinatal event as it can originate in utero late in gestation, presenting within the first 2–3 days of life [32].

At presentation, thrombus extension into the IVC was seen in 43.7–60% of the cases, less commonly affecting other vessels and very rarely leading to renal artery thrombosis, arterial ischemic stroke, sinus thromboembolism and pulmonary embolism [14,28]. Furthermore, adrenal hemorrhage was present in 14.8% of RVT cases, usually the result of extension of thrombus into the adrenal vein, with subsequent adrenal vein stasis, venous hypertension, thrombosis and infarction.

Diagnosis

Radiologic findings

Greyscale ultrasound is the radiologic imaging test of choice mainly due to its sensitivity to early renal changes with RVT, wide availability, non-invasiveness and lack of any potential side effects [33]. In general, magnetic resonance imaging (MRI) and computed tomography (CT) are seldom needed to make a diagnosis of RVT and the utility of these expensive imaging modalities has not been fully evaluated. Moreover, contrast exposure in the setting of a potentially progressive renal injury may further aggravate the glomerular homeostasis, limiting the utility of such imaging modalities. Contrarily, imaging and Doppler ultrasound features have been well described allowing early diagnosis of RVT, particularly in neonates without the cardinal clinical findings of enlarged flank mass, thrombocytopenia and hematuria [18,33,34].

Cremin et al. first proposed a staging system for RVT based on sequential ultrasound evaluations in affected children, acknowledging the likely overlap in the first two stages [18] (see Table 5.2). Initial key features of RVT in the first week of presentation, often corresponding with the first week of life, are the following: (1) renal enlargement, (2) loss of corticomedullary differentiation, (3) overall increased echogenicity and

Table 5.2 Ultrasound appearance of the kidney in the setting of RVT

Early renal changes (first week)
- Renal enlargement
- Loss of corticomedullary differentiation
- Overall increased echogenicity
- Transient perivascular echogenic interlobular/interlobar streaks

Intermediate renal changes (second week)
- Continued renal enlargement
- Continued loss of corticomedullary differentiation
- Hyperechoic foci (edema/hemorrhage)
- Hypoechoic foci indicating resolving hemorrhage or edema
- Echogenic rings around affected renal pyramids (fibrosis)

Late renal changes (> 2 weeks)
- Resolution of renal enlargement
- Calcification of thrombus
- Fibrotic scarring around renal pyramids
- Progression to atrophy

Modified from Cremmin et al. 1991 [18].

(4) transient perivascular echogenic interlobular/interlobar streaks [18,33]. The perivascular echogenic streaks are pathognomonic for RVT and indicate an originating point within the arcuate or interlobular veins. Prompt imaging of suspected neonates with RVT is critical since this "streak" finding is often transient and not visualized by the end of the first week [34]. In the second week following development of RVT, the following ultrasound features are seen: (1) prominent renal enlargement, (2) hyperechoic foci indicating edema or hemorrhage, (3) hypoechoic foci indicating resolving hemorrhage or edema, (4) worsening loss of corticomedullary differentiation and (5) echogenic rings around the affected renal pyramids indicating renal tubular damage and fibrosis [18,34]. In the final or "late" stage of RVT occurring after the second week following development of the RVT, the following findings are noted: (1) calcification of thrombus, (2) resolution of renal enlargement and progression to atrophy and (3) continued fibrotic scarring typically in the apex of affected renal pyramids [18,35].

Doppler ultrasound has been recently used in the diagnosis of RVT, particularly in the early stages. Three studies evaluated the utility of Doppler ultrasound in early diagnosis of RVT in the setting of kidney transplant and in the neonatal period in native kidneys [36–38]. Although a small total number of patients were analyzed, a typical finding of absent intrarenal and renal venous blood flow with reversal of diastolic arterial flow was seen in the first week following development of RVT. Laplante and coworkers only found this reduced or absent intrarenal blood flow and reversal of arterial flow in the early phase following kidney transplant in children and not in native kidneys in the neonatal period. Further, a greater than 10% increase in the resistance index of the vessels in the affected kidney was noted in 6 of 7 neonatal patients evaluated [37]. Based on these findings, Doppler ultrasound may be useful in the early evaluation of RVT, particularly those with transplanted kidneys but likely has a very limited diagnostic and prognostic role following the first week in all cases of RVT in children. Moreover, Doppler ultrasound may support the findings of IVC thrombi associated with RVT by determining the extent of flow interruption and demonstrating severity of occlusiveness [33].

In addition to diagnosis of RVT, ultrasound may have a role in predicting long-term outcomes. Although not externally validated, data reported by Winyard et al. suggested that increasing renal length at presentation correlates with a worse renal outcome [29]. In this study, any kidney greater than 6 cm had a poor renal outcome as determined by renal insufficiency or atrophy. Moreover, every 1 mm increase in renal length at presentation correlated with a mean fall in GFR by 3ml/min/1.73m^2 [29]. However, a subsequent study did not corroborate these findings but rather found that echogenic irregular pyramids, severely decreased renal perfusion, subcapsular fluid collections and patchy renal cortex echogenicity were predictors of poor long-term renal outcome [39]. Larger prospective studies will be needed to validate potential predictors of poor renal outcome to guide the choice and intensity of initial antithrombotic therapy.

Acute management

Since the acute and chronic management of RVT is complex, it is recommended that each institution form a multidisciplinary team including neonatologists, nephrologists, interventional radiologists and hematologists to develop a local management strategy [40]. Again, in the largest review available to date, Lau et al. compiled English language case series over a 15-year period showing no difference in renal outcomes in children with RVT when comparing supportive care alone with anticoagulation using unfractionated heparin therapy (UFH) and/or low molecular weight heparin (LMWH) strategies [28]. This provided the context for the basis of the American College of Chest Physicians (ACCP) Evidence-Based Clinical Practice

Guidelines regarding antithrombotic therapy in children [8].

The 2012 ACCP guidelines are shown schematically in Figure 5.3 [8]. For unilateral RVT with no renal insufficiency and no thrombus extension into the IVC, either observation (with radiologic monitoring) or UFH/LMWH are equally supported options. The duration of therapy with systemic anticoagulation ranges from 6 weeks to 3 months, with no high-quality data as yet to support a specific length of time. For unilateral RVT with thrombus extension into the IVC, systemic anticoagulation with UFH/LMWH for 6 weeks to 3 months is recommended [8]. Finally for bilateral RVT with renal insufficiency, thrombolytic therapy should be considered followed by UFH/LMWH for 6 weeks to 3 months [8]. The ACCP does not address management guidance in children with bilateral RVT without renal insufficiency and whether potential modifiers such as hematuria, thrombocytopenia and intracranial hemorrhage alter management recommendations [8].

In addition, the ACCP does not offer guidance on tPA dosing, route of administration, duration of therapy or use of adjuvant UFH [41,42]. Both systemic tPA and catheter-directed tPA require local expertise and typically the catheter size precludes use in neonates [41]. Raffini summarized thrombolytic regimens with a low-dose regimen starting dose of 0.06mg/kg/h in neonates and 0.03mg/kg/h in older children escalating the dose every 12–24 hours for no longer than 96 hours [41]. The concomitant use of UFH continues to be controversial, likely reducing the risk of thrombus propagation while perhaps increasing bleeding risk [42]. tPA should be avoided in children with recent major surgery (< 10 days), active bleeding, recent intracranial hemorrhage (< 30 days), recent seizures (< 48 hours), inability to maintain fibrinogen activity > 100mg/dl or platelet count < 75 000/ul and uncontrolled hypertension [41]. Other chapters offer a detailed discussion of thrombolytic modalities, including indications and contraindications..

In contrast to the ACCP recommendations, the British guidelines on management of VTE in children are more conservative with no specific recommendation for RVT and reserving support for thrombolytic therapy if there is "extensive thrombosis" extending into the IVC and in RVT cases associated with massive PE [9].

Since the ACCP and British guidelines are not risk-based, it is not surprising that there continues to be controversy in RVT management. In general, pediatric

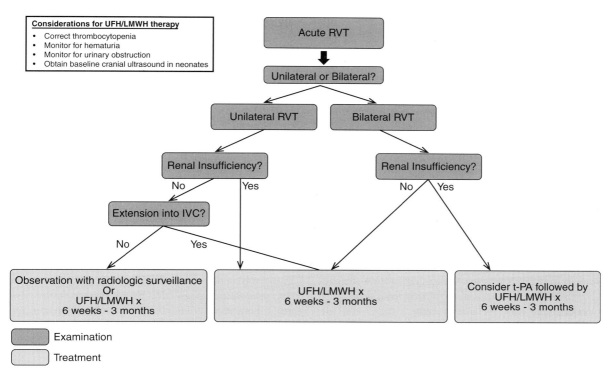

Figure 5.3 Acute RVT management algorithm. Treatment recommendations based mostly on ACCP guidelines. IVC: Inferior vena cava. UFH: Unfractionated heparin. LMWH: Low molecular weight heparin. tPA: Tissue plasminogen activator. RVT: Renal vein thrombosis.

hematologists lean toward observation when there is a unilateral RVT with hematuria, regardless of platelet count, as well when there is a grade II or higher intracranial hemorrhage [40], while considering anticoagulation for bilateral RVT and unilateral RVT with IVC thrombus extension [40].

Long-term sequelae

Following recovery from acute RVT, complications such as renal atrophy, renal insufficiency, functional loss, hypertension and post-thrombotic syndrome (in cases of IVC involvement) can persist. Studies reporting the long-term evaluation of renal outcomes and thrombosis recurrence rates are lacking due to inconsistent reporting, although the recurrence rate clinically appears to be very low [28]. The goal of antithrombotic therapy in RVT is prevention of renal atrophy, hypertension and renal insufficiency; data on improved renal outcomes with anticoagulation are conflicting [8]. Marks *et al.* reviewed outcomes of 23 newborns with RVT treated over a 21-year period, noting that 33% of newborns with RVT who received UFH had renal atrophy compared to 100% of

newborns with RVT who did not receive UFH [26]. This was not corroborated by a study of 33 newborns with RVT and the large 15-year systematic review by Lau *et al.* [25,28].

Irreversible functional loss in the affected kidney occurs in up to 70.6% of neonates with RVT regardless of the acute intervention strategy [28]. Chronic hypertension persists in 19.3% of neonates with RVT ranging from 18.9% in unilateral RVT compared to 21.7% in bilateral RVT. Long-term follow-up focusing on physical growth, blood pressure trends and laboratory surveillance of renal function is recommended. Surveillance of renal function should include BUN, creatinine, urine microalbumin and protein- and urine-specific gravity [32]. In addition to laboratory and physical exam surveillance, serial renal ultrasound with Doppler should be considered until the age of 1 year, after which further atrophy or hypertrophy is unlikely. However, onset of hypertension can be delayed by years following RVT, and long-term monitoring is important. Currently there are only expert opinion-based recommendations to guide timing and frequency of laboratory monitoring, physical exam or imaging in long-term management of RVT and the authors recommend discussion with pediatric nephrologists to tailor assessment for an individual child.

Once the neonate has reached at least 4–6 months of age or following return to a steady state in older children, inherited and acquired thrombophilia evaluation may be performed [21]. Such a strategy is based on the potential recurrent VTE risk in children with a prothrombotic abnormality in the setting of a RVT reported by the German cohort study (~ 4% recurrence rate, which occurred only during adolescence) [25]. As discussed previously the thrombophilia evaluation includes evaluation of proteins S and C activity, antithrombin activity, PT 20210 gene mutation, FVL mutation, FVIII activity, lipoprotein(a) and antiphospholipid antibodies [26,28]. Coagulation study interpretation is complex and should be done by an experienced pediatric hematologist or pathologist. Development of a prospective pediatric RVT registry would likely be useful in determining long-term renal outcomes and VTE recurrence risk.

Isolated adrenal vein thrombosis

Adrenal vein thrombosis (AVT) is common in the setting of adjacent RVT, where it usually presents with hemorrhage into an infarcted adrenal gland.

Isolated AVT is a rare diagnosis in both the adult and pediatric population. Due to its rarity and no specific ICD-9 code for AVT, there are no references to AVT in any published pediatric registries or retrospective reviews [10,13,23,43,44]. The causes of venous infarction or thrombosis of the adrenal gland are varied and include, based on the small number of cases described, DIC/sepsis, hypothermia, venous anatomical variants and abdominal pathology, typically adrenal neoplasia or bulky metastatic disease [45–47]. The Waterhouse–Friderichsen syndrome is a finding of adrenal hemorrhage and infarction in the setting of septic shock and disseminated intravascular coagulation; adrenal vein thrombus is rarely identified in this setting. In the setting of adrenal neoplasia, Osman *et al.* estimated a 2.9% incidence of AVT with the tumor pathology ranging widely from neuroblastoma, pheochromocytoma, sarcoma and adrenocortical carcinoma [45]. There does not seem to be a gender predilection as the few studies of AVT associated with adrenal tumors had contradictory findings [45,46,48]. There does appear to be a right-sided predilection although the case numbers are too small to definitively verify this. Furthermore, a physiologic shorter adrenal vein could

explain this laterality as well as the predilection for AVT to extend into the IVC [45,46]. There are no data published on the association of inherited or acquired thrombophilia with AVT.

Diagnostic evaluation of AVT is complex compared to RVT. In general, the recommended imaging modality is multimodal. Ultrasound is helpful in demonstrating caval extension, although viewing is limited by abdominal gas and obesity [45,49]. While CT scan is widely used to stage most abdominal tumors, MRI is likely better at demonstrating the extent of thrombus burden [50]. Since most AVT are associated with a primary or metastatic abdominal tumor, primary surgical resection may preclude the need for systemic anticoagulation or thrombolytic therapy. In general there are no data on anticoagulation or thrombolytic therapy for intraabdominal thrombosis other than RVT. Therefore, thrombolytic therapy is not recommended while standard systemic anticoagulation with UFH/LMWH for 3–6 months is recommended, particularly when surgical resection is not indicated for the tumor [8].

Conclusion

Despite improvement in understanding of the etiology of pediatric RVT as well as overall improved medical care, this thrombotic complication continues to pose a diagnostic and management challenge to clinicians and practitioners. The pathophysiology of RVT involves reduced intrarenal perfusion and the likely site of RVT originates in the arcuate and interlobular veins. Overall survival approaches 100% and rare deaths are usually related to coexisting comorbidities such as multiorgan failure, sepsis, meningitis and respiratory failure [28]. The classic triad seen with RVT, thrombocytopenia, abdominal mass and macroscopic hematuria, has been well described with < 25% presenting with all cardinal signs. Renal vein thrombosis most often is unilateral, left-sided, more common in males and presents in the first days of life in term infants. Greyscale ultrasound is the radiologic imaging test of choice mainly due to its sensitivity to early renal changes with RVT, wide availability, non-invasiveness and lack of any potential side effects, with a limited and undefined role for CT or MRI. Since the current literature, albeit limited, suggests a lack of difference in renal outcomes in children with RVT when comparing supportive care alone with anticoagulation using UFH and/or LMWH, acute management is controversial. Currently, supportive care with or without UFH/

LMWH is recommended in RVT when there is unilateral presentation without IVC extension, UFH/LMWH when there is unilateral RVT with IVC thrombus extension or bilateral RVT, and consideration of thrombolytic therapy when there is bilateral involvement of the renal veins with renal insufficiency. A thoughtful long-term multidisciplinary management approach involving the hematologist and nephrologist is critical as > 70% of neonates will have loss of renal function regardless of intervention or laterality and nearly 20% will have chronic hypertension. With regard to isolated AVT, pediatric literature is limited, but risk factors may include DIC/sepsis, hypothermia, venous anatomical variants and tumor involvement of the adrenal. Magnetic resonance imaging is a preferred imaging modality, and anticoagulant management as per other types of VTE is considered the standard of care. Due to the relative rarity of RVT and AVT, it may be difficult to develop prospective studies to definitively determine whether inherited/acquired thrombophilia, intense anticoagulation or thrombolytic therapy, thrombus burden or organ insufficiency modify the short- and long-term outcomes in these thrombotic disorders.

References

1. Beaufils F, Schlegel N, Brun P, Loirat C. Treatment of renal vein thromboses in the newborn. Annals of Pediatrics (Paris). 1993;**40**(2):57–60.

2. Clifford SH, Butler AM, et al. Renal-vein thrombosis in the newborn infant. The New England Journal of Medicine. 1950;**242**(3):100–4.

3. Rayer PFO. Traite des maladies des reins. Paris. 1837–1841.

4. Hutinel V. Les Maladies des Enfants. Asselin Houzeau. 1909.

5. Morison JE. renal venous thrombosis and infarction in the newborn. Arch Dis Childhood. 1945;**20**:129.

6. Barenberg L, Greenstein N, Levy W, Rosenbluth S. Renal thrombosis with infarction complicating diarrhea of the newborn. Arch Pediatr Adolesc Med. 1941;**62**(2):362–72.

7. McClelland CQ, Hughes JP. Thrombosis of the renal vein in infants. J Pediatr. 1950;**36**(2):214–27.

8. Monagle P, Chan AK, Goldenberg NA, Ichord RN, Journeycake JM, Nowak-Gottl U, et al. Antithrombotic therapy in neonates and children: Antithrombotic Therapy and Prevention of Thrombosis, 9th edn: American College of Chest Physicians Evidence-Based Clinical Practice Guidelines. Chest. 2012;**141**(2 Suppl):e737S-801S.

9. Chalmers E, Ganesen V, Liesner R, Maroo S, Nokes T, Saunders D, et al. Guideline on the investigation, management and prevention of venous thrombosis in children. British Journal of Haematology. 2011;**154**(2):196–207.

10. van Ommen CH, Heijboer H, Buller HR, Hirasing RA, Heijmans HS, Peters M. Venous thromboembolism in childhood: a prospective two-year registry in The Netherlands. The Journal of Pediatrics. 2001;**139**(5):676–81.

11. Raffini L, Huang YS, Witmer C, Feudtner C. Dramatic increase in venous thromboembolism in children's hospitals in the United States from 2001 to 2007. Pediatrics. 2009;**124**(4):1001–8.

12. Wright JM, Watts RG. Venous thromboembolism in pediatric patients: epidemiologic data from a pediatric tertiary care center in Alabama. Journal of Pediatric Hematology/Oncology. 2011;**33**(4):261–4.

13. Schmidt B, Andrew M. Neonatal thrombosis: report of a prospective Canadian and international registry. Pediatrics. 1995;**96**(5 Pt 1): 939–43.

14. Kuhle S, Massicotte P, Chan A, Mitchell L. A case series of 72 neonates with renal vein thrombosis. Data from the 1–800-NO-CLOTS Registry. Thrombosis and Haemostasis. 2004;**92**(4):729–33.

15. Llach F, Papper S, Massry SG. The clinical spectrum of renal vein thrombosis: acute and chronic. The American Journal of Medicine. 1980;**69**(6):819–27.

16. Singhal R, Brimble KS. Thromboembolic complications in the nephrotic syndrome: pathophysiology and clinical management. Thrombosis Research. 2006;**118**(3):397–407.

17. Seikaly M, Ho PL, Emmett L, Tejani A. The 12th Annual Report of the North American Pediatric Renal Transplant Cooperative Study: renal transplantation from 1987 through 1998. Pediatric Transplantation. 2001;**5**(3):215–31.

18. Cremin BJ, Davey H, Oleszczuk-Raszke K. Neonatal renal venous thrombosis: sequential ultrasonic appearances. Clinical Radiology. 1991;**44**(1):52–5.

19. Kenet G, Aronis S, Berkun Y, Bonduel M, Chan A, Goldenberg NA, et al. Impact of persistent antiphospholipid antibodies on risk of incident symptomatic thromboembolism in children: a systematic review and meta-analysis. Seminars in Thrombosis and Hemostasis. 2011;**37**(7):802–9.

20. McDonald RA, Smith JM, Stablein D, Harmon WE. Pretransplant peritoneal dialysis and graft thrombosis following pediatric kidney transplantation: a NAPRTCS report. Pediatric Transplantation. 2003;**7**(3):204–8.

21. Andrew M, Paes B, Johnston M. Development of the hemostatic system in the neonate and young infant.

The American Journal of Pediatric Hematology/Oncology. 1990;**12**(1):95–104.

22. Corrigan JJ, Jr., Sleeth JJ, Jeter M, Lox CD. Newborn's fibrinolytic mechanism: components and plasmin generation. The American Journal of Hematology. 1989;**32**(4):273–8.

23. Heller C, Schobess R, Kurnik K, Junker R, Gunther G, Kreuz W, et al. Abdominal venous thrombosis in neonates and infants: role of prothrombotic risk factors – a multicentre case-control study. For the Childhood Thrombophilia Study Group. British Journal of Haematology. 2000;**111**(2):534–9.

24. Young G, Albisetti M, Bonduel M, Brandao L, Chan A, Friedrichs F, et al. Impact of inherited thrombophilia on venous thromboembolism in children: a systematic review and meta-analysis of observational studies. Circulation. 2008;**118**(13):1373–82.

25. Kosch A, Kuwertz-Broking E, Heller C, Kurnik K, Schobess R, Nowak-Gottl U. Renal venous thrombosis in neonates: prothrombotic risk factors and long-term follow-up. Blood. 2004;**104**(5):1356–60.

26. Marks SD, Massicotte MP, Steele BT, Matsell DG, Filler G, Shah PS, et al. Neonatal renal venous thrombosis: clinical outcomes and prevalence of prothrombotic disorders. The Journal of Pediatrics. 2005;**146**(6):811–6.

27. Goldenberg NA, Knapp-Clevenger R, Manco-Johnson MJ. Elevated plasma factor VIII and D-dimer levels as predictors of poor outcomes of thrombosis in children. The New England Journal of Medicine. 2004;**351**(11):1081–8.

28. Lau KK, Stoffman JM, Williams S, McCusker P, Brandao L, Patel S, et al. Neonatal renal vein thrombosis: review of the English-language literature between 1992 and 2006. Pediatrics. 2007;**120**(5):e1278–84.

29. Winyard PJ, Bharucha T, De Bruyn R, Dillon MJ, van't Hoff W, Trompeter RS, et al. Perinatal renal venous thrombosis: presenting renal length predicts outcome. Archives of Disease in Childhood: Fetal and Neonatal Edition. 2006;**91**(4):F273–8.

30. Zigman A, Yazbeck S, Emil S, Nguyen L. Renal vein thrombosis: a 10-year review. Journal of Pediatric Surgery. 2000;**35**(11):1540–2.

31. O'Dea MJ, Malek RS, Tucker RM, Fulton RE. Renal vein thrombosis. The Journal of Urology. 1976;**116**(4):410–4.

32. Brandao LR, Simpson EA, Lau KK. Neonatal renal vein thrombosis. Seminars in Fetal & Neonatal Medicine. 2011;**16**(6):323–8.

33. Elsaify WM. Neonatal renal vein thrombosis: grey-scale and Doppler ultrasonic features. Abdominal Imaging. 2009;**34**(3):413–8.

34. Hibbert J, Howlett DC, Greenwood KL, MacDonald LM, Saunders AJ. The ultrasound appearances of neonatal renal vein thrombosis. The British Journal of Radiology. 1997;**70**(839):1191–4.

35. Wright NB, Blanch G, Walkinshaw S, Pilling DW. Antenatal and neonatal renal vein thrombosis: new ultrasonic features with high frequency transducers. Pediatric Radiology. 1996;**26**(9):686–9.

36. Alexander AA, Merton DA, Mitchell DG, Gottlieb RP, Feld RI. Rapid diagnosis of neonatal renal vein thrombosis using color Doppler imaging. Journal of Clinical Ultrasound. 1993;**21**(7):468–71.

37. Laplante S, Patriquin HB, Robitaille P, Filiatrault D, Grignon A, Decarie JC. Renal vein thrombosis in children: evidence of early flow recovery with Doppler US. Radiology. 1993;**189**(1):37–42.

38. Parvey HR, Eisenberg RL. Image-directed Doppler sonography of the intrarenal arteries in acute renal vein thrombosis. Journal of Clinical Ultrasound. 1990;**18**(6):512–16.

39. Kraft JK, Brandao LR, Navarro OM. Sonography of renal venous thrombosis in neonates and infants: can we predict outcome? Pediatric Radiology. 2011;**41**(3):299–307.

40. Brandao LR, Dix D, David M, Israels S, Massicotte MP, Williams S, et al. An attempt to reach consensus regarding management of neonatal renal vein thrombosis: The Canadian Pediatric Hemostasis and Thrombosis Network Experience. Blood. 2004;**104**:92b.

41. Raffini L. Thrombolysis for intravascular thrombosis in neonates and children. Current Opinion in Pediatrics. 2009;**21**(1):9–14.

42. Albisetti M. Thrombolytic therapy in children. Thrombosis Research. 2006;**118**(1):95–105.

43. Stein PD, Kayali F, Olson RE. Incidence of venous thromboembolism in infants and children: data from the National Hospital Discharge Survey. The Journal of Pediatrics. 2004;**145**(4):563–5.

44. Kuhle S, Massicotte P, Chan A, Adams M, Abdolell M, deVeber G, et al. Systemic thromboembolism in children. Data from the 1–800-NO-CLOTS Consultation Service. Thrombosis and Haemostasis. 2004;**92**(4):722–8.

45. Osman Y, Haraz A, El-Mekresh M, Gomha AM, El-Ghar MA, Eraky I. Adrenal tumors with venous thrombosis: a single-institution experience. Urologia Internationalis. 2011;**87**(2):182–5.

46. Figueroa AJ, Stein JP, Lieskovsky G, Skinner DG. Adrenal cortical carcinoma associated with venous tumour thrombus extension. British Journal of Urology. 1997;**80**(3):397–400. Epub 1997/10/06.

47. Godine LB, Berdon WE, Brasch RC, Leonidas JC. Adrenocortical carcinoma with extension into

inferior vena cava and right atrium: report of 3 cases in children. Pediatric Radiology. 1990;**20**(3):166–8; discussion 9.

48. Ortiz Gorraiz M, Tallada Bunuel M, Vicente Prados FJ, Rodriguez Herrera F, Rosales Leal JL, Honrubia Vilchez B, et al. Left adrenal carcinoma with caval thrombosis. Archivos Espanoles de Urologia. 2003;**56**(5):485–9.

49. Didier D, Racle A, Etievent JP, Weill F. Tumor thrombus of the inferior vena cava secondary to malignant abdominal neoplasms: US and CT evaluation. Radiology. 1987;**162**(1 Pt 1):83–9.

50. Ryan MF, Murphy JP, Jay R, Callum J, MacDonald D. MRI diagnosis of bilateral adrenal vein thrombosis. The British Journal of Radiology. 2003;**76**(908):566–9.

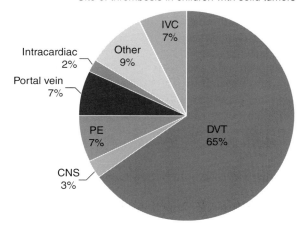

Chapter 6

Cancer and thrombosis

Uma Athale

Introduction

The association of cancer and thrombosis was first described by Armand Trousseau in 1865.[1,2] Almost 150 years later, we are still struggling to understand the pathophysiology, management and prevention of this potentially fatal complication in patients with cancer.

Thromboembolism (TE) is a major complication in adults with cancer, leading to significant morbidity and mortality, especially in the hospitalized population and patients receiving chemotherapy.[3–7] The incidence of TE in clinical studies varies from 4% to 20%, whereas autopsy rates of TE are as high as 50%, indicating that even in the adult cancer population the incidence of TE is underestimated.[6,8,9] Further, over recent years the incidence of TE in adult cancer patients has increased substantially and development of TE is identified as an independent predictor of poor survival.[4–6] A recent prospective study documented 9% of deaths secondary to venous and arterial TE in ambulatory cancer patients receiving chemotherapy.[4] The estimated direct medical care cost of adult TE in the USA is ~$600 million/year.[10] Although similar estimates are unavailable for children, development of TE undoubtedly adds to the cost of therapy for children with cancer.

Unlike adults, children in general are physiologically protected from spontaneous development of TE.[11] However, with recent advances in management of complex pediatric problems including cancer, the incidence of TE in North American children, including those with cancer, is increasing.[12,13] Recent studies report up to 10% prevalence of symptomatic TE and up to 40% asymptomatic TE in children with cancer.[14–20] Hence, it is important to understand the epidemiology, risk factors and management of cancer-associated thrombosis in children.

Cancer-specific thrombosis

The type of cancer affects the clinical presentation of thrombosis including the site of TE. This mostly is related to the biology of the disease and the therapy used. Although acute lymphoblastic leukemia (ALL) is the most frequently reported pediatric cancer in association with thrombosis, recent reports indicate that children with other types of cancer, including solid tumors, are also at higher risk for TE.[13–22] The sites of thrombosis in children with solid tumors are shown in Figure 6.1.

Hematologic malignancies

Most of the information regarding thrombosis in hematologic malignancies in children is based on studies conducted in children with ALL.[14,15,21,22] However,

Site of thrombosis in children with solid tumors

Figure 6.1 Reported sites of thrombosis in children with solid tumors, based on literature review. IVC = inferior vana cava; DVT = deep venous thrombosis; CNS = central nervous system; PE = pulmonary embolism.

Pediatric Thrombotic Disorders, ed. Neil A. Goldenberg and Marilyn J. Manco-Johnson. Published by Cambridge University Press. © Cambridge University Press 2015.

children with acute myeloid leukemia and lymphoma are also at equal risk for developing TE.[13,15,17,18] Deep venous thrombosis (DVT), especially central venous line (CVL)-related DVT, is the most commonly reported type of TE in children with hematological malignancy.[14,21,22] Because of the preference of CVL placement in upper venous system veins (such as subclavian or internal jugular veins [internal or external long term catheters], or in brachialis or basilic veins [peripherally inserted central catheters or PICC]), DVT are frequently detected in the upper venous system.[14–16,21] A CVL also predisposes children to develop right atrial clots. Children with lymphoma and a large mediastinal mass are probably at higher risk of CVL-related TE.[20] However not all thromboses are CVL-related. Acute leukemia and its therapy induce a systemic hypercoagulable state.[14,16,21,22] This is evident from non-CVL related TE observed in this population. Lower limb DVT, not related to CVL, are reported in ~25% of children with hematologic malignancies who develop TE.[15,18,21] However, the most characteristic site for TE in children with ALL, particularly during treatment with asparaginase (Asp), is cerebral sinovenous thrombosis (CSVT).[14,15,21,22]

Coagulaopathy in acute promyelocytic leukemia

Due to its association with disseminated intravascular coagulaopathy (DIC) at diagnosis, acute promyelocytic leukemia (APML or AML M3), poses a special challenge of diagnosis and management of TE and hence deserves special mention. The incidence of APML varies according to the ethnicity; APML accounts for approximately 4–7% of AML in North American children compared with 20–32% of AML in South American, Italian and African children.[23,24] APML is characterized by chromosomal translocation t(15:17) resulting in formation of fusion proteins PML-RARα or PLZF-RARα, which block the differentiation of myeloid cells and cause an arrest in cellular differentiation at the promyelocytic phase.[25] All transretinoic acid (ATRA), by inducing dissociation of nuclear coexpressors, enables transcriptional activation and cell differentiation.[25,26] The biological targeted response of ATRA translates into high remission rates and cure rates in APML patients and, thus, forms the mainstay of therapy.[20,25,26]

Coagulopathy characterized by hemorrhage and thrombosis is one of the hallmarks of the disease.[15,25–28] Most of the information regarding coagulopathy in APML is derived from studies in adults.[15,27,28] Bleeding, especially parenchymal intracranial and intra-abdominal hemorrhage, is common at diagnosis and a major cause of early death;[15,25–28] DIC seems to be the major cause of bleeding. About 4% of adult patients with APML present with TE at diagnosis and a cumulative incidence of TE during therapy is ~8–9%.[28] Thrombosis presents as pulmonary embolism (PE), DVT, cardiac chamber thrombosis or intracranial TE. The etiology of thrombosis in APML is multifactorial and is driven by the biology of the leukemic blasts and the effect of ATRA. Although ATRA therapy leads to resolution of coagulopathy and hemorrhage induced by DIC at initial presentation of APML, it may paradoxically lead to imbalance of hemostasis toward a procoagulant state resulting in TE.[26–28] ATRA-associated TE usually occur 1–3 weeks following the therapy, when usually the hyperleukocytosis and the APML-associated coagulopathy are resolved, and it is distinct from APML differentiation syndrome. This life-threatening entity is characterized by unexplained fever, edema, hypoxia, interstitial pulmonary infiltrates, serositis leading to pleuropericardial effusion, hypotension and renal dysfunction.[25,26] ATRA-associated TE can affect multiple organs including heart, brain, lungs and spleen. Table 6.1 describes the postulated prothrombotic effects of APML and ATRA. Prior to the ATRA era, antifibrinolytic agents like epsilon-aminocaproic acid and tranexamic acid had been advocated for the management of APML. However, the concurrent use of ATRA and antifibrinolytic agents is hypothesized to exacerbate the risk of thrombosis.[26,28] Hence, in absence of clear evidence of benefit, routine use of antifibrinolytic agents outside of clinical trials is not recommended.

Solid tumors

Children with solid tumors may develop thrombosis of the vessels in the vicinity of the tumor either because of the pressure by the tumor leading to venous stasis or by direct tumor invasion. The vessels affected by tumor invasion depend on the type and site of cancer. For example, children with hepatoblastoma tend to have portal vein thrombosis, children with Wilms tumor tend to have renal vein and inferior vena cava (IVC) thrombosis, and children with extremity tumors like sarcoma may develop extremity DVT.[18,19,29,30] Apart from the anatomical effect and tumor invasion, children with a solid tumor also develop TE away from the site of

Table 6.1 Proposed prothrombotic effects of acute promyelocytic leukemia and its therapy

	Process	Mechanism	Markers
Disease related	Promyeloblast-related procoagulants	Cancer procoagulant factor, TF	Increased TAT, FPA, prothrombin fragment F1.2, D-dimer
	Endothelial damage	Activation of inflammatory cytokines	IL-6, TNF-α, TF
Therapy related	ATRA	Induction of apoptosis, up-regulation of adhesive molecules and increased production of cytokines lead to development of imbalance, favoring procoagulant activity	-

Abbreviations: ATRA = all trans retinoic acid; TAT = thrombin–antithrombin complex; FPA = fibrinopeptide A; IL = interleukin; TNF = tumor necrosis factor; TF = tissue factor.

the disease secondary to a hypercoagulable state related to cancer.[19,29,30] Children with sarcomas and other solid tumors are shown to have activation of the coagulation system.[31] Figure 6.1 describes the location of TE reported in children with solid tumors.[18,19,29,31–34]

TE in children with brain tumor

Adult patients with malignant brain tumors are at increased risk for TE including DVT and PE.[35,36] The 1-year cumulative rate of symptomatic venous TE is reported to be in the range of 20–30%, especially in adults with malignant gliomas.[35,37] Development of TE is associated with a 30% increased risk of death compared to those without TE.[38] The etiology of TE in this patient population is multifactorial. In addition to surgery, neurological weakness, immobility and CVL, activation of coagulation by tumor-induced tissue factor, endothelial damage and/or activation by chemotherapy and radiation therapy have been thought to play an important role in pathogenesis of VTE in patients with malignant glioma.

In contrast, children with brain tumors seem to have a very low prevalence of TE. To date three retrospective studies have reported cumulative prevalence of symptomatic VTE, ranging from 0.5% to 3.2% in children with brain tumors.[18,39,40] The retrospective nature of the studies may have underestimated the true risk of thrombosis in children with brain tumors. However, a similar study design has identified a significantly higher prevalence of TE in children with non-central nervous system cancers compared to those with brain tumors.[18] The etiology of the low prevalence of TE in children with brain tumors compared to adults with brain tumors or children with other types of cancer is unknown. This may partly be related to the different biology of

pediatric brain tumors; glioblastoma multiforme, which is common in adults, is rarely reported in the pediatric population.[35,38]

Use of aggressive therapies including stem cell transplantation (SCT) and antiangiogenic agents may change the epidemiology of thrombosis in association with pediatric brain tumors in the future.[40–42] The report of fatal PE in a child receiving autologous SCT for brain tumor highlights the importance of a high index of suspicion of TE to avoid delay in diagnosis and reduce morbidity and mortality related to TE in children with cancer.[42]

Risk factors predisposing children to cancer-associated thrombosis

Cancer-associated TE is a complex phenomenon resulting from the interaction of various factors inherent to the patient, the cancer and cancer therapy. The risk factors predisposing children to the development of thrombosis while undergoing cancer therapy are not well defined. Table 6.2 outlines the known risk factors identified in children with cancer-associated TE.

Types of thrombosis peculiar to children with cancer

Tumor thrombosis

Vascular invasion by tumor and tumor thrombosis can occur in children with solid tumors. Wilms tumor, neuroblastoma, osteosarcoma and hepatoblastoma are associated with vascular tumors invasion.[43] Tumor thrombi are shown to affect vessels including

Table 6.2 Risk factors predisposing children with cancer to development of thrombosis

Type of risk factor	Risk factor	Comments
Patient-related risk factors		
	Age	Children with ALL older than 10 years of age are shown to be at increased risk of developing TE.[15–17] Similarly, adolescents and young adults with solid tumors are at higher risk of developing TE compared to younger children[13,18,19]
	Thrombophilia	Although some studies have shown increased risk of TE in patients with inherited or acquired thrombophilia, the exact role of thrombophilia in the development of cancer-associated TE in children is unknown[14–17,22]
Disease-related risk factors		
	Type of cancer	Type of cancer is shown to be an independent predictor of TE in children[13,18]
	Cancer stage or risk category	Children with high-risk ALL and those with metastatic solid tumors are shown to have increased risk of TE[18,19,21,22]
	Site of cancer	Vascular invasion or compression by tumor may lead to development of TE in the vicinity of solid tumor[19,20,30,32]
Therapy-related risk factors		
	Central venous line	CVL is a well-known risk factor for development of thrombosis in children[16]
	Chemotherapy	Chemotherapeutic drugs like Asp, steroids, ATRA may induce procoagulant state[14,15,21,26–28]

Abbreviations: ALL = acute lymphoblastic leukemia; TE = thromboembolism; Asp = asparaginase; ATRA = all transretinoic acid.

the IVC, common iliac vein and right atrium resulting in PE.[30,34,43–45]

Wilms tumor is the most commonly reported pediatric malignancy in association with tumor thrombosis in the IVC. This may be related to direct drainage of the renal vein into the IVC. About 4% to 18% of children with Wilms tumor have IVC involvement by the tumor.[30,44] In a recent study of 165 patients with Wilms tumor and vascular invasion, the level of extension was IVC in 134 (81%) patients and RA in 31 (19%).[44] Other tumors such as neuroblastoma, hepatoblastoma and hepatocellular carcinoma also tend to have cardiovascular invasion.[3,45] Tumor thrombosis in the IVC and extension to the RA present a challenge in initial surgical management of the tumor. The presence of RA thrombus requires a combined thoracoabdominal approach with cardiopulmonary bypass.[30,44] Some investigators prefer preoperative chemotherapy to reduce the extent of tumor thrombus and facilitate resection. However, development of symptomatic PE has been reported following initiation of cytotoxic therapy.[34,44]

Although the role of anticoagulation therapy in the management of tumor thrombosis is unclear, prophylactic LMWH has been used to prevent PE from IVC thrombi.[34]

Cerebral sinovenous thrombosis (CSVT)

Compared to the general pediatric population, CSVT is frequent in children with cancer. The Canadian Pediatric Stroke Registry reported an incidence of 0.7 per 100,000 children per year.[46] In contrast, Wermes *et al.* reported ~6% incidence of CSVT in children with ALL treated on the Berlin–Frankfurt–Munster (BFM) ALL 90/95 protocol.[33] Cerebral sinovenous thrombosis is commonly reported in association with ALL and may reflect the use of Asp in most ALL therapy protocols. Approximately 50% children with ALL and symptomatic thrombosis have CNS thrombosis and over half of these CNS thromboses occur in the cerebral sinuses.[21,22,47] However, CSVT is also reported in other types of cancer in children, including neuroblastoma and non-Hodgkin's lymphoma (NHL). It is estimated that ~1% to 3% of patients with advanced stage NHL may develop CSVT irrespective of Asp therapy.[48,49]

The etiology of CSVT in association with cancer in children appears to be multifactorial and may be related to direct tumor invasion, tumor or tumor therapy (e.g., Asp)-induced hypercoagulability, or associated complications like dehydration.[22,47] Underlying prothrombotic disorders may increase the risk of CSVT.[50,51] The clinical presentation of CSVT

Table 6.3 Differential diagnosis of new-onset neurological symptoms in a child with cancer

Malignant invasion (e.g., leukemic meningoencephalitis or chloroma, metastatic lesions)

Drug toxicity (e.g., methotrexate-induced posterior reversible encephalopathy syndrome)

Hypertensive encephalopathy

Cerebrovascular events including arterial/ischemic stroke, CSVT

Infection (meningitis, abscess)

CNS hemorrhage due to thrombocytopenia or coagulopathy

Radiation-induced vascular or cortical damage

Metabolic derangement (e.g., SIADH, hypoglycemia)

Abbreviations: CSVT = cerebrosinovenous thrombosis; CNS = central nervous system; SIADH = syndrome of inappropriate antidiuretic hormone secretion.

depends on the age of the patient, acuity of thrombotic process and extent of the thrombosis and is similar to that seen in the general pediatric population.[46] The median duration of symptoms prior to presentation is reported to be ~ 5 days with a range of 12 hours to 120 days.[46] Headache, seizure (generalized or partial) and vomiting are reported to be common presenting symptoms. Since these symptoms may also result from other comorbidities (e.g., chemotherapy, hypertension) common in children receiving cancer therapy, a high index of suspicion is required for diagnosis of CSVT.[52] Table 6.3 outlines the differential diagnoses of new-onset neurological symptoms in patients with acute leukemia.

Hepatic sinusoidal obstruction syndrome (SOS)

Hepatic sinusoidal obstruction syndrome (SOS), previously known as veno-occlusive disease (VOD), is a serious and potentially fatal complication associated with conventional and high-dose chemotherapy in children with hematological malignancies and certain solid tumors.[53] Originally described in patients undergoing autologous or allogeneic SCT, it is also observed in patients receiving conventional chemotherapy with dactinomycin for Wilms tumor, neuroblastoma and rhabdomyosarcoma or thioguanine for ALL.[54–56] SOS is seen in 10–60% of patients undergoing SCT and is thought to be related to agents like busulphan, melphalan, cyclophosphamide

and total body irradiation, whereas non-SCT SOS is seen with such agents as dactinomycin and thioguanine.[57] The clinical constellation of hyperbilirubinemia (> 2 mg/dl), painful hepatomegaly, fluid retention with ascites and unexplained weight gain (> 5%) is pathognomonic for SOS. Thrombocytopenia unresponsive to transfusion is an early sign of SOS. Diagnosis is supported by Doppler ultrasonography showing reversal of portal blood flow (hepatofugal).

SOS associated with SCT tends to be more severe and rapidly progressive than that associated with conventional chemotherapy. The exact pathogenesis of this entity is still under evaluation but seems to be multifactorial; the central event appears to be sinusoidal endothelial damage resulting from toxic metabolites of chemotherapeutic agents along with cytokine activation, immune dysregulation and prothrombotic coagulopathy.[53] Derangement of several coagulation proteins have been noted in association of SOS, including reduction in protein C, protein S, factor VII and factor X and elevated levels of plasminogen activator inhibitor (PAI)-1. The presence of low protein C levels prior to initiation of the SCT conditioning regimen has been shown to be a risk factor for SOS.[53,54,58]

Although the role of coagulation protein deficiencies in the pathogenesis of SOS is unclear, abnormalities of the same led to several trials with antithrombin (AT) supplementation, steroids, unfractionated heparin (UFH) and low molecular weight heparin (LMWH) in the prevention of SOS.[53,58] Ursodeoxycholic acid had been shown to have benefit in the prevention of SOS.[53,55,56] Defibrotide, a deoxyribonucleic acid derivative from bovine and porcine mucosa, has been shown to be effective in prophylaxis of SOS by modulating hepatic sinusoidal endothelium. Defibrotide has anti-inflammatory, anti-ischemic and antithrombotic properties but lacks systemic anticoagulant effects, which explain the desirable absence of hemorrhagic side effects.[53–56]

Standard treatment of SOS requires close monitoring, supportive care with strict fluid restriction and diuresis. Various agents including high-dose methylprednisolone, AT and activated protein C have been used with variable success.[53,54] Fibrinolytic therapy with and without anticoagulation is effective, especially in early stages of disease.[53] Although recombinant human tissue plasminogen activator (tPA) in a dose of 0.2 mg/m^2/day as a 4-hour infusion has been shown to be effective in established SOS, further studies are warranted.[53] Serious hemorrhage is a major side effect especially in patients with multiorgan failure; hence tPA is recommended only in initial stages of VOD. Defibrotide is emerging as a relatively safe and effective agent in children even in those with severe SOS. The recommended dose of defibrotide is 10–60 mg/kg/day IV given in four divided doses.[53–56]

Pulmonary embolism

About 30% of adult patients with upper extremity DVT are reported to develop PE. Although CVL-related TE and upper venous system DVT are common in children with ALL, PE is reported in only 1–2% of children with ALL and symptomatic TE.[21,22] A recent meta-analysis reports ~10% incidence of PE in adult patients with lymphoma, whereas a retrospective cohort study reported ~2.5% children with lymphoma with symptomatic PE.[20,59] This may be a reflection of relative infrequency of PE in children compared to adults. However, careful evaluation for PE in patients with suspected or proven TE elsewhere in the body may be warranted.

Special considerations for anticoagulation management in children undergoing cancer therapy

The general principles of anticoagulation therapy for children with cancer are similar to those for the general pediatric population as described in current American College of Chest Physicians (ACCP) guidelines[60] and are reviewed in Chapter 1 on extremity and caval DVT, Chapter 15 on new anticoagulants and Chapter 14 on thrombolysis. Hence, this chapter will focus on special considerations for anticoagulation management in children receiving cancer chemotherapy.

Anticoagulation therapy in patients undergoing cancer chemotherapy is challenging due to the inherent increased risk of bleeding associated with thrombocytopenia and other coagulopathies as a result of cancer and its therapy.[14,15,17,61] The optimization of anticoagulation therapy is further limited by the frequent invasive procedures (e.g., lumbar puncture [LP] for intrathecal medication or tumor surgery) that require interruption of anticoagulation. Currently, even in the adult literature, there are no evidence-based guidelines for management of TE in patients undergoing cancer chemotherapy and at risk for thrombocytopenia or other coagulopathies.[3,62–66]

The following recommendations are derived from consensus-based guidelines and expert opinions.[62–67]

Who should be treated with systemic anticoagulation therapy, and for how long?

In adults with cancer, the development of TE is associated with high morbidity and mortality and hence adults with cancer and TE (irrespective of symptomatic or asymptomatic) are almost always treated.[62] However, similar evidence to identify children with cancer and TE who might benefit from anticoagulation therapy is not available. Due to the documented higher recurrence rate, the current recommendation suggests that children with symptomatic TE be treated with anticoagulation for at least 3 months or until the perceived triggers (i.e., Asp, active cancer) are no longer present.[60] The role of anticoagulation therapy for children with asymptomatic TE, especially CVL-related TE, is unclear. Ruud et al. have shown that the majority of asymptomatic CVL-related TE is transient, indicating that such TE may not require to be treated.[68] However, in view of the clinical implications of CVL-related TE (namely high risk of sepsis, PE and loss of venous access), ACCP guidelines suggest to treat all episodes of radiologically documented CVL-related TE.[60]

Which is the preferred anticoagulant agent?

Although oral vitamin K antagonists (VKA) are inexpensive and easy to administer, the management of anticoagulation with these agents is difficult in children and particularly those with cancer.[14,15,17,60,61] This is because of poor oral intake, especially in younger children, unpredictable endogenous and exogenous availability of vitamin K in the presence of mucositis, antibiotic therapy altering gut flora, or need for parenteral nutrition and potential interactions with chemotherapeutic agents.[69–71] Further, the longer half-life of VKA complicates anticoagulation management around intermittent thrombocytopenia and/or need for procedures.

Studies in adults with cancer have shown that LMWH is more efficacious than VKA, safe and likely to have additional survival benefit relative to VKA.[3,6,62–64,72,73] Similar information is not available for children with cancer. However, due to the comparable safety and efficacy to unfractionated heparin (UFH), minimal drug interactions and shorter half-life than VKA, allowing ease of management around elective invasive procedures, LMWH is the preferred anticoagulant in children with cancer, despite the need for daily subcutaneous injections.[60,74–79]

How should LMWH dose be adjusted in patients with thrombocytopenia?

Frequent development of thrombocytopenia related to myelosuppressive chemotherapy poses a major challenge in management of effective, yet safe, anticoagulation in patients with cancer. This is further complicated by lack of evidence, both in pediatric and adult literature, regarding safe and effective dosing of anticoagulants in patients with thrombocytopenia.[76,80–87] Most recommendations are based on expert opinions. Current practice is either to use platelet transfusion, tailor anticoagulation intensity to platelet count or to reduce or withhold anticoagulation for severe thrombocytopenia. The underlying presumption for the latter practice is that thrombocytopenia likely has a "protective" effect against thrombus progression. However, this effect has not been proven and hence, the impact of reducing anticoagulation intensity (to reduce bleeding risk) on thrombus resolution especially in severe TE (like PE or CNS-TE) is unknown. Further, the practice of platelet transfusion vs. LMWH dose reduction and the platelet trigger for the same are variable.[83–86] There are no specific suggestions regarding platelet transfusion and most of the available guidelines suggest that this decision be individualized.[60,64,65] However, in order to maximize anticoagulation therapy in the initial or acute stage of thrombus formation, the preference is toward platelet transfusion for severe thrombocytopenia ($< 50 \times 10^9$/l) rather than dose adjustment of LMWH. As regards dose adjustment based on platelet count, there seems to be a consensus to give full dose LMWH for a platelet count above 50×10^9/l and withhold anticoagulation if the platelet count is less than or equal to 20×10^9/l.[3,15,20,87] The practice of LMWH dose adjustment is variable between the platelet counts of 20 and 50×10^9/l. Close monitoring of patients for any signs of bleeding and platelet count is recommended.

How to adjust LMWH dose for patients undergoing invasive procedures?

Despite limited evidence of safety and efficacy, the current recommendation is to hold LMWH for 24 hours prior to invasive procedures to avoid bleeding complications.[60,88–90] Following an uncomplicated minor procedure (like LP), LMWH can be resumed immediately. However, following a more invasive procedure (like surgery) anticoagulation can be restarted only when the risk of bleeding is deemed to be minimal or nonexistent. The decision of resuming anticoagulation should be in consultation with surgical colleagues and other specialties involved (e.g., intensive care unit).

What is the role of antithrombin (AT) replacement for prevention or treatment of TE?

Antithrombin (AT) deficiency is thought to be the central mechanism of the prothrombotic state in patients receiving Asp therapy.[49,91,92] Hence several investigators evaluated the role of direct or indirect (through fresh frozen plasma [FFP]) AT replacement on the risk of development of symptomatic or asymptomatic TE. These studies have shown mixed results and there is no conclusive evidence supporting AT replacement in treatment of TE in children with cancer.[16,93–99] Thus, routine FFP or AT replacement is not recommended. Additionally, the consequence of acquired AT deficiency (e.g., with Asp therapy) on therapeutic LMWH levels has not been evaluated. Studies evaluating FFP failed to show any beneficial effect in restoring the natural anticoagulant factor deficiency, whereas studies evaluating AT supplementation showed some restoration of AT and hemostatic abnormality associated with Asp therapy.[16,93–99] However, the clinical benefit of AT supplementation in prevention of TE is yet to be proven. The PARKAA study showed a non-significant trend toward reduction of CVL-related TE with prophylactic AT concentrate.[16] A retrospective study of 214 adult patients with ALL and lymphoma (CAPELAL) showed a significant reduction in TE in patients receiving AT supplements compared to those without AT supplements during induction therapy using the BFM protocol (4.8% vs. 12.2% p = 0.04).[100] Based on the available data, routine use of AT supplements for prevention of TE in children receiving Asp is not recommended. Despite lack of evidence, several institutions supplement FFP and/or AT for prevention of TE while receiving Asp. This practice may lead to unnecessary exposure of patients to blood products and an increase in the cost of care. In addition, the presence of free asparagine in FFP may reduce the antileukemic efficacy of Asp.[101,102]

Asparaginase therapy after TE: to start or not to start? When to start?

Asparaginase is an important antileukemic agent with an impact on the survival of children with ALL. Asparaginase is a mainstay of combination chemotherapy. It acts by depleting exogenous asparagine and thereby selectively killing leukemic blasts.[103] Depletion of asparagine also results in reduced synthesis of hemostatic proteins such as protein C, protein S and AT.[91] Two studies have shown that suboptimal Asp therapy is an independent predictor of poor outcome. The Dana-Farber Cancer Institute ALL Consortium 91–001 protocol showed that 5-year event-free survival (EFS) of patients who required early discontinuation of Asp was 73% (±7%) compared to 90% (±2%) in those who received at least 25 doses of the scheduled 30 Asp doses (p < 0.01).[104] Similarly the CAPELAL study showed that ~ 50% of adult patients discontinued Asp due to TE and the overall survival (OS) and disease-free survival (DFS) of patients with TE and early discontinuation of Asp was significantly reduced compared to those with full dose Asp (19 vs. 53 months of OS and 14 vs. 58 months of DFS).[100] These data highlight the importance of continuation of Asp therapy for control of leukemia and lymphoma.

There are no evidence-based guidelines for management of Asp therapy in children who develop thrombosis and are receiving anticoagulation therapy. To avoid a persistent prothrombotic state and progression of the thrombotic process, Asp therapy is usually discontinued at the time of diagnosis of TE because of the fear of progression of TE. With stabilization of clinical status and therapeutic anticoagulation (usually after the initial 10–12 days), it is feasible to reintroduce Asp even in the context of CSVT. Recent studies have shown that reintroduction of Asp in children with TE is safe without any further thrombotic events.[15,105,106] This strategy requires close monitoring of patients with imaging studies.

When to use an IVC filter?

The use of IVC filters for prevention of PE in adults is well documented.[107] However, the information regarding vena caval filters in the pediatric age group is limited and originates from small case series.[108,109] Studies in adult cancer patients have shown that vena caval filters in patients with advanced cancer are safe, well tolerated and effective.[110] Similar experience regarding the utility and safety of vena caval filters in children with cancer is lacking.

Based on available data in the general pediatric population, the ACCP guidelines suggest the use of a retrievable filter in children with body weight > 10 kg, lower extremity TE and a contraindication to anticoagulation.[60] The weight restriction is due to the size of the IVC and that of available filters. Such a procedure should be undertaken by a skilled pediatric interventional radiologist trained in endovascular procedures with experience in filter placement. In addition to the procedural complications (e.g., bleeding, pneumothorax, IVC injury or thrombosis), filter-related complications include clot extension in the IVC, filter migration, filter fracture, thrombosis of the filter basket and IVC perforation. There is currently no evidence to support prophylactic use of IVC filters even in adult patients.[3]

Can children with brain tumors get anticoagulation therapy?

Children with brain tumors can be treated with anticoagulation therapy successfully. However, due to rarity of this event, the reported experience of anticoagulation therapy in children with brain tumors is limited. The ACCP guidelines recommend keeping the platelet count > 50×10^9/l in adults with brain tumors receiving anticoagulation therapy.[3]

What is the role of thromboprophylaxis in children with cancer?

Primary thromboprophylaxis

Although studies in the adult population support the use of primary thromboprophylaxis in select groups of patients (e.g., patients who are hospitalized or post-surgical), primary thromboprophylaxis of children with cancer is not currently recommended.[3,62] Indeed currently there are no reliable indicators to stratify pediatric patients according to the risk of TE.

Several investigators have evaluated the role of primary prophylaxis with AT, FFP, VKA or LMWH either as a single agent or in combination (Table 6.4). All studies have shown lack of benefit of AT and FFP supplements for prevention of TE or correction of biochemical abnormalities related to Asp therapy. Two cohort studies have shown a benefit of LMWH. Small sample sizes, variability in

Table 6.4 Summary of studies evaluating thromboprophylaxis in children with cancer

Study	Study design	Population	Population with prophylaxis	Intervention	Timing of intervention	Outcome measure	Results
PARKAA[16]	Prospective cohort	Children with ALL (> 6 mo– < 18 yrs) (n = 109)	Patients receiving induction therapy with Asp and have CVL (n = 37)	Once weekly AT supplementation vs. no supplementation	During induction therapy on days 1, 8, 15, 22	Clinically symptomatic or asymptomatic TE at any location	Incidence of TE in patients treated with AT (28%; 95% CI: 12.1–49.4%) and in non-AT arm (36.7%; 95% CI: 24.4–48.8%). No difference between development of TE in treated and untreated arms (p = 0.43)
Ruud et al.[68]	RCT	Children with newly diagnosed cancer (n = 73)	Children with cancer, jugular CVL and at least 6 mo of therapy	Low-dose warfarin with intended INR between 1.3–1.9 vs. no warfarin		CVL-related TE diagnosed by ultrasonography	48% vs. 36% TE in patients with and without warfarin (p = 0.44). Very few patients had INR in the desired range.
Harlev et al.[82]	Retrospective cohort	Children with ALL (n = 80)	Patients older than 1 year with FVL and PT mutation (n = 18)	LMWH 1 mg/kg Q daily SC	Induction and reinduction with Asp (from the days of start of Asp till 1 week after last dose)	Symptomatic and asymptomatic TE	Overall TE 7.5%; patients without thrombophilia and prophylaxis (4.5%) and those with thrombophilia and prophylaxis (16.6%) (p = 0.124)
Elhasid et al.[81]	Prospective cohort	Children with ALL	Patients with inherited thrombophilia (n = 41)	LMWH			
Halton et al.[93]	Prospective cohort	Children with ALL	During consolidation therapy (n = 8)	FFP at 20 ml/kg	Consolidation therapy	Coagulation proteins and biochemical markers of thrombin generation	No difference following FFP supplementation
Zaunschirm et al.[98]	Prospective cohort	Children with ALL	Children with ALL with low AT (< 80% of normal) and fibrinogen (< 100 mg/dl) (n = 13)	FFP 3 times per day and/or AT concentrate as continuous infusion in doses adjusted according to AT and fibrinogen levels	First remission induction (n = 11); second induction (n = 2); reinduction with prior cerebral hemorrhage (n = 1)	APTT, thrombin time, AT, fibrinogen levels and factors II, V, VIII	Expected AT and fibrinogen levels (> 80% of normal and > 100 mg/dl) were achieved within 24-48 hrs after start of replacement therapy

Study	Study design	Population	Subgroup	Intervention	Timing	Outcome measure	Results
Nowak-Gottl et al.[96]	Prospective cohort	Children with ALL (n = 42)	Patients with fibrinogen < 60 mg/dl and prolonged APTT (n = 20)	FFP median 10 ml/kg (range 5–20 ml/kg)	During ALL induction therapy	Fibrinogen, coagulation proteins and markers of thrombin generation	No effect of FFP on fibrinogen, coagulation proteins or parameters of thrombin generation.
Abdelkefi et al.[111]	RCT	Patients with cancer 4–60 years of age with CVL (n = 108; 74 with cancer)	Patients prior to subclavian CVL insertion	Continuous infusion of UFH 100 IU/kg/day (maximum 10,000 IU/day) (n = 55 with 65 CVLs) vs. 50 ml/day of normal saline (n=53 with 63 CVLs)	While in hospital. All CVLs were removed prior to discharge	CVL-related TE documented by ultrasonography and bleeding	CVL-related TE occurred in 1 of 65 CVLs (1.5%) in UFH group compared to 8 or 63 (12.6%) in control group (p = 0.03). No difference in bleeding risk (p = 0.18)
Meister et al.[95]	Prospective cohort study	Children with ALL (n = 112)	Patients with AT < 50% received AT supplementation	Combination of AT supplementation and enoxaparin (1 mg/kg/ day) (n = 41) vs. AT alone (non-contemporaneous control group) (n = 71)	During induction therapy	Symptomatic TE anytime during 240 days of follow-up	12.7% (95% CI 6.0–22.7) of children with AT alone compared to no TE (95% CI 0–8.6%) in children with combined prophylaxis (p < 0.05)
Abbott et al.[94]	Retrospective comparative cohort	Children with ALL (n = 719)	Patients with low AT and fibrinogen (n = 240)	FFP and/or cryoprecipitate to replace low AT and fibrinogen	ALL induction therapy	CNS thrombosis or hemorrhage	No effect of prophylactic FFP and cryo on the risk of development of CNS TE

Abbreviations: PARKAA = Prophylactic Antithrombin Replacement in Kids with Acute Lymphoblastic Leukemia Treated with Asparaginase Group; RCT = randomized control trial; ALL = acute lymphoblastic leukemia; ASP = asparaginase; CVL = central venous line; AT = antithrombin; TE = thromboembolism; CI = confidence interval; INR = international normalization ratio; FVL = factor V Leiden; PT = prothrombin; LMWH = low molecular weight heparin; FFP = fresh frozen plasma; APTT = activated partial thromboplastin time; UFH = unfractionated heparin; CNS = central nervous system.

primary outcome (CVL-related TE, symptomatic vs. asymptomatic TE) as well as patient population (children with ALL vs. all cancers, those with thrombophilia) are major limitations of the studies evaluating thromboprophylaxis.

Abdelkefi *et al.* reported a RCT comparing a continuous infusion of UFH vs. normal saline and showed a statistically significant benefit of UFH in the prevention of CVL-related TE in patients with hematological disorders (68% with malignant disorders).[111] Results of this study are difficult to adopt for the pediatric oncology population since the study was comprised of a wide age range (4–60 years) without separate breakdown of pediatric age group, mix of malignant and non-malignant conditions and use of short-term external CVLs. Harlev *et al.* evaluated the role of LMWH (1 mg/kg subcutaneous daily) given from start of Asp therapy until 1 week after discontinuation for children detected to have either FVL and/or prothrombin (PT) gene mutation (n = 18; 22.5% of the total study population of 80 children). Three of 18 (16.6% of) children (all three with PT mutation) developed TE (all three CVL-related and two symptomatic); 2 of 18 (11%) children developed TE while receiving LMWH prophylaxis, whereas 3 of 62 (4.5%) children without prophylaxis developed TE (p = 0.124).[82]

Secondary thromboprophylaxis

There are no evidence-based recommendations for secondary thromboprophylaxis for children with cancer. As in adults, children with cancer and TE are shown to have increased risk of TE recurrence, especially with recurrence of cancer or risk factor (e.g., Asp).[12,15,18] Hence, secondary prophylaxis may be justified in children with cancer who have re-exposure to the identified risk factor. For example, secondary prophylaxis may be used when the patient is re-exposed to Asp therapy as in the reinduction or consolidation phase or relapse/recurrence of cancer. The role of prolonged thromboprophylaxis in CVL-related TE where CVL remains *in situ* for a prolonged period of time (e.g., 2 years) is unclear.

Conclusion

Cancer, especially hematologic malignancy, appears to be a potent risk factor for TE in children. Solid tumors are also associated with TE sometimes direct tumor invasion into large veins. Although the majority of TE in children with cancer is CVL related, distant TE are not uncommon. Two types of TE peculiar to this group include CSVT, common with ALL and Asp

therapy, and SOS – related either to chemotherapy or SCT. The etiology of TE in children with cancer is multifactorial and risk factors include prothrombotic coagulopathies induced by the malignancy itself, use of CVL and endothelial damage from surgery, chemotherapy and CVL. Current areas of controversy include: (1) use and intensity of anticoagulation in children with thrombocytopenia; (2) the duration of secondary prophylaxis in children with cancer and TE following primary therapy; and (3) indications, if any, for primary prophylaxis of TE. Prospective cohort studies and RCTs are needed to provide evidence upon which to base clinical decision-making around the prevention and treatment of TE in children with cancer.

References

1. Varki A. Trousseau's syndrome: multiple definitions and multiple mechanisms. Blood 2007;**110**:1723–1729.

2. Khorana AA. Malignancy, thrombosis and Trousseau: the case for an eponym. J Thromb Haemost 2003;**1**:2463–2465.

3. Lyman GH, Khorana AA, Falanga A, et al. American Society of Clinical Oncology guideline: recommendations for venous thromboembolism and treatment in patients with cancer. J Clin Oncol 2007;**25**:1–16.

4. Khorana AA, Francis CW, Culakova E, et al. Thromboembolism is a leading cause of death in cancer patients receiving outpatient chemotherapy. J Thromb Haemost 2007;**5**:632–634.

5. Khorana AA, Francis CW, Culakova E, et al. Thromboembolism in hospitalized neutropenic cancer patients. J Clin Oncol 2006;**24**:484–490.

6. Lee AYY, Levine MN. Venous thromboembolism and cancer: risks and outcome. Circulation 2003;**107**:I-17–I-21.

7. Stein PD, Beemath A, Meyers FA, et al. Incidence of thromboembolism in patients hospitalized with cancer. Am J Med 2006;**119**:60–68.

8. Rickles FR, Levine MN. Epidemiology of thrombosis in cancer. Acta Haematol 2001;**106**:6–12.

9. Kwaan HC, Vicuna B. Incidence and pathogenesis of thrombosis in hematologic malignancies. Semin Thromb Hemost 2007;**33**:303–312.

10. Bulland MF, Willey V, Hauch O, Wygent G, Spyroupolous AC, Hoffman L. Longitudinal evaluation of health plan cost per venous thromboembolism or bleed event in patients with prior venous thromboembolism event during hospitalization. J Manag Care Pharm 2005;**11**:663–673.

11. Andrew M, Vegh P, Johnston M, Bowker J, Ofosu F, Mitchell L. Maturation of the hemostatic system during childhood. Blood 1992;**80**:1998–2005.

12. Raffini L, Huang Y-S, Witmer C, Feudtner C. Dramatic increase in venous thromboembolism in U.S. Children's Hospitals from 2001–2007. Pediatrics 2009;**124**:1001–1008.

13. O'Brien SH, Klima J, Termuhlen AM, Kelleher KJ. Venous thromboembolism and adolescent and young adult oncology inpatients in US Children's Hospitals, 2001 to 2008. J Pediatr 2011;**159**:133–137.

14. Nowak-Gottl U, Kenet G, Mitchell LG. Thrombosis in childhood acute lymphoblastic leukemia: epidemiology aetiology, diagnosis, prevention and treatment. Best Pract Res Clin Haematol 2009;**22**:104–114.

15. Athale UH, Chan AKC. Thromboembolic complications in children with hematologic malignancies. Semin Thromb Hemost 2007;**33**(4):416–426.

16. Mitchell LG, Andrew M, Hanna K, et al. A prospective cohort study determining the prevalence of thrombotic events in children with acute lymphoblastic leukemia and a central venous line who are treated with L-asparaginase. Results of the Prophylactic Antithrombin Replacement in Kids with Acute Lymphoblastc Leukemia Treated with Asparaginase (PARKAA) study. Cancer 2003;**97**:508–516.

17. Bajzar L, Chan AKC, Massicotte MP, Mitchell LG. Thrombosis in children with malignancy. Curr Opin Pediatr 2006;**18**:1–9.

18. Athale UH, Siciliano S, Thabane L, Pai N, Cox S, Lathia A, Khan AA, Armstrong A, Chan AKC. Epidemiology and clinical risk factors predisposing to thromboembolism in children with cancer. Pediatr Blood Cancer 2008;**51**:792–797.

19. Paz-Priel I, Long L, Helman LJ, Mackall CL, Wayne AS. Thromboembolic events in children and young adults with pediatric sarcoma. J Clin Oncol 2007;**25**:1519–1524.

20. Athale UH, Nagel K, Khan A, Chan AKC. Thromboembolism in children with lymphoma. *Thromb Res* 2008;**122**:459–465.

21. Athale UH, Chan AKC. Thrombosis in children with acute lymphoblastic leukemia Part I: Epidemiology of thrombosis in children with acute lymphoblastic leukemia. Thromb Res 2003;**111**:125–131.

22. Caruso V, Lacoviello L, Castelnuovo AD, Storti S, Mariani G, Gaetano GD, Donati MB. Thrombotic complications in childhood acute lymphoblastic leukemia: a meta-analysis of 17 prospective studies comprising 1752 patients. Blood 2006;**108**:2216–2222.

23. Behm F. Manifestations of the bone marrow. In Parham D, ed. Pediatric Neoplasia: Morphology and Biology. Philadelphia: Lippincott-Raven; 1996: pp. 449–504.

24. Maule MM, Dama E, Mosso ML, Magnani C, Pastero G, Merletti F. High incidence of acute promyelocytic leukemia in children in northwest Italy, 1980–2003: a report from the Childhood Cancer Registry of Piedmont. Leukemia 2008;**22**:439–441.

25. Tallman MS, Altman JK. How I treat acute promyelocytic leukemia. Blood 2009;**114**:5126–5135.

26. Zakarija A, Kwaan HC. Adverse effects of hemostatic function of drugs used in hematologic malignancy. Semin Thromb Hemost 2007;**33**:355–364.

27. Tallman MS, Abutalib SA, Altman JK. The double hazard of thrombophilia and bleeding in acute promyelocytic leukemia. Semin Thromb Hemost 2007;**33**:330–338.

28. Choudhry A, DeLoughery TG. Bleeding and thrombosis in acute promyelocytic leukemia. Am J Hematol 2012;**87**:596–603.

29. Unal S, Varan A, Yalcan B, Buyukpamukcu M, Gurgey A. Evaluation of thrombotic children with malignancy. Ann Hematol 2005;**84**:395–399.

30. Kim S, Chung DH. Pediatric solid malignancies: neuroblastoma and Wilms' tumor. Surg Clin North Am 2006;**86**(2):469–487.

31. Schiavetti A, Foco M, Chiriaco D, Iacobini M, Varrasso G, Ingrosso A, Conti L. Venous thrombosis and procoagulant factors in high-risk neuroblastoma. J Pediatr Hematol/Oncol 2010;**32**:93–96.

32. Schiavetti A, Foco M, Ingrosso A, Bonci E, Conti L, Matrunola M. Venous thrombosis in children with solid tumors. J Pediatr Hematol/Oncol 2008;**30**:148–152.

33. Wermes C, Fleischhack G, Junker R, Schobess R, Schwabe D, Sykora KW, Nowak-Gottle U. Cerebral venous sinus thrombosis in children with acute lymphoblastic leukemia carrying MTHFR TT677 genotype and further prothrombotic risk factors. Klin Pediatr 1999;**211**(4):211–214.

34. Bagatell R, Morgan E, Cosentino C, Whitesell L. Two cases of pediatric neuroblastoma with tumor thrombus in inferior vena cava. J Pediatr Hematol/Oncol 2002;**24**:397–400.

35. Jenkins EO, Schiff D, Mackman N, Key NS. Venous thromboembolism in malignant gliomas. J Thromb Haemost 2010;**8**:221–227.

36. Perry JR. Anticoagulation of malignant glioma patients in the era of novel antiangiogenic agents. Curr Opin Neurol 2010;**23**:592–596.

37. Perry JR, Julian JA, Laperriere NJ, Geerts W, Agnelli G, Rogers LR, Malkin MG, Sawaya R, Baker R, Falanga A, Parpia S, Finch T, Levine MN. PRODIGE: a randomized placebo-controlled trial of dalteparin low molecular weight heparin thromboprophylaxis in

patients with newly diagnosed malignant glioma. J Thromb Haemost 2010;**8**:1959–1965.

38. Semrad TJ, O'Donnell R, Wun T, Chew H, Harvey D, Zhou H, White RH. Epidemiology of venous thromboembolism in 9489 patients with malignant glioma. J Neurosurg 2007;**106**:601–608.

39. Tabori U, Beni-Adani L, Dvir R, et al. Risk of venous thromboembolism in pediatric patients with brain tumors. Pediatr Blood Cancer 2004;**43**:633–636.

40. Deitcher SR, Gajjar A, Kun L, et al. Clinically evident venous thromboembolism in children with brain tumors. J Pediatr 2004;**145**:848–850.

41. MacDonald TJ, Stewart CF, Kocak M, Ellenbogen RG, Phillps P, Lafond D, Poussaint TY, Kieran MW, Boyett JM, Kun LE. Phase I clinical trial of cilengitide in children with refractory brain tumors: pediatric brain tumor consortium study PBTC-012. J Clin Oncol 2008;**26**:919–924.

42. Kounami S, Aoyagi N, Nakayama K, Yoshiyama M, Boshi H, Sakiyama M, Takeuchi T, Yoshikawa N. Fatal pulmonary thromboembolism after a second course of high-dose chemotherapy with autologous peripheral blood stem cell transplant. Pediatr Transplantation 2003;**7**:400–403.

43. Kirkwood I, McCarville M, Baharami A, Shulkin B. [F-18]FDG PET/CT appearance of tumor thrombi in pediatric solid tumors. J Nucl Med 2012;**53**(Suppl 1): 2193.

44. Shamberger RC, Ritchey ML, Haase GM, Bergemann MS, et al. Intravascular extension of Wilms' tumor. Ann Surg 1001;**234**:116–121.

45. Wang JN, Chen JS, Chuang HY, Yang YJ, Chang KC, Wu J-M. Invasion of the cardiovascular system in childhood malignant hepatic tumors. J Pediatr Hematol/Oncol 2002;**24**:436–439.

46. deVeber G, Andrew M, Adam C, Bjorson B, Booth F, Buckley DJ, et al. Cerebral sinovenous thrombosis in children. New Eng J Med 2001;**345**:417–423.

47. Mitchell LG, Sutor AN, Andrew M. Hemostasis in childhood acute lymphoblastic leukemia: coagulopathy induced by disease and treatment. Semin Thromb Hemostasis 1995;**21**:390–401.

48. Reddingius RE, Patte C, Couanet D, Kalifa C, Lemerle J. Dural sinus thrombosis in children with cancer. Med Ped Oncol 1997;**29**:296–302.

49. Legrand I, Lalande G, Neuenschwander S, Dulac O, Kalifa LG. Thrombosis du sinus longitudinal superior au cours du treatment de lymphoma hez l'enfant. J Radiol 1986;**67**:595–600.

50. Dlamini N, Billinghurst L, Kirkham FJ. Cerebral venous sinus (sinovenous) thrombosis in children. Neurosurg Clin North Am 2010;**21**:511–27.

51. Kennet G, Lutkhoff LK, Albisetti M, Bernard T, Bonduel M, et al. Impact of thrombophilia on risk of arterial ischemic stroke or cerebral sinouvenous thrombosis in neonates and children: a systematic review and metanalyses of observational studies. Circulation 2010;**121**:1838–1847.

52. Sebire G, Tabarki B, Saunders DE, Leroy I, Liesner R, Saint-Martin C, Husson B, Williams AN, Wade A, Kirkham FJ. Cerebral venous sinus thrombosis in children: risk factors, presentation, diagnosis and outcome. Brain 2005;**128**:477–489.

53. Cefalo MG, Maurizi P, Arlotta A, Scalzone M, Attina G, Ruggiero A, Riccardi R. Hepatic veno-occlusive disease. A chemotherapy-related toxicity in children with malignancy. Pediatric Drugs 2010;**12**:277–284.

54. Haussman U, Fischer J, Eber S, Scherer F, Serger R, Gungor T. Hepatic veno-occlusive disease in pediatric stem cell transplantation: impact of preemptive antithrombin III replacement and combined antithrombin III/defibrotide therapy. Haematologica 2006;**91**:795–800.

55. Quereshi A, Marshall L, Lancaster D. Defibrotide in the treatment and prevention of veno-occlusive disease in autologous and allogeneic stem cell transplantation in children. Pediatr Blood Cancer 2008;**50**:831–832.

56. Del Toro G. Defibrotide in sinusoidal obstruction syndrome: mounting evidence in pediatric patients. Pediatr Blood Cancer 2008;**50**:735–736.

57. Stork LC, Matloub Y, Broxson E, La M, Yanofsky R, Sather H, Hutchinson R, Heerema NA, Sorrell AD, Masterson M, Bleyer A, Gaynon PS. Oral 6-mercaptopurine versus oral 6-thioguanine and veno-occlusive disease in children with standard-risk acute lymphoblastic leukemia: report of the Children's Oncology Group CCG-1952 clinical trial. Blood 2010;**115**:2740–2748.

58. Iguchi A, Kobayaschi R, Kaneda M, Kobayaschi A. Plasma protein C is a useful clinical marker for hepatic veno-occlusive disease (VOD) in stem cell transplantation. Pediatr Blood Cancer 2010;**54**:437–443.

59. Caruso V, Castelnuovo AD, Meschengieser S, Lazzari MA, Gaetano GD, Storti S, Lacoviello L, Donati MB. Thrombotic complications in adult patients with lymphoma a meta-analysis of 29 independent cohorts including 18 018 patients and 1149 events. Blood 2010;**115**:5322–5328.

60. Monagle P, Chan AKC, Goldenberg NA, Ichord RN, Journeycake JM, Nowak-Gottl U, Vesely, SK. Antithrombotic Therapy in Neonates and Children: Antithrombotic Therapy and Prevention of Thrombosis, 9th edn: American College of Chest Physicians Evidence-Based Clinical Practice Guideline. Chest 2012;**141**:e737S–801S.

61. Wiernikowaski J, Athale UH. Thromboembolic complications in children with cancer. Thromb Res 2006;**118**:137–152.

62. Khorana AA, Streiff MB, Farge D, Mandala M, Debourdeau P, Cajfinger F, Marty M, Falanga A, Lyman GH. Venous thromboembolism prophylaxis and treatment in cancer: a consensus statement of major guidelines panel and call to action. J Clin Oncol 2009;**27**:4919–4926.

63. Panova-Novea, Falanga A. Treatment of thromboembolism in cancer patients. Exp Op Pharmacotherapy 2010;**11**:2049–2058.

64. Kearon C, Elie AKL, Comerota AJ, Prandoni P, Bounameaux H, Goldhaber SZ, Nelson ME, Wells PS, Gould MK, Dentali F, Crowther M, Kahn SR. Antithrombotic Therapy for VTE Disease: Antithrombotic Therapy and Prevention of Thrombosis, 9th edn: American College of Chest Physicians Evidence-Based Clinical Practice Guidelines. Chest 2012;**141**;e419S–494S.

65. Mandala M, Falanga A, Roila F, on behalf of the ESMO Guidelines Working Group. Management of venous thromboembolism in cancer patients: ESMO clinical recommendations. Ann Oncol 2009;**20**:182–184.

66. Streif MB, Bockenstedt PL, Cataland SR, Chesney C, Eby C, Fogarty PF, Gao S, Garcia-Aguilar J, Goldhaber SZ, Hassoun H, Hendrie P, Holmstron B, Jones KA, Kuderer N, Lee JT, Milleson MM, Neff AT, Ortel TL, Smith JL, Yee GC, Zakarija A. Venous thromboembolic disease. J Nat Compr Canc Netw 2011;**9**:714–777.

67. Chalmers E, Ganesen V, Liesner R, Maroo S, Nokes T, Saunders D, Williams M. Guidelines on the investigation, management and prevention of venous thrombosis in children. Br J Haematol 2011;**154**:196–201.

68. Ruud E, Holmstrome H, De Lange C, Hogstad EM, Wesenberg F. Low-dose warfarin for the prevention of central line-associated thrombosis in children with malignancy – a randomized controlled study. Acta Paediatrica 2006;**95**:1053–1059.

69. Streif W, Andrew M, Marzinotto V, Massicotte P, Chan AK, Julian JA, Mitchell L. Analysis of warfarin therapy in pediatric patients: A prospective cohort study of 319 patients. Blood 1999;**94**:3007–3014.

70. Andrew M, Monagle P, Brooker L. Oral anticoagulant therapy in pediatric patients. Thromboembolic Complications During Infancy and Childhood. Hamilton: B.C. Decker Inc; 2000: pp. 321–356.

71. Buck ML. Anticoagulation with warfarin in infants and children. Ann Pharmacother 1996;**30**:1316–1322.

72. Lee AYY, Levine MN, Baker RI, Bowden C, Kakkar AK, Prins M, Rickles FR, Julian JA, Haley S, Kovacs MJ, Gent M. Low molecular-weight heparin versus a coumarin for the prevention of recurrence venous thromboembolism in patients with cancer. N Eng J Med 2003;**349**:146–153.

73. Kuderer NM, Ortel TL, Francis CW. Impact of venous thromboembolism and anticoagulation on cancer and cancer survival. J Clin Oncol 2009;**27**:4902–4911.

74. Revel-Vilk S, Chan AKC. Anticoagulation therapy in children. Sem Thromb Hemost 2003;**29**:425–432.

75. Gould MK, Dembitzer AD, Doyle RL, Hastie TJ, Garber AM. Low-molecular-weight heparins compared with unfractionated heparin for treatment of acute deep venous thrombosis. A meta-analysis of randomized, controlled trials. Ann Intern Med 1999;**130**:800–809.

76. Massicotte P, Adams M, Marzinotto V, Brooker LA, Andrew M. Low-molecular-weight heparin in pediatric patients with thrombotic disease: a dose finding study. J Pediatr 1996;**128**:313–318.

77. Albisetti M, Andrew M. Low molecular weight heparin in children. Eur J Pediatr 2002;**161**:71–77.

78. Dix D, Andrew M, Marzinotto V, et al. The use of low molecular weight heparin in pediatric patients: a prospective cohort study. J Pediatr 2000;**136**:439–445.

79. Nohe N, Flemmer A, Rumler R, Praun M, Auberger K. The low molecular weight heparin dalteparin for prophylaxis and therapy of thrombosis in childhood: a report on 48 cases. Eur J Pediatr 1999;**158**(Suppl 3): S134–139.

80. Ibrahim RB, Peres E, Dansey R, Abidi MH, Abella EM, Gumma MM, Milan N, Smith DW, Heilbrun LK, Klein J. Safety of low-dose low-molecular-weight-heparins in thrombocytopenic stem cell transplantation patients: a case series and review of the literature. Bone Marrow Transpl 2005;**35**:1071–1077.

81. Elhasid R, Lanir N, Sharon R, Arush M, Weyl B, Levin C, Potovsky S, Barak AB, Brenner B. Prophylactic therapy with enoxaparin during L-asparaginase treatment in children with acute lymphoblastic leukemia. Blood Coagul Fibrinolysis 2001;**12**:367–370.

82. Harlev D, Zaidman I, Sarig G, Arush MWB, Brenner B, Elhasid R. Prophylactic therapy with enoxaparin in children with acute lymphoblastic leukemia and inherited thrombophilia during L-asparaginase treatment. Thromb Res 2010;**126**:93–97.

83. Stine KC, Saylors RL, Saccente CS, Becton DL. Treatment of deep venous thrombosis in pediatric cancer patients receiving chemotherapy. Clin Appl Thromb Hemost 2007;**13**:161–165.

84. Tousovska K, Zapletal O, Skotakova J, Bukac J, Sterba J. Treatment of deep venous thrombosis with low molecular weight heparin in pediatric cancer patients: safety and efficacy. Blood Coagul Fibrinolysis 2009;**20**:583–589.

85

85. Imberti D, Vallisa D, Anselmi E, Moroni CF, Berte R, Lazzaro A, Bernuzzi P, Arcari AL, Cavanna L. Safety and efficacy of enoxaparin treatment in venous thromboembolic disease during acute leukemia. Tumori 2004;**90**:390–393.

86. Akasheh MS, Abu-Hajir M. The safety of enoxaparin in patients older than 60 years with acute myelogenous leukemia or high risk myelodysplastic syndrome undergoing chemotherapy. Bah Med Bull 2001;**24**:66–68.

87. Falanga A, Marchetti M. Venous thromboembolism in hematologic malignancies. J Clin Oncol 2009;**27**:4848–4485.

88. Dix D, Charpentier K, Sparling C, Massicotte MP. Determination of trough anti-factor Xa levels in pediatric patients on low molecular weight heparin (LMWH). J Pediatr Hematol/Oncol 1998;**20**:398, Abstract no. 667.

89. Avila LR, Shaik F, Macartney C, Williams S, Brandao L. The effect of therapeutic anticoagulation on the risk of traumatic lumbar punctures in children with acute lymphoblastic leukemia. J Thromb Haemost 2011;**9**(Suppl 2):1–1055, Abstract no. O-TU-043.

90. Moruf A, Spyropoulus AC, Schardt TQ, Gibson E, Manco-Johnson MJ, Wang M, Goldenberg NA. Peri-procedural bridging with low molecular weight heparin in patients receiving warfarin for venous thromboembolism: A pediatric experience. Thromb Res 2012;**130**:612–615.

91. Mitchell L, Hoogendoorn H, Giles AR, Vegh P, Andrew M. Increased endogenous thrombin generation in children with acute lymphoblastic leukemia: risk of thrombotic complications in L-Asparaginase-induced antithrombin III deficiency. Blood 1994;**83**:386–391.

92. Hongo T, Okada S, Ohzeki T, Ohta H, Nishimura S, Hamamoto K, Yagi K, Misu H, Eguchi N, Suzuki N, Horibe K, Ueda K. Low plasma levels of hemostatic proteins during the induction phase in children with acute lymphoblastic leukemia: A retrospective study by the JACLS: Japan Association of Childhood Leukemia Study. Pediatr Int 2002;**44**:293–299.

93. Halton JM, Mitchell LG, Vegh P, Eves M, Andrew ME. Fresh frozen plasma has no beneficial effect on the hemostatic system in children receiving L-asparaginase. Am J Hematol 1994;**47**:157–161.

94. Abbott LS, Deevska M, Fernandez CV, Dix D, Price VE, Wang H, Parker L, Yhap M, Fitzgerald C, Barnard DR, Berman JN. The impact of prophylactic fresh-frozen plasma and cryoprecipitate on the incidence of central nervous system thrombosis and hemorrhage in children with acute lymphoblastic leukemia receiving asparaginase. Blood 2009;**114**:5146–5151.

95. Meister B, Kropshofer G, Klein-Franke A, Strasak AM, Hager J, Streif W. Comparison of low-molecular-weight heparin and antithrombin versus antithrombin alone for the prevention of symptomatic venous thromboembolism in children with acute lymphoblastic leukemia. Pediatr Blood Cancer 2008;**50**:298–303.

96. Nowak-Gottl U, Rath B, Binder M, Hassel JU, Wolff J, Husemann S, Ritter J. Inefficacy of fresh frozen plasma in the treatment of L-asparaginase-induced coagulation factor deficiencies during ALL induction therapy. Haematologica 1995;**80**:451–453.

97. Gugliotta L, D'Angelo A, Mattioli Belmonte M, Vigano-D'Angelo S, Colombo G, Catani L, Gianni L, Lauria F, Tura S. Hypercoagulability during L-asparaginase treatment: the effect of antithrombin III supplementation in vivo. Br J Haematol 1990;**74**:465–470.

98. Zaunschirm A, Muntean W. Correction of hemostatic imbalances induced by L-asparaginase therapy in children with acute lymphoblastic leukemia. Pediatr Hematol Oncol 1986;**3**:19–25.

99. Nowak-Gottl U, Kuhn N, Wolff JE, Boos J, Kehrel B, Rath B, Jurgens H. Inhibition of hypercoagulation by antithrombin substitution in E. coli L-asparaginase-treated children. Eur J Haematol 1996;**56**:35–38.

100. Hunault-Berger M, Chevallier P, Delain M, et al. Changes in antithrombin and fibrinogen levels during induction chemotherapy with L-asparaginase in adult patients with acute lymphoblastic leukemia or lymphoblastic lymphoma: use of supportive coagulation therapy and clinical outcome. Haematologica 2008;**93** (10):1488–1494.

101. Steiner M, Attarbaschi A, Hass OA, Kastner U, Gadner H, Mann G. Fresh frozen plasma contains free asparagine and may replace the plasma asparagine pool during L-asparaginase therapy. (Letter to the Editor.) Leukemia 2008;**22**:1290.

102. Zuckerman T, Ganzel C, Tallman MS, Rowe JM. How I treat hematologic emergencies in adults with acute leukemia. Blood 2012;**120**(10):1993–2002.

103. Muller HJ, Boos J. Use of L-asparaginase in childhood ALL. Crit Rev Oncol Hematol 1998;**28**:97–113.

104. Silverman LB, Gelber RD, Dalton VK, Asselin BL, Barr RD, Clavell LA, Hurwitz CA, Moghrabi A, Samson Y, Schorin MA, Arkin S, Declerck L, Cohen HJ, Sallan SE. Improved outcome of children with acute lymphoblastic leukemia: results of Dana-Farber consortium protocol 91–01. Blood 2001;**97**:1211–1217.

105. Qureshi A, Mitchell C, Richards S, Vora A, Goulden N. Asparaginase-related venous thrombosis in UKALL 2003 – re-exposure to asparaginase is feasible and safe. Br J Haematol 2010;**149**:410–413.

106. Grace RF, Dahlberg SE, Neuberg D, Sallan SE, Connor JM, Neufeld EJ, Deangelo DJ, Silverman LD. The

frequency and management of asparaginase-related thrombosis in paediatric and adult patients with acute lymphoblastic leukemia treated on Dana-Farber Cancer Institute Consortium protocols. Br J Haematol 2011;**152**(4):452–459.

107. Crowther MA. Inferior vena cava filters in the management of venous thromboembolism. Am J Med 2007;**120**:S13–S17.

108. Raffini L, Cahill AM, Hellinger J, Manno C. A prospective observational study of IVC filters in pediatric patients. Pediatr Blood Cancer 2008;**51**(4):517–520.

109. Kukareja KU, Gollamudi J, Patel MN, Johnson ND, Racadio JM. Inferior vana caval filters in children: our experience and suggested guidelines. J Pediatr Hematol/Oncol 2011;**33**(3):334–338.

110. Schwarz RE, Marrero AM, Conlon KC, Burt M. Inferior vena caval filters in cancer patients: indications and outcome. J Clin Oncol 1996;**14**(2):652–657.

111. Abdelkefi A, Othman TB, Kammoun L, Chelli M, Romdhan NB, Kriaa A, Ladeb S, Torjman L, Lakhal A, Achour W, Hassen AB, Hsairi M, Ladeb F, Abdeladhim AB. Prevention of central venous line-related thrombosis by continuous infusion of low-dose unfractionated heparin in patients with hemato-oncological disease. Thromb Haemost 2004;**92**:654–661.

Epidemiology, etiology, and pathophysiology of infection-associated venous thromboembolism in children

Anjali A. Sharathkumar, Neil A. Goldenberg, and Anthony K.C. Chan

Introduction

Venous thromboembolic events (VTE) are increasingly being recognized in children. The clinical spectrum of VTE constitutes deep venous thrombosis (DVT) and pulmonary embolism (PE). Unlike in adults, VTE in children is usually secondary to complications of a primary illness like sepsis, cancer or treatment of primary illness including placement of central venous lines (CVLs) and surgical intervention for correction of underlying diseases [1]. The reported incidence of VTEs in children ranges from 5.4 [2] to 9.7 [3] per 10,000 hospital admissions. Although the presence of CVLs accounted for 95% of thromboembolic events in hospitalized children [4], it is becoming clear that underlying infection in itself predisposes for the development of thrombosis [1,2,4–13]. A key reason is the intricate relationship between the coagulation system and the immune system [14].

The coagulation system is one of the primitive components of the host defense against bacterial infection [15]. Local thrombosis can serve as a part of the first line of host defense against bacterial invasion in vertebrates and non-vertebrates. An interesting example of the interaction between the host coagulation system and pathogens is the horseshoe crab, which uses endotoxin to trigger a clotting response that presumably walls off the bacteria, providing an initial defense against invasion [16]. The clotting system of the horseshoe crab consists of three serine proteases and one clottable protein that are functionally similar to mammalian fibrinogen and share some sequence homology with primate fibrinopeptide B [16]. This coagulation response to bacterial infections also appears to be preserved in mammals, in which infections trigger tissue factor

(TF) expression on the surface of monocytes, which in turn initiates the coagulation cascade (Figure 7.1). To combat the host immune response, bacteria have developed virulence strategies to interact with host hemostatic factors such as plasminogen and fibrinogen in order to achieve widespread dissemination. Many investigators around the world are extensively studying the potential link between bacterial infections and thrombosis, and knowledge in this area is growing.

In order to survey published studies and reviews on the epidemiology of VTE in various infections in children, we performed a Medline search via Ovid, using keywords "infection and thrombosis," "infection and DVT," "infection and VTE," "bacteria and thrombosis," "fungal infection and thrombosis," "viral infection and thrombosis," and "children/newborns/neonates/adolescents." The search was limited from 1990 to March 2013. Search results were reviewed for inclusion of VTE-related reports in the summary tables of the manuscript.

Overview of coagulation

The primary function of the coagulation system is to achieve hemostasis and initiate wound healing. Hemostasis is a process that halts bleeding from a damaged vessel. Hemostasis is often divided into primary and secondary components. Primary hemostasis involves the activation, adhesion, and aggregation of platelets with the help of von Willebrand factor (vWF). Secondary hemostasis involves the coagulation system and consists of a cascade of linked reactions in which a serine protease, once activated, is capable of activating its downstream substrate, culminating in a fibrin clot.

Pediatric Thrombotic Disorders, ed. Neil A. Goldenberg and Marilyn J. Manco-Johnson. Published by Cambridge University Press. © Cambridge University Press 2015.

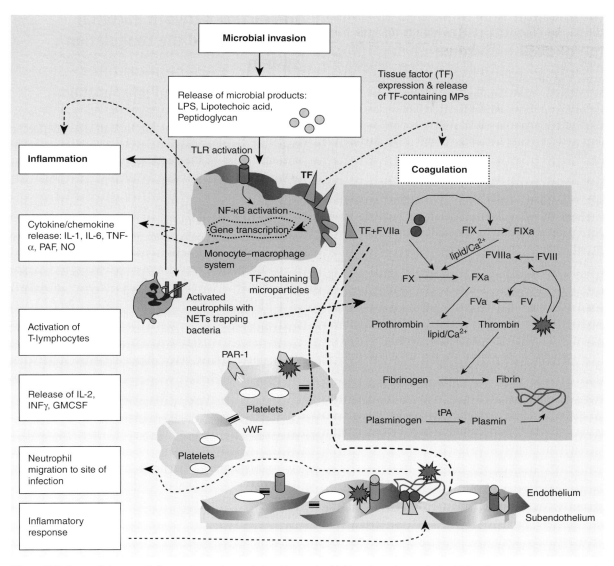

Figure 7.1 Cross-talk between inflammation and coagulation: Upon microbial invasion, release of microbial antigens activate monocytes/macrophages via toll-like receptors. Activated monocytes/macrophages release cytokines/chemokines and tissue factor containing microparticles. Tissue factor serves as an interface between inflammation and coagulation; it activates factor VII, which in turn activates the coagulation cascade leading to thrombin generation. Inflammatory cytokines cause neutrophil migration at the site of inflammation. These cytokines mount an inflammatory response, which in turn increases tissue factor expression and activation of coagulation. Thrombin generation causes platelet activation through PAR-1 receptors and further amplifies the coagulation cascade. Endothelium secretes von Willebrand factor and causes platelet adhesion and aggregation. The activated platelets and damaged endothelium provide a phospholipid surface for the deposition of coagulation cascade. Additionally activated neutrophils develop neutrophil extracellular traps, which help with trapping bacteria and causing neutrophil apoptosis.
Abbreviations IL: Interleukin; INFγ: Interferon gamma; PAF: Platelet activating factor; NO: Nitric oxide; NET: Neutrophil extracellular trap; vWF: von Willebrand factor; PAR-1:protease activated receptor-1. (A black and white version of this figure will appear in some formats. For the colour version of this figure, please refer to the plate section.)

Primary and secondary hemostasis are integrally linked in both time and space.

In general, secondary hemostasis is triggered if mechanisms of primary hemostasis fail to control bleeding. In the event of damage to vascular endothelium, TF normally sequestered in the subendothelial layer is exposed. TF binds and activates circulating factor VII (FVII). The TF and activated FVII (FVIIa) complex activates factor X (FX) from the common pathway and factor IX (FIX) from the intrinsic pathway. Activated FX (FXa) in combination with activated factor V (FVa), phospholipids, and calcium forms a prothrombinase complex, which then cleaves prothrombin to thrombin. Thrombin cleaves fibrinogen to form fibrin. Fibrin forms a blood clot, the end result of coagulation, which seals the injured endothelium and prevents bleeding. Factor XIII strengthens the fibrin clot. Factor IX activation also amplifies the clotting reaction through interaction with activated factor VIII (FVIIIa), which accelerates FX activation and thrombin generation. Thrombin generation amplifies the coagulation cascade at multiple levels. Uncontrolled thrombin generation can cause widespread systemic thrombosis leading to "disseminated intravascular coagulation (DIC)" and multiorgan failure [17]. To avoid this deleterious complication, the coagulation cascade is kept in check by anticoagulation systems. The major anticoagulants include antithrombin (AT), tissue factor pathway inhibitor (TFPI), and activated protein C (APC). Antithrombin is produced by the liver and inhibits several coagulation factors such as thrombin, FVIIa, FIXa, and FXa. TFPI is a serine protease that inhibits FVIIa. In the presence of FXa, TFPI also inhibits the TF–FVIIa complex. Protein C is an inactive plasma serine protease. When thrombin is produced, it binds to thrombomodulin present on the vascular endothelial surface. The thrombin/thrombomodulin complex can then cleave protein C into APC; APC generation is enhanced by the endothelial cell protein C receptor (EPCR) on the endothelial surface. In combination with cofactor protein S (PS), APC can cleave and inactivate FVa and FVIIIa to negatively regulate coagulation.

The fibrinolytic system functions to break down existing fibrin clots. The major protease of the fibrinolytic system is plasmin. Plasminogen is the inactive form of plasmin and circulates in the plasma. Plasminogen is activated by tissue-type plasminogen activator (tPA) and urokinase-type plasminogen activator (u-PA). This system can be inhibited by plasminogen activator inhibitor-1 (PAI-1), which inhibits both tPA and u-PA, or by α_2-antiplasmin, which inhibits plasmin. Together, coagulation, anticoagulation, and fibrinolysis maintain a hemostatic balance of the host. Developmental aspects of hemostasis relevant to pediatrics are discussed in Chapters 8 and 9.

Interaction between bacterial pathogens and the coagulation system

Bacterial invasion and inflammation

The infectious process starts with the first contact between the bacteria and the human host. Different bacterial species gain access to the human body through different sites, such as the skin, nasopharynx, lungs, gastrointestinal, or urogenital tract. Bacterial invasion is generally mediated by the bacterial surface and secreted products that can counteract the host's defense systems. Both the ability to produce invasive molecules and to counteract host defenses are critical to bacterial pathogenesis in systemic diseases.

Gram-positive and Gram-negative organisms are common pathogens in children. The most common Gram-positive organisms include staphylococcus and streptococcus, while the most common Gram-negative organisms include *E. coli*, pseudomonas and enterobacter. Gram-positive organisms release lipoproteins and superantigens, while Gram-negative organisms release lipopolysaccharide (LPS). Exposure to these bacterial ligands or pathogen-associated molecular patterns is recognized by toll-like receptors (TLRs) from the monocyte/macrophage system [18,19]. Intracellular receptors with ligand-sensing leucine-rich repeat regions linked to signaling components, known as nucleotide binding oligomerization domains, also play a role in bacterial ligand recognition [20]. The receptor/ligand interaction triggers a range of signaling pathways that result in transcription of an array of genes associated with both inflammation and immunity. These signaling pathways eventually converge to promote NF-kB-mediated gene transcription, which drives transcription of a range of important proinflammatory cytokine and chemokine genes, such as tumor necrosis factor alpha (TNF-α) and inteleukins (IL-1, IL-6, IL-8, and IL-12), which in turn produce an inflammatory response. These chemical mediators of inflammation produce autocrine loops that further amplify the inflammatory cascade.

Interplay between inflammation and coagulation

Bacterial invasion induces an inflammatory response. Inflammation-induced cellular and humoral modulation leads to activation of coagulation. Inflammation impacts the initiation, propagation, and the inhibitory phases of blood coagulation. Inflammatory mediators like bacterial ligands (lipoproteins and LPS) and TNF-α induce the expression of TF on monocytes and macrophages. The endothelium responds to these mediators with structural changes, such as cytoplasmic swelling and detachment, and also with functional changes, such as the expression of adhesion molecules like P-selectin. This results in increased platelet adhesion, leukocyte trafficking, and expression of TF from the subendothelium [21]. Inducible TF is stimulated by the presence of platelets and granulocytes in a P-selectin-dependent manner [21–23].

Under normal circumstances, negatively charged membrane surfaces limit amplification of coagulation loops so that, even if some activated coagulation factors are generated, propagation of coagulation is minimal. Complement activation, however, or exposure of subendothelial collagen in combination with thrombin, provides a potent stimulus eliciting the exposure of negatively charged phospholipid membrane surfaces. Natural anticoagulant mechanisms limit the thrombotic response, but these pathways are depressed by inflammatory mediators. The protein C pathway is one of the major targets. Thrombomodulin (TM) and the endothelial protein C receptors (EPCR) are both required for optimal protein C activation. Both these receptors are expressed on vascular endothelium and both are down-regulated by inflammatory mediators. Furthermore, free PS levels often decrease, due to the reduced levels of PS, resulting in impaired anticoagulant function of the APC that is generated. In plasma, 60% of the cofactor PS is complexed to a complement regulatory protein, C4b binding protein (C4bBP). Increased plasma levels of C4bBP as a consequence of the acute-phase reaction in inflammatory diseases may result in a relative deficiency of protein S. This together with protein C deficiency, contributes to a procoagulant state during sepsis.

Disease states that are associated with autoimmunity produce antiphospholipid antibodies. These antibodies may severely impair the protein C pathway. In addition, inflammation affects the fibrinolytic pathway by elevating levels of PAI-1, thereby decreasing fibrinolysis and hence clot lysis. The procoagulant impact of inflammation can also be seen at the cellular level. Inflammatory mediators like IL-6 increase both platelet count and their responsiveness to agonists such as thrombin [24]. All of these events tend to shift the hemostatic balance in favor of clot formation or thrombosis.

Activation of coagulation and subsequent fibrin deposition are essential components of the host defense against infectious agents in an attempt to limit the invasion of microorganisms and the occurrence of a subsequent inflammatory response [25,26]. An exaggerated response, however, can lead to a situation in which coagulation itself contributes to disease in its most severe form causing microvascular thrombosis and organ dysfunction, in DIC [17]. Microvascular thrombosis also causes syndromes known as hemolytic uremic syndrome (HUS) and thrombotic thrombocytopenic purpura (TTP). This is a particular form of thrombotic microangiopathy typically characterized by microangiopathic hemolytic anemia, thrombocytopenia, renal failure, and diffuse fibrin deposition in the renal glomeruli initiated by shiga toxin released during infection with *E. Coli* O157 or *Shigella dysenteriae*. TTP is a particular form of thrombotic microangiopathy typically characterized by microangiopathic hemolytic anemia, profound peripheral thrombocytopenia, and a severe deficiency of the von Willebrand factor-cleaving protease ADAMTS13 (A disintegrin and metalloproteinase with thrombospondin-1 motifs [13th member of the family]) [27–30]. Because HUS, while infection-associated, is not associated with thromboembolism, and because TTP is not commonly infection-associated, neither of these thrombotic microangiopathies is further discussed in this chapter.

Components of the coagulation system are able to modulate the inflammatory response [31]. Thrombin exerts proinflammatory activity by cleaving mainly protease activating receptor (PAR)-1 and -2 on platelets and the monocyte/macrophage system, while APC cleaves PAR-1 in an EPCR-dependent manner and thereby modulates inflammation and apoptosis [32]. It is also becoming evident that leukocytes, specifically monocytes and neutrophils, play a crucial role in creating a prothrombotic milieu during inflammation. Monocytes and macrophages release phophatidyl serine and TF-containing microparticles (MPs), while neutrophils produce "neutrophil extracellular traps (NETs)" [33,34]. Both TF-containing MPs and NETs disseminate procoagulant potential. Like phagocytosis, formation of NETs is important for neutophil bacteriocidal activity [35–38]. These NETs are complex structures composed of smooth "threads," which are formed by nucleosomes from unfolded chromatin, histones and neutrophil granules. Upon activation (by IL-8, LPS, bacteria, fungi, activated platelets, or toll-like receptors [TLRs]), neutrophils start a program that leads to their death and the formation of NETs [35,37,38]. In vivo studies in mice showed that monocytes and platelets cooperate to form NETs and create a procaogulant milieu [39]. Laboratory studies have shown that Gram-positive bacteria (*Staphylococcus aureus*, Group A streptococcus) and Gram-negative bacteria (*Shigella fexneri* and *Salmonella typhimurium*) as well as fungi (*Candida albicans*) bind to NETs [35,37]. In in vitro studies, NETs were shown to be prothrombotic and procoagulant [40,41]. Extracellular histones also promote thrombin generation through platelet-dependent mechanisms via involvement of platelet TLR2 and TLR4 [42,43].

In summary, TF expression, impairment of the PC pathway, down-regulation of fibrinolysis, leukocyte activation, MPs formation of procoagulant microparticles and NETs, release of cytokines and involvement of PARs and TLRs, all play vital roles in the cross-talk between inflammation and coagulation during bacterial invasion. These processes are summarized and depicted in Table 7.1 and Figures 7.1 and 7.2.

The evolutionary link between inflammation and coagulation

The extensive cross-talk between the coagulation and inflammation/immune response suggests an evolutionary link between coagulation and inflammation. The structural homology among various coagulation proteins and inflammatory proteins further substantiates this notion. Important examples of this homology include the following observations: (1) TF, the initiator of coagulation, has structural homology to the cytokine receptors [44]; (2) the lectin domain of TM has homology to the selectins involved in leukocytes adhesion [45]; and (3) EPCR shares approximately 20% sequence identity with the major histocompatibility complex class 1/CD1 family of molecules [46]. In addition, complement molecules, which are crucial for mounting an initial immune response against bacteria, are directly linked to the coagulation system through binding with anticoagulant protein PS, suggesting a coevolutionary the process [47].

Infection in the context of Virchow's triad

Virchow's triad is an important concept which helps to understand the etiology and pathogenesis of VTE [48]. The important elements of this triad include: (1)

altered blood flow characteristics (stasis); (2) hypercoagulability, and (3) endothelial damage. Infection likely mediates each component of the triad. As mentioned previously, the inflammatory organisms blunt the anticoagulant response, thus mediating hypercoagulability. In addition, pathogen invasion mounts local tissue inflammation leading to the disturbance of normal functioning of the organ. This can temporarily alter the blood flow characteristics contributing to thrombosis. For example, in patients with osteomyelitis of the hip, immobility of the limb could contribute to venous stasis leading to thrombosis. Pathogen invasion can cause direct damage to the endothelium, initiating local hemostasis. Also, inflammation in contiguous tissues could cause direct damage to the vascular endothelium, contributing to thrombus formation. For example in Lemierre's syndrome [6] or osteomyelitis [6], pathogen induced inflammatory response in the oropharynx and joint, respectively, are thought to cause inflammation in the contiguous venous segment and initiate thrombosis. Figures 7.1 and 7.2 illustrate the relationship between infection and Virchow's triad.

Sepsis treatment by restoration of physiologic anticoagulant pathways

Based on the pathophysiology of sepsis, there is conceptual justification for the repletion of physiologic anticoagulants in patients with severe sepsis and coagulopathy [49,50]. Numerous preclinical studies in different models of sepsis and DIC conducted in multiple animal species have demonstrated the efficacy of PC concentrates, AT concentrates, recombinant TFPI, and soluble TMs in the treatment of experimental sepsis.

PC concentrates and AT concentrates have been used in adults and in a few pediatric trials of DIC in general or meningococcemia-associated DIC in particular [51–58]. In 2001, Protein C Worldwide Evaluation in Severe Sepsis (PROWESS), the first double-blind, placebo-controlled trial with recombinant human APC (rhAPC, Drotecogin-α activated, Xigris, Eli Lilly), showed a significant reduction (6.4%) in overall mortality in adult sepsis, with a relative risk reduction of approximately 20%, specifically in poor-risk patients [59]. Despite the favorable results of the PROWESS study, other studies in different populations failed to show a favorable risk/benefit profile [60]. Furthermore, the recent randomized multinational PROWESS-shock trial

Table 7.1 Summary of cross-talk between hemostasis, bacterial invasion (infection), and inflammation

Constituents	Primary function in hemostasis	Alterations with bacterial invasion and inflammation
Primary hemostasis		
Platelet	• Form of platelet plug with the help of vWF to stop bleeding • Provide phospholipid surface for coagulation cascade • Provide coagulation proteins (TF, FV, vWF, FVIII, PF4, PDGF) • Release tissue factor-containing microparticles	• Express TLR-like receptors, which interact with bacterial superantigens • Thrombin-activated platelets express CD40L, which induces expression of proinflammatory cytokines (IL-1, IL-6, and IL-8) and adhesion molecules (ICAM-1, VCAM-1, and E-selectin) • P-selectin and E-selecting receptors on platelets interact with neutrophils and enhance netrophil recruitment at the site of injury
Secondary hemostasis		
Procoagulant proteins (factors I through XIII) and Proteins of contact system	Generate thrombin and form fibrin clot at the site of vessel injury	• Contact system (Kallikrein/HMWM, FXII) releases bradykinin and causes local inflammation • Bacterial products (M proteins) bind with fibrinogen and interfere with phagocytosis while fibrin clot creates a physical barrier to microbial invasion and helps facilitate phagocytosis • Inflammatory cytokines enhance TF expression on endothelium and monocytes and amplify coagulation • Thrombin has proinflammatory effects on endothelial cells, smooth muscle cells, and platelets
Anticoagulant proteins		
Protein C system (thrombomodulin, protein C & protein S)	Degrade FVa and FVIIa & down-regulate coagulation cascade	• APC binds to monocyte/macrophage blocks NF-kB nuclear translocation down-regulates proinflammatory cytokine and adhesive molecules production
Antithrombin	Inhibit thrombin generation	• AT binding to endothelial cells produces prostacycline release which: (1) inhibits platelets (2) blocks neutrophil tethering to blood vessels (3) decreases endothelial cell production of various cytokines/chemokines
Tissue factor pathway inhibitor (TFPI)	Inhibit TF-induced coagulation	• Blocks inflammation-induced thrombin generation

Table 7.1 (cont.)

Constituents	Primary function in hemostasis	Alterations with bacterial invasion and inflammation
Fibrinolytic pathway (Plasminogen, tPA, u-PA, PAI-1, alpha-2 antiplasmin)	Prevent thrombus propagation through direct lysis of fibrin clot	• Bacteria produce plasminogen activators, plasminogen receptors, and plasmin generation to enhance bacterial invasion
Leukocytes		
Monocyte–macrophage system	Enhance platelet adhesion & leukocyte rolling Release tissue factor containing microparticles and create procoagulant milieu	• Releases inflammatory mediators (IL-1, IL-6, TNF-∞) and contributes to inflammatory response • Kills bacteria by phagocytosis
Neutrophils	Form neutrophil extracellular traps (NETs) and create procoagulant milieu	• Release inflammatory mediators & contribute to inflammatory response • Kill bacteria by phagocytosis • Prevent invasion of bacteria by creating mechanical barrier with NETs

Abbreviations: vWF: von Willebrand's factor; TF: Tissue factor; F: Factor; PF4: Platelet factor 4; PDGF: Platelet-derived growth factor; CD40L: CD40 ligand; HMWK: High molecular weight kininogen; ICAM: Intercellular adhesion molecule; VCAM: Vascular cell adhesion protein; NF-kB: Nuclear factor kappa B; TFPI: Tissue factor pathway inhibitor; tPA: tissue-type plasminogen activator; u-PA: uroplasminogen activator; PAI-1: Plasminogen activator inhibitor-1; IL: Interleukin; TNF: Tumor necrosis factor; NETs: Neutrophil extracellular traps; TLR: Toll-like receptor; APC: activated PC (protein C); AT: antithrombin.

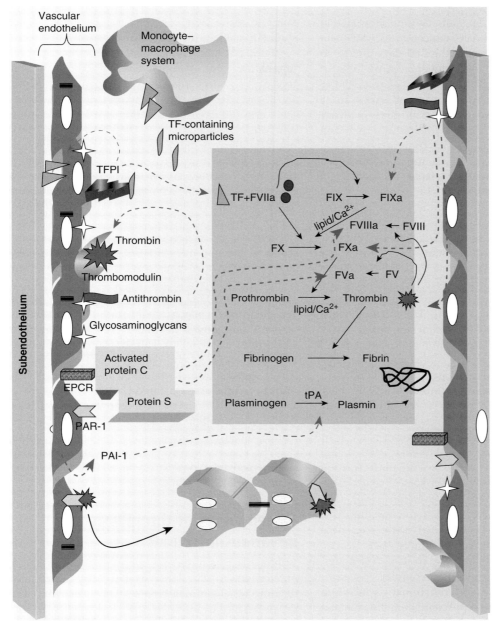

Figure 7.2 Schematic representation of the role of endothelium in hemostasis. Vascular endothelium serves anticoagulant and procoagulant functions. On the anticoagulant side, it expresses TFPI (**T**issue **F**actor **P**athway **I**nhibitor), thrombomodulin, EPCR (**E**ndothelial **P**rotein **C** **R**eceptors), glycosaminoglycans and PAI-1(plasminogen activator inhibitor-1). On the procoagulant side endothelial cells synthesize vWF (von Willebrand factor), TF (tissue factor), thrombin receptor or **P**roease **A**ctivated **R**eceptor-1 (PAR1). Red lines represent anticoagulant/inhibition loops while black lines represent procoagulant/activation loops. (A black and white version of this figure will appear in some formats. For the colour version of this figure, please refer to the plate section.)

found no significant reduction in mortality in patients treated with rhAPC compared to placebo, and subsequent to these study findings rhAPC was removed from the market by November 2011 [61]. A large-scale randomized clinical trial in children with sepsis, Researching severe Sepsis and Organ Dysfunction in Children: a global perspective (RESOLVE), recruited 477 children with sepsis (ages, 28 days to 17 years), and showed no benefit of rhAPC concentrates. The subanalyses showed that the safety profile of rhAPC concentrates was unacceptable in infants younger than 60 days due to an increased incidence of intracranial bleeding [57]. An observational study by Decembrino et al. recruited 18 neonates (12 preterm and 6 full term, ages 1 to 28 days) with sepsis and suggested preliminary evidence of safety of rhAPC in this population [62]. A recent meta-analysis reviewed all the trials of rhAPC in adults and children with sepsis and concluded that there was no evidence suggesting the benefit of rhAPC for treating patients with severe sepsis or septic shock and rhAPC should not be used for the treatment of sepsis outside of clinical trials [63]. In a somewhat analagous setting, high-purity, plasma-derived, vapor-treated human PC concentrate (Ceprotin®, Baxter AG, Vienna, Austria) has shown efficacy in newborns with severe PC deficiency and life-threatening purpura fulminans and/or thrombosis associated with DIC [62,64]. This concentrate is approved for congenital PC deficiency, but its use in acquired deficiency states is not approved. Several case series and retrospective cohort studies describing beneficial effects of zymogen protein C concentrate in infectious purpura fulminans and DIC have been published [65]. A phase II dose-finding study randomized 40 children with severe meningococcal sepsis and pupura fulminans to receive placebo or human PC concentrate (200 IU/kg/day, 400 IU/kg/day or 600 IU/kg/day) and assessed the activation process of PC by measuring markers of coagulation activation and inflammatory cytokines [66]. The results of this study showed that the baseline APC levels were positively correlated with sequential organ failure assessment, mortality risk scores, and makers of coagulation activation (D-dimer, PAI-1, thrombin-antithrombin complex, plasmin-antiplasmin complex) and inflammation (TNF-α, IL-1, IL-6, IL-8). These reports indicate thus far that PC concentrate has an acceptable safety profile including no reports of drug interactions, blood-borne infections, bleeding or prothrombotic complications. The PC concentrates have received regulatory agency approvals for use in meningococcal septicemia. Although the data on efficacy and safety of PC concentrates in DIC and other coagulopathies are not robust, it may be reasonable to consider off-label use of human PC concentrates in these settings as well.

Clinical trials of AT concentrates in adults have failed to show clear benefit in sepsis. Early clinical studies in adults with DIC showed benefit of AT concentrates, but these studies were non-randomized and non-blinded [68]. A double-blind, placebo-controlled trial of AT concentrates in adult patients with septic shock and DIC showed reduced mortality in the treatment arm (28-day ICU mortality 28% in intervention arm versus 50% mortality in non-intervention arm), but this difference did not reach statistical significance [60]. A similar study by Eisele et al. showed relative reduction in mortality by 39% with AT concentrates (30 day all-cause mortality 25% in intervention arm versus 41% in non-intervention arm) without statistical significance. The same study also showed that patients in the intervention group developed less organ failure compared to the non-intervention group [68]. An early study by Hanada et al. used AT concentrates with or without heparin infusion in six children (1 month to 5 years old) with DIC and showed benefit [69]. Kreuz et al. performed a pilot feasibility study of treating sepsis with AT concentrates in children beyond infancy and recruited 29 children [70]. This study provided preliminary data on safety and efficacy of AT concentrates, which warrant further evaluation in large-scale trials prior to routine usage in clinical care.

Similar to PC and AT concentrates, recombinant TFPI and recombinant soluble TM concentrates are being evaluated in clinical studies in adult populations [71–75]. These early reports are inconclusive regarding efficacy and additional study in adults is warranted prior to performing clinical trials in pediatrics.

Epidemiology of thrombosis in various infections

Although across numerous cohort study and registry publications to date infection has been consistently identified as a common risk factor for pediatric VTE, the prevalence of infection at VTE diagnosis in children has varied considerably (Table 7.2). Systemic infections cause widespread activation of coagulation leading to thromboembolic complications involving multiple organs, while local infections primarily cause thrombophlebitis of adjacent or contiguous veins. Depending on the extent of organ involvement the clinical spectrum ranges from local DVT to multi-organ failure. The subsequent section will discuss the available literature on systemic and locoregional infections and VTE.

Table 7.2 Prevalence of infection as a risk factor for VTE in children at time of VTE diagnosis, across published cohort studies and registries

First author	Publication year	Total number of patients (n)	Prevalence of infection at VTE diagnosis (%)	Reference #
Andrew M	1994	137	7%	1
Massicotte P*	1998	244	20%	4
van Ommen CH	2003	100	45%	12
Goldenberg NA	2004	82	13%	7
Oren H	2005	271	29%	8
Newall F	2006	95	NR	11
Sirachainan N**	2007	24	21%	9
Sandoval JA	2008	358	15%	3

* Study population consisted of children with central venous catheter-associated VTE.
** Study design was retrospective. NR = not reported.

Systemic infections and thromboembolic complications

I. DIC and purpura fulminans

Disseminated intravascular coagulation (DIC) is a severe complication of cancer, sepsis, and certain other toxin-associated conditions in which diffuse endothelial injury (mediated by endotoxin, cytokines, and other less well-characterized endothelially active factors) incite coagulopathy on multiple levels. The final common pathway is consumption of procoagulant factors, intrinsic anticoagulants, fibrinogen, and platelets. This frequently manifests with spontaneous hemorrhage, but may also be complicated by thrombosis. Indeed, microvascular thrombosis (through a pathophysiological process that is likely similar to that which occurs in purpura fulminans associated with PC and PS deficiencies) causes end-organ dysfunction (Figure 7.3a and b). In severe cases, this results in coagulopathy and/or cytokine storm and multisystem organ failure, which portends a high risk of death.

Besides meningococcal infection, Gram-positive bacteria (methicillin resistant *Staphylococcus aureus* [MRSA], methicillin sensitive *Staphylococcus aureus* [MSSA], and *Streptococcus*), Gram-negative bacteria (*E. coli*, pseudomonas, klebsiella, enterobacter and anaerobes are known to cause DIC and septic shock syndrome [8,76,77]. The mortality in children with DIC is associated with its severity and age of the patients [78,79]. Patients with DIC scores ≥ 5 (overt DIC) had a 50% mortality rate, compared to 20% for patients with DIC scores < 5, in one report [79]. In patients with meningococcemia, the mortality rate was higher in children younger, versus older, than 3.1 years (40% versus 13% respectively) [78].

The primary therapy for DIC with sepsis is antimicrobial treatment of the infection and intensive supportive care. The role of PC concentrates and AT concentrates for the treatment of DIC is discussed above.

II. Acquired antiphospholipid antibody syndrome (APS)

Antiphospholipid antibody (APA)-mediated coagulopathy is not necessarily associated with thrombosis. Evidence and experience in pediatric VTE indicate that APA are highly prevalent at VTE diagnosis. In one cohort study, 43% of children were acutely positive for the lupus anticoagulant, as measured by dilute Russell viper venom time [7]. Relatively little prospective data is available regarding the proportion of children with VTE who have persistent APA at 12 weeks or more following initial testing, and hence meet current consensus criteria for APS. Furthermore, the proportion of pediatric APS cases that may be acquired secondary to infection – i.e., that have developed in association with acute infection and appear unrelated to an underlying rheumatologic condition – remains poorly understood.

III. *Burkholderia cepacia* infection and cystic fibrosis

Raffini *et al.* studied the rate of VTE in children with cystic fibrosis (CF) and observed that bacterial colonization with *Burkholderia cepacia* (*B. cepacia*) predisposes to development of VTE [80]. Their center's CF registry contained 284 patients. During a 2.3-year

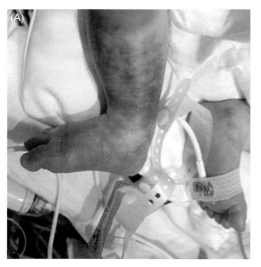
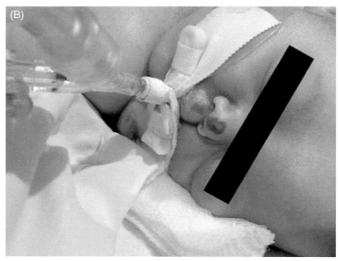

Figure 7.3 An infant with fulminant sepsis showing acquired pupura fulminans over the legs (A) and tip of the nose (B).

period (January 2003 through April 2005), there were 401 hospital admissions in 162 patients for pulmonary exacerbation; 72 of these admissions were in 18 patients colonized with *B. cepacia*. Over 95% of patients had CVLs (PICC or Mediport) during their course of therapy. Less than 4% of 162 patients with CF exacerbation had symptomatic VTE, whereas this rate was 27% among18 CF patients colonized with *B. cepacia*. Notably, most VTEs were CVC-associated, rather than pulmonary.

Locoregional infections and VTE

I. Head and neck infections and VTE

Otitis media, sinusitis, mastoiditis, orbital cellulitis, and pharyngitis are commonly encountered infections in the head and neck area that are associated with DVT in intracranial and extracranial veins. Thrombophlebitis of the internal jugular vein, commonly known as Lemierre's syndrome, is an example of extracranial DVT while cerebral sinus venous thrombosis (CSVT) is an example of intracranial DVT that can occur in relation to head and neck infections.

(a) Lemierre's syndrome (thrombophlebitis of the internal jugular vein) [7]

Jugular thrombophlebitis in Lemierre's syndrome is related to pharyngeal infection and infection within tonsilar fossa. Presentation includes high-grade fever, throat pain, neck pain, and malaise, ultimately progressing to respiratory insufficiency and hypotension related to sepsis. Prothrombotic mechanisms in Lemierre's syndrome are incompletely understood, but are likely to represent both direct angioinvasiveness of the *Fusobacterium necrophorum* (classical Lemierre's) or other (non-classical) organisms, as well as periinfectious/proinflammatory coagulation activation. In addition, in vitro studies have suggested that *Fusobacterium necrophorum* can mediate platelet aggregation in vitro [81]. Observations of the influence of *Fusobacterium necrophorum* on clot-based assays in animal models have been conflicting, however.

Several pediatric case series of Lemierre's syndrome have been published in recent decades [7,82, 83]. In addition to classical Lemierre's syndrome, cases of a so-called otogenic variant have been described, involving *Fusobacterium* otitis media complicated by mastoiditis and cavernous sinus thrombosis, with or without associated meningitis [84]. Thrombophilic abnormalities were characterized in one report [7]. Thrombophilia was disclosed in all investigated cases, most of which was acquired and transient. Specifically, APA and elevated FVIII activity levels were commonly present at presentation but rarely persisted upon re-evaluation 2 to 6 months post-diagnosis.

In rare cases, isolated jugular vein thrombosis (without cerebral sinovenous involvement) has been described in the setting of mastoiditis, in the absence of Lemierre's syndrome [85,86]. Presumably, in such cases, the pathophysiology involves direct extension of infection/inflammation from the mastoid to the jugular bulb.

(b) Cerebral sinus venous thrombosis (CSVT)

Cerebral sinus venous thrombosis is a rare but serious disorder in children. The common clinical presentation in children with CSVT includes seizures, diffuse neurological symptoms, and focal neurological symptoms [13]. The report from the Canadian Ischemic Stroke Registry provided the most comprehensive experience on CSVT in children. This study included 160 children (from 36 weeks of gestation through 18 years of age) from 12 tertiary care pediatric centers in Canada over a period of 6 years (January 1992 through December 1997) [13]. Among these 160 children, 18% (28/160) of events occurred due to head and neck infections. The majority of these subjects were non-neonates (21/28). In addition to head and neck infections, 9% (15/160) of children had documented bacterial sepsis. This observation further underscores the association between bacterial invasion and CSVT.

Cerebral sinovenous thrombosis is an underemphasized complication of mastoiditis [87]. In a recent analysis from a tertiary referral center, the Children's Hospital of Philadelphia, 87 cases of mastoiditis were treated by the otolaryngology service in a 7-year period, with sigmoid sinus thrombosis identified as a complication in 16% [86]. The pathophysiology of otogenic CSVT is thought to involve direct extension of infection/inflammation from the mastoid to the sigmoid sinus; thrombosis can often extend to involve multiple segments of the cerebral sinovenous circulation.

Infection has been identified as a predisposing condition in 17–88% of neonates and older children at diagnosis of CSVT [13,88–93]. The prevalence of mastoiditis in particular at time of CSVT diagnosis in children has ranged from 30% [93,94]. In a recent single-institutional retrospective analysis in the United Kingdom in which cases of CSVT were identified by ICD-9 code, otitis media (OM) was the most common risk factor, occurring in 62% [95]. A recent retrospective analysis from five pediatric centers in the USA found infection as a risk factor in 40% of 70 children with CSVT, with OM comprising 15% overall [96].

A particularly important complication of mastoiditis is Gradenigo's syndrome, characterized by diplopia and lateral rectus muscle weakness from cranial nerve VI palsy, as well as facial pain in a trigeminal nerve distribution. Approximately 50 cases have been reported in the literature, mostly pediatric [98]. Gradenigo's syndrome is pathophysiologically related to extension of infection from the mastoid to the petrous apex of the temporal bone, adjacent to which lay the trigeminal ganglion and cranial nerve VI. When Gradenigo's syndrome is complicated by CSVT, it has been argued that, in addition to adequate anticoagulation and antimicrobial therapy, acute otolaryngological intervention (mastoidectomy with surgical decompression of the temporal bone) optimizes the potential for recanalization of the cerebral sinovenous system.

Other causes of CSVT include meningitis and head and neck cellulitis. In a recent retrospective analysis from five pediatric centers in the USA, meningitis was recognized as a predisposing condition in 3% of 70 children with CSVT [96]. A retrospective review of 147 cases of head and neck cellulitis seen over a 15-year period at an Hawaiian community hospital reported CSVT in one patient (a case of cavernous sinus thrombosis) [98].

II. Abdominal infections and intra-abdominal thrombosis

Portal vein thrombosis, splenic vein thrombosis, hepatic vein thrombosis (Budd–Chiari syndrome), mesenteric vein thrombosis, renal vein thrombosis, and inferior vein thrombosis are intra-abdominal thrombotic events observed in children. Presentations vary by site, but commonly include organ dysfunction and organomegaly. There is a paucity of literature addressing associations between infection and various types of abdominal thrombosis. A report by Muorah et al. studied 15 children (median age: 10 years) with pyogenic liver abscess and four of them (37.5%) developed portal vein thrombosis [99]. Thromboses of the visceral vasculature are discussed in detail in other chapters.

III. Pelvic infections

Pelvic infections with anaerobic organisms like *Bacteroides fragilis* are associated with thrombophlebitis of uterine veins, ovarian veins, and iliofemoral veins. This complication is commonly described in adult females during the puerperium and post-partum period [100–102]. The most common clinical presentation includes high-grade fevers, vaginal discharge, and swelling of lower extremities. Although there are no reports in the pediatric population, the authors have treated adolescents with locoregional VTE as a complication of pelvic infections involving anaerobic organisms like *Bacteroides fragilis*.

IV. Musculoskeletal infections (MSI)

In patients with musculoskeletal infections, especially osteomyelitis of the long bones, bedrest, along with the presence of infection, create a prothrombotic milieu for the development of deep venous thrombosis (DVT). A recent literature review by Mantadakis *et al.* showed that the incidence of DVT as a complication of MSI is underappreciated because the symptoms of DVT overlap with deep-seated MSI [103]. This report included 28 retrospective studies and identified 93 children with MSIs who developed DVT. The majority were boys. Data regarding the type and location of MSIs were available for 74 (80%) of the 93 evaluated patients. Osteomyelitis was the most frequently observed type of MSI (69/74, 93%) followed by pyomyositis (n = 4), or septic arthritis (n = 1). *Staphylococcus aureus* was the predominant pathogen (83/93, 89%); 61% of these isolates were MRSA. Pulmonary involvement, presumably due to septic emboli, was observed in 65% of the included children. Four children died due to multiple organ failure and two due to respiratory distress. A recent single-center retrospective review from Children's Medical Center in Dallas identified 11 cases of deep venous thrombosis among 212 children with osteomyelitis [5] Principal organisms identified were MRSA (consistent with other reports) [104–106].

Thromboembolism in viral and fungal infections

Unlike bacterial pathogens, the role of non-bacterial pathogens such as viruses and fungi in thrombogenesis has not been systematically studied. There are reports of thromboembolic events complicating viral and fungal infections and attempts have been made to evaluate the role of these infections on coagulation activation. Considering the close relationship between inflammation and thrombosis, it is intuitive that these infections can trigger thrombosis. It is important to underscore that serious infections with non-bacterial pathogens like viruses and fungi commonly occur in immunocompromised children such as children with congenital or acquired immunodeficiency disorders including chronic granulomatous disease (CGD) and immunosuppression for stem cell or solid organ transplantation. It is likely that the development of thromboembolism in the context of fungal and viral infections in such children has a multifactorial etiology.

Viral infections and venous thromboembolism

A number of viruses have been investigated for prothrombotic effects and/or described in case reports/ series of VTE. Studies in mouse models of viral myocarditis (infected with coxackie B3 virus) showed that viral myocarditis creates a hypercoagulable state through increased expression of myocardial TF expression and activity [106]. This infection-associated hypercoagulability can be superimposed upon a clinical TE risk factor of venous stasis (low-flow state) in the setting of myocarditis-induced heart failure.

In other work, human cytomegalovirus-infected endothelial cells were found to enhance platelet adhesion and aggregation after 7 days of infection and create a procoagulant milieu [107]. Antiphospholipid antibodies have been documented in patients with hepatitis B and human immunodeficiency virus infection [108,109]. Elevated levels of TNF are reported in patients with dengue hemorrhagic fever. A case of sigmoid sinus thrombosis has been reported in a 5-year-old boy with cytomegalovirus-associated otitis media [110]. Systemic varicella has been described to induce acquired purpura fulminans due to transient autoimmune protein S deficiency [111,112]. Beyond purpura fulminans, systemic varicella has been associated with deficiencies of both PC and PS and a high frequency of the lupus anticoagulant [111–113]. Another virus, dengue, is known to cause consumptive coagulopathy, and mortality in children aged 6–12 years has been associated with development of DIC [114–115].

Fungal infections and venous thromboembolism

There is a paucity of literature on fungal infection and thromboembolism. Thrombosis occurs in association with fungal infection of blood vessels, and this is almost exclusively limited to immune-compromised hosts such as children receiving chemotherapy or following organ transplantation [116, 117]. Cavernous sinus thrombosis has been reported in two children undergoing therapy for acute lymphoblastic leukemia who suffered from rhinocerebral zygomycosis [118]. Poorly controlled diabetes mellitus is a risk factor for cerebral *mucorales* and associated CSVT [119]. Pathogenesis with regard to hypercoagulability and inflammation is generally poorly understood. However, in chronic necrotizing pulmonary aspergillosis, a single study has reported elevated systemic biomarkers of inflammation (IL-6, IL-8, RANTES, TNF-α, and ICAM-1) and proinflammatory markers of endothelial activation, coagulation activation, and fibrinolytic inhibition (vWF, TF and PAI-1)[120].

Infection and recurrence of VTE

The overall estimates for recurrence for VTE in children range from 80 to 21% in published studies with heterogeneous follow-up periods [1,12]. The VTE recurrence risk remains largely unknown for infection-associated VTE with respect to local versus systemic infection, as well as for specific infectious etiologies. Crary *et al.* [5] observed that children with osteomyelitis-associated DVT did not experience recurrence. On the contrary, Raffini *et al.* [80] observed that children with cystic fibrosis, especially those who have respiratory colonization with *B. cepacia*, are at increased risk for VTE recurrence compared to children with CF without *B. cepacia* colonization. This may suggest that the risk of recurrent DVT is low in children with transient bacterial infection, while this risk is higher in children with chronic diseases who have colonization of bacterial pathogens.

Conclusions and future directions

During the last two decades, significant advances have been made in understanding the cross-talk between infection, inflammation, and coagulation. Under normal physiological circumstances, coagulation activation is kept in check by anticoagulant proteins and fibrinolysis. During localized or systemic infections, bacterial proteins induce a prothrombotic state by interfering with natural anticoagulant and fibrinolytic mechanisms and triggering excessive tissue factor-mediated thrombin generation. Various local and systemic infections in children have been associated with VTE. Efforts are underway to translate this knowledge to clinical practice for prevention and treatment of VTE. Inflammatory and procoagulant biomarkers (e.g., platelet count, C-reactive protein, levels of interleukins and P-selectins, coagulation proteins, intensity of thrombin generation, simultaneous thrombin and plasmin generation, measurement of tissue-factor-containing microparticles) are being evaluated for early detection of a prothrombotic state and prediction of clinical TE events. Given the role of anticoagulant pathways in infection-associated TE, concentrates of APC, PC, and AT are available for use in children under specific circumstances (albeit often off-label). There remains an urgent need for additional study of whether anticoagulant interventions may safely improve outcomes in pediatric sepsis. Meanwhile, novel anticoagulant drugs are being evaluated in clinical trials in pediatric VTE, and will include settings of infection-associated thromboembolism.

References

1. Andrew M, David M, Adams M, Ali K, Anderson R, Barnard D, et al. Venous thromboembolic complications (VTE) in children: first analyses of the Canadian Registry of VTE. Blood. 1994;**83**(5):1251–7.

2. Monagle P, Adams M, Mahoney M, Ali K, Barnard D, Bernstein M, et al. Outcome of pediatric thromboembolic disease: a report from the Canadian Childhood Thrombophilia Registry. Pediatr Res. 2000;**47**(6):763–6.

3. Sandoval JA, Sheehan MP, Stonerock CE, Shafique S, Rescorla FJ, Dalsing MC, et al. Incidence, risk factors, and treatment patterns for deep venous thrombosis in hospitalized children: an increasing population at risk. J Vasc Surg. 2008;**47**(4):837–43.

4. Massicotte MP, Dix D, Monagle P, Adams M, Andrew M. Central venous catheter related thrombosis in children: analysis of the Canadian Registry of Venous Thromboembolic Complications. J Pediatr. 1998;**133**(6):770–6.

5. Crary SE, Buchanan GR, Drake CE, Journeycake JM. Venous thrombosis and thromboembolism in children with osteomyelitis. J Pediatr. 2006;**149**(4):537–41.

6. Goldenberg NA, Knapp-Clevenger R, Hays T, Manco-Johnson MJ. Lemierre's and Lemierre's-like syndromes in children: survival and thromboembolic outcomes. Pediatrics. 2005;**116**(4):e543–8.

7. Goldenberg NA, Knapp-Clevenger R, Manco-Johnson MJ, Mountain States Regional Thrombophilia G. Elevated plasma factor VIII and D-dimer levels as predictors of poor outcomes of thrombosis in children. [Erratum appears in N Engl J Med. 2005;352(20):2146]. New Engl J Med. 2004;**351**(11):1081–8.

8. Oren H, Cingoz I, Duman M, Yilmaz S, Irken G. Disseminated intravascular coagulation in pediatric patients: clinical and laboratory features and prognostic factors influencing the survival. Pediatr Hematol Oncol. 2005;**22**(8):679–88.

9. Sirachainan N, Chuansumrit A, Angchaisuksiri P, Pakakasama S, Hongeng S, Kadegasem P. Venous thromboembolism in Thai children. Pediatr Hematol Oncol. 2007;**24**(4):245–56.

10. Gunes AM, Baytan B, Gunay U. The influence of risk factors in promoting thrombosis during childhood: the role of acquired factors. Pediatr Hematol Oncol. 2006;**23**(5):399–410.

11. Newall F, Wallace T, Crock C, Campbell J, Savoia H, Barnes C, et al. Venous thromboembolic disease: a single-centre case series study. J Paediatr Child Health. 2006;**42**(12):803–7.

12. van Ommen CH, Heijboer H, van den Dool EJ, Hutten BA, Peters M. Pediatric venous thromboembolic disease in one single center: congenital prothrombotic

disorders and the clinical outcome. J Thromb Haemost. 2003;**1**(12):2516–22.

13. deVeber G, Andrew M, Adams C, Bjornson B, Booth F, Buckley DJ, et al. Cerebral sinovenous thrombosis in children. New Engl J Medicine. 2001;**345**(6):417–23.

14. Esmon CT, Xu J, Lupu F. Innate immunity and coagulation. J Thromb Haemost. 2011;**9** Suppl 1:182–8.

15. Iwanaga S, Lee BL, Iwanaga S, Lee BL. Recent advances in the innate immunity of invertebrate animals. J Biochem Molec Biol. 2005;**38**(2):128–50.

16. Iwanaga S, Miyata T, Tokunaga F, Muta T. Molecular mechanism of hemolymph clotting system in Limulus. Thromb Res. 1992;**68**(1):1–32.

17. Levi M, Ten Cate H. Disseminated intravascular coagulation [see comment]. New Engl J Med. 1999;**341**(8):586–92.

18. Takeuchi O, Sato S, Horiuchi T, Hoshino K, Takeda K, Dong Z, et al. Cutting edge: role of toll-like receptor 1 in mediating immune response to microbial lipoproteins. J Immunol. 2002;**169**(1):10–14.

19. Hopkins PA, Sriskandan S. Mammalian toll-like receptors: to immunity and beyond. Clin Exp Immunol. 2005;**140**(3):395–407.

20. Inohara, Chamaillard, McDonald C, Nunez G, McDonald C, Nunez G. NOD-LRR proteins: role in host-microbial interactions and inflammatory disease. Ann Rev Biochem. 2005;**74**:355–83.

21. McGregor L, Martin J, McGregor JL. Platelet-leukocyte aggregates and derived microparticles in inflammation, vascular remodelling and thrombosis. Front Biosci. 2006;**11**:830–7.

22. Osterud B. Tissue factor: a complex biological role. Thromb Haemost. 1997;**78**(1):755–8.

23. Osterud B. Tissue factor expression by monocytes: regulation and pathophysiological roles. Blood Coag Fibrinol. 1998;**9** Suppl 1:S9–14.

24. van der Poll T, Levi M, Hack CE, Ten Cate H, van Deventer SJ, Eerenberg AJ, et al. Elimination of interleukin 6 attenuates coagulation activation in experimental endotoxemia in chimpanzees. J Exp Med. 1994;**179**(4):1253–9.

25. Opal SM, Esmon CT, Opal SM, Esmon CT. Bench-to-bedside review: functional relationships between coagulation and the innate immune response and their respective roles in the pathogenesis of sepsis. Crit Care (London, England). 2003;**7**(1):23–38.

26. Opal SM, Opal SM. Interactions between coagulation and inflammation. Scand J Infect Dis. 2003;**35**(9):545–54.

27. Booth KK, Terrell DR, Vesely SK, George JN. Systemic infections mimicking thrombotic thrombocytopenic purpura. Am J Hematol. 2011;**86**(9):743–51.

28. Douglas KW, Pollock KGJ, Young D, Catlow J, Green R. Infection frequently triggers thrombotic microangiopathy in patients with preexisting risk factors: a single-institution experience. J Clin Apheresis. 2010;**25**(2):47–53.

29. Kiki I, Gundogdu M, Albayrak B, Bilgic Y. Thrombotic thrombocytopenic purpura associated with Brucella infection. Am J Med Sci. 2008;**335**(3):230–2.

30. Lin C-Y, Lin S-H. Fatal thrombotic throbmocytopenic purpura coexisting with bacterial infection: a case report. Acta Neurol. 2008;**17**(1):42–6.

31. Esmon CT. The interactions between inflammation and coagulation. Brit J Haematol. 2005;**131**(4):417–30.

32. Bae JS, Yang L, Manithody C, Rezaie AR, Bae J-S, Yang L, et al. The ligand occupancy of endothelial protein C receptor switches the protease-activated receptor 1-dependent signaling specificity of thrombin from a permeability-enhancing to a barrier-protective response in endothelial cells. Blood. 2007;**110**(12):3909–16.

33. Delabranche X, Berger A, Boisrame-Helms J, Meziani F. Microparticles and infectious diseases. Med Mal Infect. 2012;**42**(8):335–43.

34. Satta N, Toti F, Feugeas O, Bohbot A, Dachary-Prigent J, Eschwege V, et al. Monocyte vesiculation is a possible mechanism for dissemination of membrane-associated procoagulant activities and adhesion molecules after stimulation by lipopolysaccharide. J Immunol. 1994;**153**(7):3245–55.

35. Brinkmann V, Reichard U, Goosmann C, Fauler B, Uhlemann Y, Weiss DS, et al. Neutrophil extracellular traps kill bacteria. Science. 2004;**303**(5663):1532–5.

36. Brinkmann V, Laube B, Abu Abed U, Goosmann C, Zychlinsky A. Neutrophil extracellular traps: how to generate and visualize them. J Vis Exp. 2010;**36**: pii:1724, doi: 10.3791/1724.

37. Brinkmann V, Zychlinsky A. Beneficial suicide: why neutrophils die to make NETs. Nat Rev Microbiol. 2007;**5**(8):577–82.

38. Clark SR, Ma AC, Tavener SA, McDonald B, Goodarzi Z, Kelly MM, et al. Platelet TLR4 activates neutrophil extracellular traps to ensnare bacteria in septic blood. Nature Medicine. 2007;**13**(4):463–9.

39. von Bruhl M-L, Stark K, Steinhart A, Chandraratne S, Konrad I, Lorenz M, et al. Monocytes, neutrophils, and platelets cooperate to initiate and propagate venous thrombosis in mice in vivo. J Exp Med. 2012;**209**(4):819–35.

40. Massberg S, Grahl L, von Bruehl ML, Manukyan D, Pfeiler S, Goosmann C, et al. Reciprocal coupling of coagulation and innate immunity via neutrophil serine proteases. Nature Medicine. 2010;**16**(8):887–96.

41. Ermert D, Urban CF, Laube B, Goosmann C, Zychlinsky A, Brinkmann V. Mouse neutrophil extracellular traps in microbial infections. J Innate Immun. 2009;**1**(3):181–93.

42. Ammollo CT, Semeraro F, Xu J, Esmon NL, Esmon CT. Extracellular histones increase plasma thrombin generation by impairing thrombomodulin-dependent protein C activation. J Thromb Haemost. 2011;**9**(9):1795–803.

43. Semeraro F, Ammollo CT, Morrissey JH, Dale GL, Friese P, Esmon NL, et al. Extracellular histones promote thrombin generation through platelet-dependent mechanisms: involvement of platelet TLR2 and TLR4. Blood. 2011;**118**(7):1952–61.

44. Morrissey JH, Gregory SA, Mackman N, Edgington TS. Tissue factor regulation and gene organization. Oxford Surveys on Eukaryotic Genes. 1989;**6**:67–84.

45. Sadler JE. Thrombomodulin structure and function. Thromb Haemost. 1997;**78**(1):392–5.

46. Oganesyan V, Oganesyan N, Terzyan S, Qu D, Dauter Z, Esmon NL, et al. The crystal structure of the endothelial protein C receptor and a bound phospholipid. J Biol Chem. 2002;**277**(28):24851–4.

47. Dahlback B. Protein S and C4b-binding protein: components involved in the regulation of the protein C anticoagulant system. Thromb Haemost. 1991;**66**(1):49–61.

48. Dickson B. Venous thrombosis: on the history of Virchow's triad. UTMJ. 2004;**81**:166–71.

49. Mammen EF. Perspectives for the future. Intensive Care Med. 1993;**19** Suppl 1:S29–34.

50. Cunnington A, Nadel S. New therapies for sepsis. Curr Top Med Chem. 2008;**8**(7):603–14.

51. Hellgren M, Javelin L, Hagnevik K, Blomback M. Antithrombin III concentrate as adjuvant in DIC treatment. A pilot study in 9 severely ill patients. Thromb Res. 1984;**35**(4):459–66.

52. von Kries R, Stannigel H, Gobel U. Anticoagulant therapy by continuous heparin-antithrombin III infusion in newborns with disseminated intravascular coagulation. Eur J Pediatr. 1985;**144**(2):191–4.

53. Kreuz WD, Schneider W, Nowak-Gottl U. Treatment of consumption coagulopathy with antithrombin concentrate in children with acquired antithrombin deficiency – a feasibility pilot study. Eur J Pediatr. 1999;**158** Suppl 3:S187–91.

54. Ettingshausen CE, Veldmann A, Beeg T, Schneider W, Jager G, Kreuz W. Replacement therapy with protein C concentrate in infants and adolescents with meningococcal sepsis and purpura fulminans. Semin Thromb Hemost. 1999;**25**(6):537–41.

55. Rivard GE, David M, Farrell C, Schwarz HP. Treatment of purpura fulminans in meningococcemia with protein C concentrate. J Pediatr. 1995;**126**(4):646–52.

56. Goldstein B, Nadel S, Peters M, Barton R, Machado F, Levy H, et al. ENHANCE: results of a global open-label trial of drotrecogin alfa (activated) in children with severe sepsis. Pediatr Crit Care Med. 2006;**7**(3):200–11.

57. Nadel S, Goldstein B, Williams MD, Dalton H, Peters M, Macias WL, et al. Drotrecogin alfa (activated) in children with severe sepsis: a multicentre phase III randomised controlled trial. Lancet. 2007;**369**(9564):836–43.

58. Fourrier F, Chopin C, Huart JJ, Runge I, Caron C, Goudemand J. Double-blind, placebo-controlled trial of antithrombin III concentrates in septic shock with disseminated intravascular coagulation. Chest. 1993;**104**(3):882–8.

59. Bernard GR, Vincent JL, Laterre PF, LaRosa SP, Dhainaut JF, Lopez-Rodriguez A, et al. Efficacy and safety of recombinant human activated protein C for severe sepsis. New Engl J Med. 2001;**344**(10):699–709.

60. Ranieri VM, Thompson BT, Barie PS, Dhainaut J-F, Douglas IS, Finfer S, et al. Drotrecogin alfa (activated) in adults with septic shock. New Engl J Med. 2012;**366**(22):2055–64.

61. Silva E, de Figueiredo LFP, Colombari F. Prowess-shock trial: a protocol overview and perspectives. Shock. 2010;**34** Suppl 1:48–53.

62. Decembrino L, D'Angelo A, Manzato F, Solinas A, Tumminelli F, De Silvestri A, et al. Protein C concentrate as adjuvant treatment in neonates with sepsis-induced coagulopathy: a pilot study. Shock. 2010;**34**(4):341–5.

63. Marti-Carvajal AJ, Sola I, Gluud C, Lathyris D, Cardona AF. Human recombinant protein C for severe sepsis and septic shock in adult and paediatric patients. Cochrane Database Syst Rev. 2012;**12**:CD004388.

64. Dreyfus M, Masterson M, David M, Rivard GE, Muller FM, Kreuz W, et al. Replacement therapy with a monoclonal antibody purified protein C concentrate in newborns with severe congenital protein C deficiency. Semin Thromb Hemost. 1995;**21**(4):371–81.

65. Veldman A, Fischer D, Wong FY, Kreuz W, Sasse M, Eberspacher B, et al. Human protein C concentrate in the treatment of purpura fulminans: a retrospective analysis of safety and outcome in 94 pediatric patients. Critical Care (London, England). 2010;**14**(4):R156.

66. de Kleijn ED, de Groot R, Hack CE, Mulder PGH, Engl W, Moritz B, et al. Activation of protein C following infusion of protein C concentrate in children with severe meningococcal sepsis and purpura fulminans: a

randomized, double-blinded, placebo-controlled, dose-finding study. Crit Care Med. 2003;**31**(6):1839–47.

67. Clarke RC, Johnston JR, Mayne EE. Meningococcal septicaemia: treatment with protein C concentrate. Intens Care Med. 2000;**26**(4):471–3.

68. Eisele B, Lamy M. Clinical experience with antithrombin III concentrates in critically ill patients with sepsis and multiple organ failure. Semin Thromb Hemost. 1998;**24**(1):71–80.

69. Hanada T, Abe T, Takita H. Antithrombin III concentrates for treatment of disseminated intravascular coagulation in children. Am J Pediatr Hematol/Oncol. 1985;**7**(1):3–8.

70. Kreuz W, Schneider W, Nowak-Gottl U. Treatment of consumption coagulopathy with antithrombin concentrate in children with acquired antithrombin deficiency – a feasibility pilot study. Eur J Pediatr 1999:**158** Suppl 3:S87–91.

71. Abraham E, Reinhart K, Opal S, Demeyer I, Doig C, Rodriguez AL, et al. Efficacy and safety of tifacogin (recombinant tissue factor pathway inhibitor) in severe sepsis: a randomized controlled trial. JAMA. 2003;**290**(2):238–47.

72. de Pont ACJM, Moons AHM, de Jonge E, Meijers JCM, Vlasuk GP, Rote WE, et al. Recombinant nematode anticoagulant protein c2, an inhibitor of tissue factor/factor VIIa, attenuates coagulation and the interleukin-10 response in human endotoxemia. J Thromb Haemost. 2004;**2**(1):65–70.

73. Godoi LC, Gomes KB, Alpoim PN, Carvalho MdG, Lwaleed BA, Sant'Ana Dusse LM. Preeclampsia: the role of tissue factor and tissue factor pathway inhibitor. J Thromb Thrombolysis. 2012;**34**(1):1–6.

74. Saito H, Maruyama I, Shimazaki S, Yamamoto Y, Aikawa N, Ohno R, et al. Efficacy and safety of recombinant human soluble thrombomodulin (ART-123) in disseminated intravascular coagulation: results of a phase III, randomized, double-blind clinical trial. J Thromb Haemost. 2007;**5**(1):31–41.

75. Wunderink RG, Laterre P-F, Francois B, Perrotin D, Artigas A, Vidal LO, et al. Recombinant tissue factor pathway inhibitor in severe community-acquired pneumonia: a randomized trial. Am J Resp Crit Care Med. 2011;**183**(11):1561–8.

76. Levi M. Disseminated intravascular coagulation. Crit Care Med. 2007;**35**(9):2191–5.

77. Chuansumrit A, Hotrakitya S, Hathirat P, Isarangkura P. Disseminated intravascular coagulation in children: diagnosis, management and outcome. Southeast Asian J Trop Med Public Health. 1993;**24** Suppl 1:229–33.

78. Hazelzet JA, Risseeuw-Appel IM, Kornelisse RF, Hop WC, Dekker I, Joosten KF, et al. Age-related differences in

outcome and severity of DIC in children with septic shock and purpura. Thromb Haemost. 1996;**76**(6):932–8.

79. Khemani RG, Bart RD, Alonzo TA, Hatzakis G, Hallam D, Newth CJL. Disseminated intravascular coagulation score is associated with mortality for children with shock. Intens Care Med. 2009;**35**(2):327–33.

80. Raffini LJ, Raybagkar D, Blumenstein MS, Rubenstein RC, Manno CS. Cystic fibrosis as a risk factor for recurrent venous thrombosis at a pediatric tertiary care hospital. J Pediatr. 2006;**148**(5):659–64.

81. Forrester LJ, Campbell BJ, Berg JN, Barrett JT. Aggregation of platelets by Fusobacterium necrophorum. J Clin Microbiol. 1985;**22**(2):245–9.

82. Ramirez S, Hild TG, Rudolph CN, Sty JR, Kehl SC, Havens P, et al. Increased diagnosis of Lemierre syndrome and other Fusobacterium necrophorum infections at a Children's Hospital. Pediatrics. 2003;**112**(5):e380.

83. Alvarez A, Schreiber JR. Lemierre's syndrome in adolescent children – anaerobic sepsis with internal jugular vein thrombophlebitis following pharyngitis. Pediatrics. 1995;**96**(2 Pt 1):354–9.

84. Le Monnier A, Jamet A, Carbonnelle E, Barthod G, Moumile K, Lesage F, et al. Fusobacterium necrophorum middle ear infections in children and related complications: report of 25 cases and literature review. Pediatr Infect Dis J. 2008;**27**(7):613–7.

85. Lim S-C, Lee S-S, Yoon T-M, Lee J-K. Lemierre syndrome caused by acute isolated sphenoid sinusitis and its intracranial complications. Auris Nasus Larynx. 2010;**37**(1):106–9.

86. Redaelli de Zinis LO, Gasparotti R, Campovecchi C, Annibale G, Barezzani MG. Internal jugular vein thrombosis associated with acute mastoiditis in a pediatric age. Otol Neurotol. 2006;**27**(7):937–44.

87. Thorne MC, Chewaproug L, Elden LM. Suppurative complications of acute otitis media: changes in frequency over time. Arch Otolaryngol Head Neck Surg. 2009;**135**(7):638–41.

88. Carpenter J, Tsuchida T. Cerebral sinovenous thrombosis in children. Curr Neurol Neurosci Rep. 2007;**7**(2):139–46.

89. Huisman TA, Holzmann D, Martin E, Willi UV. Cerebral venous thrombosis in childhood. Eur Radiol. 2001;**11**(9):1760–5.

90. Heller C, Heinecke A, Junker R, Knofler R, Kosch A, Kurnik K, et al. Cerebral venous thrombosis in children: a multifactorial origin. Circulation. 2003;**108**(11):1362–7.

91. Fitzgerald KC, Williams LS, Garg BP, Carvalho KS, Golomb MR. Cerebral sinovenous thrombosis in the neonate. Arch Neurol. 2006;**63**(3):405–9.

92. Kenet G, Waldman D, Lubetsky A, Kornbrut N, Khalil A, Koren A, et al. Paediatric cerebral sinus vein thrombosis. A multi-center, case-controlled study. Thromb Haemost. 2004;**92**(4):713–18.

93. Sebire G, Tabarki B, Saunders DE, Leroy I, Liesner R, Saint-Martin C, et al. Cerebral venous sinus thrombosis in children: risk factors, presentation, diagnosis and outcome. Brain. 2005;**128**(Pt 3):477–89.

94. Carvalho KS, Bodensteiner JB, Connolly PJ, Garg BP. Cerebral venous thrombosis in children. J Child Neurol. 2001;**16**(8):574–80.

95. Mallick AA, Sharples PM, Calvert SE, Jones RWA, Leary M, Lux AL, et al. Cerebral venous sinus thrombosis: a case series including thrombolysis. Arch Dis Child. 2009;**94**(10):790–4.

96. Wasay M, Dai AI, Ansari M, Shaikh Z, Roach ES. Cerebral venous sinus thrombosis in children: a multicenter cohort from the United States. J Child Neurol. 2008;**23**(1):26–31.

97. Lutter SA, Kerschner JE, Chusid MJ. Gradenigo syndrome: a rare but serious complication of otitis media. Pediatr Emerg Care. 2005;**21**(6):384–6.

98. Kimura AC, Pien FD. Head and neck cellulitis in hospitalized adults. Am J Otolaryngol. 1993;**14**(5):343–9.

99. Muorah M, Hinds R, Verma A, Yu D, Samyn M, Mieli-Vergani G, et al. Liver abscesses in children: a single center experience in the developed world. J Pediatr Gastroenterol Nutr. 2006;**42**(2):201–6.

100. Brown CE, Lowe TW, Cunningham FG, Weinreb JC. Puerperal pelvic thrombophlebitis: impact on diagnosis and treatment using x-ray computed tomography and magnetic resonance imaging. Obstet Gynecol. 1986;**68**(6):789–94.

101. Brown CE, Stettler RW, Twickler D, Cunningham FG. Puerperal septic pelvic thrombophlebitis: incidence and response to heparin therapy. Am J Obstet Gynecol. 1999;**181**(1):143–8.

102. Wysokinska EM, Hodge D, McBane RD, 2nd. Ovarian vein thrombosis: incidence of recurrent venous thromboembolism and survival. Thromb Haemost. 2006;**96**(2):126–31.

103. Mantadakis E, Plessa E, Vouloumanou EK, Michailidis L, Chatzimichael A, Falagas ME. Deep venous thrombosis in children with musculoskeletal infections: the clinical evidence. Int J Infect Dis. 2012;**16**(4):e236–43.

104. Hollmig ST, Copley LAB, Browne RH, Grande LM, Wilson PL. Deep venous thrombosis associated with osteomyelitis in children. J Bone Joint Surg Am. 2007;**89**(7):1517–23.

105. Gonzalez BE, Teruya J, Mahoney DH, Jr., Hulten KG, Edwards R, Lamberth LB, et al. Venous thrombosis associated with staphylococcal osteomyelitis in children. Pediatrics. 2006;**117**(5):1673–9.

106. Nourse C, Starr M, Munckhof W. Community-acquired methicillin-resistant *Staphylococcus aureus* causes severe disseminated infection and deep venous thrombosis in children: literature review and recommendations for management. J Paediatr Child Health. 2007;**43**(10):656–61.

107. Antoniak S, Boltzen U, Riad A, Kallwellis-Opara A, Rohde M, Dorner A, et al. Viral myocarditis and coagulopathy: increased tissue factor expression and plasma thrombogenicity. J Mol Cell Cardiol. 2008;**45**(1):118–26.

108. Rahbar A, Soderberg-Naucler C. Human cytomegalovirus infection of endothelial cells triggers platelet adhesion and aggregation. J Virol. 2005;**79**(4):2211–20.

109. Leder AN, Flansbaum B, Zandman-Goddard G, Asherson R, Shoenfeld Y. Antiphospholipid syndrome induced by HIV. Lupus. 2001;**10**(5):370–4.

110. Yuste JR, Prieto J. Anticardiolipin antibodies in chronic viral hepatitis. Do they have clinical consequences? Eur J Gastroenterol Hepatol. 2003;**15**(7):717–19.

111. Kuczkowski J, Stankiewicz C, Izycka-Swieszewska E, Przewozny T. Sigmoid sinus thrombosis in a 5-year-old child with acute otitis media and acquired CMV infection. Otolaryngol Pol. 2006;**60**(6):923–7.

112. Josephson C, Nuss R, Jacobson L, Hacker MR, Murphy J, Weinberg A, Manco-Johnson MJ. The varicella autoantibody syndrome. Pediatr Res 2001;**50**:345–52.

113. Josephson C. Manco-Johnson M, Nuss R, Key N, Moertel C, Jacobson L, Meech S, Weinberg A, Lefkowitz J. Lupus anticoagulant and protein S deficiency in children with post-varicella purpura fulminans or thrombosis. J Pediatr 1996;**128**:324–8.

114. Canpolat C, Bakir M. A case of purpura fulminans secondary to transient protein C deficiency as a complication of chickenpox infection. Turk J Pediatr. 2002;**44**(2):148–51.

115. Lumbiganon P, Kosalaraksa P, Thepsuthammarat K, Sutra S. Dengue mortality in patients under 18 years old: an analysis from the health situation analysis of the Thai population in 2010 project. J Med Assoc Thai. 2012;**95** Suppl 7:S108–13.

116. Srichaikul T, Nimmannitya S. Haematology in dengue and dengue haemorrhagic fever. Best Pract Res Clin Haematol. 2000;**13**(2):261–76.

117. Ribes JA, Vanover-Sams CL, Baker DJ. Zygomycetes in human disease. Clin Microbiol Rev 2000;**13**:236–301.

118. del Pont MJ, De Cicco L, Gallo G, Llera J, De Santibanez, D'Angostino D. Hepatic arterial thrombosis due to Mucor species in a child following orthotopic liver transplanation. Transpl Infect Dis 2000;**2**:33–5.

119. Ryan M, Yeo S, Maguire A, Webb D, O'Marcaigh A, McDermott M, et al. Rhinocerebral zygomycosis in childhood acute lymphoblastic leukaemia. Eur J Pediatr. 2001;**160**(4):235–8.

120. Simmons JH, Zeitler PS, Fenton LZ, Abzug MJ, Fiallo-Scharer RV, Klingensmith GJ. Rhinocerebral mucormycosis complicated by internal carotid artery thrombosis in a pediatric patient with type 1 diabetes mellitus: a case report and review of the literature. Pediatr Diabetes 2005;**6**:234–8.

121. Rodland EK, Ueland T, Bjornsen S, Sagen EL, Dahl CP, Naalsund A, et al. Systemic biomarkers of inflammation and haemostasis in patients with chronic necrotizing pulmonary aspergillosis. BMC Infect Dis. 2012;**12**:144.

Developmental hemostasis I

Paul Monagle

Introduction

The hemostatic system is a complex interaction between the vasculature, cellular components and plasma proteins that interact to maintain hemostasis in the healthy body. Further, this complex interaction occurs across a variety of flow states, under variable pressure conditions. The hemostatic system on a wider scale also interplays with other physiological systems, including those that facilitate immune and inflammatory responses, angiogenesis and wound repair.

There is currently no mechanism for assessing or testing the hemostatic system in its true physiological state. All laboratory tests isolate specific components of the system, and assess those components under artificial constructs that hopefully give the clinician valuable information about the way the patient will behave. In this context, we divide the hemostatic system into primary, secondary and tertiary hemostasis to better define the interdependent mechanisms that combine to maintain overall hemostasis. Primary hemostasis describes the cellular interaction of platelets and the endothelium, and the initiation of the platelet plug that is localized to the point of injury at the vessel wall. Secondary hemostasis describes the activation of the coagulation system that is initiated, amplified and prolonged in a sequence of activations of coagulation proteins, and regulated by a series of positive and negative feedback mechanisms. Tertiary hemostasis is a description of the fibrinolytic system which regulates the breakdown of blood clots as healing vessels regain vascular integrity. In reality none of these components act in isolation. Nor do these processes act in sequential timeframes as the names would suggest. However, such terminology is useful in allowing an incredibly complex and interwoven system to be considered in a way that helps us to understand pathophysiology of diseases, explain clinical presentations and direct our currently available therapies.

Until the 1980s, the hemostatic system in children was generally presumed to be equivalent to that of adults.[1] The term "developmental hemostasis" was first introduced by Maureen Andrews in the 1980s to describe the age-related physiological changes of the coagulation system (predominantly secondary hemostasis) observed progressively over time from fetal, neonatal and pediatric to adult life.[2,3] Subsequently, the evolution of the haemostatic system was shown to continue throughout life, as evidenced by studies of the coagulation system in centenarians.[4] However the changes are most marked during childhood, and hence are of most clinical relevance during this time. Our understanding of hemostatic physiology in neonates and infants remains poor when compared with our knowledge of this subject in adults. The reasons for this deficit are several: in neonates and infants, multiple reference ranges are required because these patients have rapidly changing systems;[2,5,6] blood sampling in the young is technically difficult; only small blood samples can be obtained; microtechniques are required; and greater variability in plasma concentrations of coagulation proteins necessitates the use of large patient numbers to establish normative data.[7]

Because of these difficulties, animal models have been used to increase our understanding of developmental hemostasis.[8] The lamb has been the most frequently used model. Both the pig and sheep have similar vascular and hemostatic physiologies to that of humans. The newborn dog has been used as a model of intraventricular hemorrhage.[9] Recently, differences in response of the coagulation system to volutrauma have been demonstrated between newborn and adult rats.[10] Using targeted manipulations of the mouse genome, murine models of deficiencies in virtually every protein involved in hemostasis have been created. The information learned from these models has

Pediatric Thrombotic Disorders, ed. Neil A. Goldenberg and Marilyn J. Manco-Johnson. Published by Cambridge University Press. © Cambridge University Press 2015.

increased our understanding of the role of these proteins in fetal development.[11] Apart from secondary hemostasis, animal models have also been used to examine the impact of age on the vascular endothelium, which is difficult to study in humans for reasons of access as well.[12,13]

Given the limitations of our testing constructs, and the difficulties of performing this research in children, much about the true nature of developmental hemostasis remains to be determined. Further research is required not only to improve our clinical understanding of hemostatic disorders in children, but to improve our understanding of the basic physiology of human growth and development. This in turn will provide great insight into the multitude of diseases which present during adult life, but likely have their origins during childhood, many of which, such as cardiovascular disease, are intimately linked to the hemostatic system.

This chapter will provide an up-to-date description of our current understanding of developmental hemostasis, focusing on primary hemostasis (vascular endothelial and platelet-related changes) and secondary hemostasis (coagulation protein changes). For many of the observations described regarding development hemostasis at the individual protein level, the clinical significance for hemostasis and thrombosis in pediatrics requires further study.

Vascular endothelial changes with age

The vascular endothelium profoundly influences hemostasis due to the procoagulant and anticoagulant properties of endothelial cells and extracellular matrix components. This organ is surely one of the most complex in the body. Not only is there evidence that the arterial endothelium functions differently from the venous endothelium, which is different in turn from capillary endothelial function, but each of these vascular components likely also varies in different organs within the body.[14] The properties of the vascular endothelium would appear to be significantly influenced by age; however, this remains the least well-studied component of the hemostatic system.

Perhaps even more important than the direct age-related changes in the coagulant properties of the endothelium, is the likely role the endothelium plays in regulating the plasma coagulation proteins. A recent study demonstrated that even with a transplanted adult liver *in situ*, children maintain plasma levels of certain coagulation proteins at their expected age-specific levels.[15] Thus the liver, despite being the site of production for most of the coagulation proteins, is not the critical regulator of plasma levels. The authors of the study hypothesized hormonal control, vascular endothelial control via an as yet unidentified mechanism, or control via variable clearance. However, whatever the mechanism, the vascular endothelium seems the most likely candidate as the primary regulator. The endothelium is intimately involved with the function of the coagulation proteins.[16] Vascular endothelial dysfunction, as observed in disseminated intravascular coagulation, is usually measured by the degree of disturbance in coagulation proteins, even though it is not a primary disorder of coagulation.[17]

With respect to the direct pro- or anticoagulant effect of the vascular endothelium, studies in a rabbit venous model show that there is a significantly greater mass of glycosaminoglycans (GAGs) in inferior vena cavae (IVCs) from pups when compared with adult rabbits. The antithrombin (AT)-mediated anticoagulant activity of IVC GAGs, especially heparin sulfate, is greater in pups as compared to adult rabbits.[12] In a rabbit arterial model, total proteoglycan, chrondroitin sulfate and heparin sulfate content are increased in the intima and media of aortas from pups relative to those of adult rabbits. The AT activity in aortas of pups, due to heparin sulfate GAGs, is relatively greater.[13] The greater GAG-mediated vessel wall AT activity in pups compared with adult rabbits suggests that young blood vessels may have more antithrombotic potential. Soluble levels of endothelial cell adhesion molecules and selectins are also age-dependent, suggesting developmental differences in endothelial cell expression and secretion of these molecules.[18]

Most of the information on other changes in endothelial function during early life has come from studies on the pulmonary, intestinal, cerebral and skeletal muscle vascular beds in different animal species. With respect to nitric oxide (NO), results from studies in the different species indicate that NO becomes increasingly important with age as a contributor to endothelium-dependent dilation in the pulmonary, cerebral and skeletal muscle vascular beds. In contrast, the contribution of NO to endothelium-dependent dilation decreases developmentally in the intestinal vascular bed. Other endothelial factors that change in importance for vascular control during growth include COX metabolites, H_2O_2 and CO. For any vascular bed, the physiological impact of growth-related changes in endothelial function can be difficult to predict because these changes are sometimes superimposed on changes in vascular smooth muscle as well. As with the endothelium, these changes are usually highly species- or organ-specific. How much of these data can be extrapolated to humans is unclear. There is an urgent need to further understand the cellular and molecular mechanisms of these changes in order to provide mechanistic insight into the age-related changes in vascular endothelial function.[19]

Platelet changes with age

In comparison to vascular endothelium, much more research in humans has been done to determine the differences in platelet number, structure and function with age. Despite this, there remain many difficulties. Traditional platelet function studies in newborn infants are almost impossible due to sample volume requirements. Flow cytometry is more useful because of the small sample volume required; however, experience with this technique in neonates remains limited, and subtle changes in responses due to differences in blood collection techniques significantly hamper age-related comparative research. Many studies in the newborn age group have used cord blood; however, differences in sample timing, method of collection, and concentrations and compositions of platelet agonists certainly contribute to the conflicting reports on cord platelet function, making interpretation of the current literature very difficult. The relevance of cord blood studies to neonatal life remains questionable.

Megakaryocytopoiesis has been difficult to study in the fetus and neonate because of the intrinsic low level of megakaryocyte production in the marrow and the difficulty in accessing marrow samples on normal children to study. Platelets first appear in circulation at 5 weeks post-conception, and megakaryocytes appear in the liver at 8 weeks. Human fetal and neonatal megakaryocytes appear smaller than adult megakaryocytes.[20] Initial microassay techniques suggested that megakaryocytopoiesis is likely increased at 24 to 36 weeks' gestation versus full-term.[21]

Megakaryocytes

There are increased numbers of megakaryocyte precursors in the cord blood of preterm babies compared with term infants. In turn, compared to adults, term infants have increased circulating megakaryocyte progenitor numbers at birth correlated with platelet numbers.[22] Reticulated platelet counts in healthy neonates have variably been reported as either reduced, similar to or increased when compared to adult levels, with some studies reporting differences with gestational age.[23,24] There is no information on developmental differences of megakaryocyte and platelet precursors during childhood.

Platelet function

Traditional platelet aggregometry has not identified any substantial differences in platelet function with age. However, very recent work has suggested that there may be differences in platelet binding and cellular interactions that are age-dependent. Circulating monocyte–platelet aggregates (MPAs) are a sensitive marker of platelet activation. These aggregates are well characterized in adults, and form as a result of platelet activation-dependent surface expression of P-selectin and its binding to a constitutively expressed ligand on monocytes. In a study in which platelet activation, exocytosis and formation of MPAs in healthy children (n = 22) and adults (n = 10) was measured by whole blood flow cytometry, the number of circulating MPAs was higher in children compared to adults, with no corresponding increase in circulating platelet activation (PAC-1 binding) or exocytosis (P-selectin expression). Platelet-bound monocytes in children did not express elevated P-selectin; however, P-selectin expression could still be induced by a chemical agonist. This suggests the possibility of a novel P-selectin independent mechanism of MPA formation in children (see Figure 8.1).

Another difference in platelet surface marker expression is suggested by the observed different frequency of heparin-induced thrombocytopenia in children compared to adults, although the potential mechanisms behind this difference have not yet been explored.[25]

Coagulation protein changes with age

The defining principle of developmental hemostasis is that the functional levels of coagulation proteins change in a predictable way with age.[5] The trends in changes are consistent across multiple studies; however, the absolute values of these changes are reagent- and analyzer-dependent.[7] The results of global tests of coagulation, such as the activated partial thromboplastin time (APTT), reflect these functional changes of coagulation proteins. Other global measures of hemostasis may be more or less sensitive to age-related

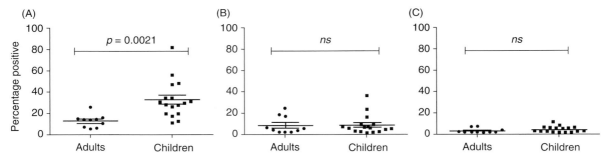

Figure 8.1 Circulating monocyte–platelet aggregates were increased in children (n = 17, age 5–14) compared to adults (n=10, age 20–43), as shown in Figure A. However, there was no corresponding increase in activation of circulating platelets in children compared to adults (Figure B), as demonstrated by PAC-1 binding and granule exocytosis (Figure C), as demonstrated by P-selectin expression. These results suggest that circulating MPAs in children are not a result of increased platelet activation, and that a P-selectin independent mechanism of MPA formation may be responsible.

changes in hemostatic proteins. For example, thromboelastography (TEG) shows little if any variation in healthy children with age.[26] Studies in this field have predominantly reported functional assays of the coagulation proteins, presumably due to the fact that these assays are commonly used in clinical practice. In fact, measurements of immunological levels of the coagulation proteins have not been reported to date.

Early evidence suggests that these age-related changes in protein concentration are not isolated to the coagulation system, but are in fact evident across multiple protein systems within the plasma proteome. Variation in the human plasma proteome with age has been examined using plasma samples collected from healthy neonates (day 1 and day 3) and adults. The study reported significant changes in number and abundance of numerous proteins in neonates compared to adults.[27]

Plasma concentrations of most coagulation proteins are measurable by approximately 10 weeks of gestational age, and they continue to increase gradually in conjunction with the gestational age.[28] Coagulation proteins are independently synthesized by the fetus and do not cross the placenta. The best estimates of normal values for fetuses are obtained from fetoscopy collections.[29] By extrapolation, these values are used to approximate normal ranges in very premature infants as well; however, true reference ranges for extremely premature infants are not available because the majority of these infants have postnatal complications. A number of studies have reported reference ranges for coagulation proteins, inhibitors of coagulation, and components of the fibrinolytic system for premature (30 to 36 weeks' gestational age) and full-term infants on day 1 of life,

as well as longitudinally over the first 6 months of life (see Table 8.1).[30,31]

There are multiple reasons for the reported variations in values for coagulation screening tests in neonates. First, some studies used cord blood samples rather than samples from infants. Second, differing ethnic populations between studies and certainly the use of different reagents impact on the absolute results. Variation in prothrombin time (PT) results can be minimized by reporting the PT as an *international normalized ratio* (INR). The INR is calculated as the patient PT/healthy adult pooled plasma control PT to the power of the *international sensitivity index* (ISI). The ISI corrects for the large variation in sensitivity of thromboplastin reagents to plasma concentrations of coagulation proteins. Unfortunately, there is no such standardization for activated partial thromboplastin times (APTT). Reference ranges for APTTs differ with each different reagent and analyzer system, often significantly. Different analyser and reagent combinations are variably sensitive to age-related changes in the global coagulation assays.[7,32]

The most studied factors in infants are the vitamin K-dependent factors, presumably driven by the clinical significance of hemorrhagic disease of the newborn (HDN). Physiologically low levels of factors (F)II, FVII, FIX and FX have been consistently reported[2,5,6] and were measured in infants who received vitamin K prophylaxis at birth. The levels of the VK-dependent factors and the contact factors (FXI, FXII, prekallikrein and high molecular weight kininogen) gradually increase to values approaching adult levels by 6 months of life.[2,5,6] Some authors suggest that the prolonged activated partial thromboplastin time (APTT) during the first months of life is in

Table 8.1 Studies reporting age-related differences in coagulation assays or proteins during healthy childhood

Author	Year	Assays/proteins reported	Age groups	N
Perlman, M et al.[80]	1975	PT, TT, APTT, fibrinogen, FDP, platelet count, hematocrit, FV, FVIII, plasminogen, hemoglobin	Healthy infants Small-for-dates infants Post-mature infants	n = 35 n = 26 n = 30
Beverley, DW et al.[31]	1984	APTT, FII-VII-X, fibrinogen, α_2-antiplasmin, platelet count, MPV, megathrombocyte index, plasminogen	Cord blood Newborns (48 hours)	n = 80
Andrew, M et al.[2]	1987	PT, APTT, TCT, fibrinogen, FII, FV, FVII, FVIII, vWF, FIX, FX, FXI, FXII, PK, HMWK, FXIIIa, FXIIIb, plasminogen, antithrombin, α_2M, α_2-AP, C_1E-INH, α_1-AT, HCII, protein C, protein S	Day 1 newborn Day 5 newborn Day 30 newborn Day 90 newborn Day 180 newborn Adult	28–75 samples per age group
Andrew, M et al.[6]	1988	PT, APTT, TCT, fibrinogen, FII, FV, FVII, FVIII, vWF, FIX, FX, FXI, FXII, PK, HMWK, FXIIIa, FXIIIb, plasminogen, antithrombin, α_2M, α_2-AP, C_1E-INH, α_1-AT, HCII, protein C, protein S	Premature newborns (30–36 weeks' gestation) Day 1 Day 5 Day 30 Day 90 Day 180	23–67 samples per age group
Andrew, M et al.[3]	1992	PT/INR, APTT, bleeding time, fibrinogen, FII, FV, FVII, FVIII, vWF, FIX, FX, FXI, FXII, PK, HMWK, FXIIIa, FXIIIs, plasminogen, tPA, PAI, antithrombin, α_2M, α_2-AP, C_1E-INH, α_1-AT, HCII, protein C, protein S (total and free)	1–5 years 6–10 years 11–16 years Adults	20–50 samples per age group
Reverdiau-Moalic, P et al.[28]	1996	PT/INR, APTT TCT, FI, FII, FVII, FVII, FIX, FX, FV, FVIII, FXI, FXII, PK, HMWK, AT, HCII, TFPI, protein C (Ag, Act), protein S (free and total), C4b-BP	Fetuses 19–23 24–29 30–38 wks' gestation Newborns (immediately after delivery) Adults	n = 20 n = 22 n = 22 n = 60 n = 40
Carcao, MD et al.[81]	2002	PFA100 Hb Platelet count	Neonates Children Adults	n = 17 n = 57 n = 31
Salonvaara, M et al.[82]	2003	FII, FV, FVII, FX, APTT, PT/INR, platelet count	Premature infants 24–27 weeks 28–30 weeks 31–33 weeks 34–36 weeks	n = 21 n = 25 n = 34 n = 45
Flanders, M et al.[83]	2005	PT, APTT, FVIII, FIX, FXI, RCF, vWF,	7–9 years 10–11 years 12–13 years 14–15 years 16–17 years Adults	n = 245 n = 164 n = 164 n = 164 n = 150 n = 120
Flanders, M et al.[84]	2006	FII, FV, FVII, FX, fibrinogen, α_2-AP, plasminogen, AT, PC, PS	7–9 years 10–11 years 12–13 years 14–15 years 16–17 years Adults	n = 245 n = 164 n = 164 n = 164 n = 150 n = 120
Monagle, P et al.[7]	2006	APTT (4 reagents), PT/INR, fibrinogen, TCT, FII, FV, FVII, FVIII, FIX, FX, FXI, FXII, antithrombin, protein C, protein S, D-dimers, TFPI (free and total), endogenous thrombin potential	Day 1 Day 3 < 1 year 1–5 years 6–10 years 11–16 years Adults	minimum 20 samples per age group

Table 8.1 (cont.)

Author	Year	Assays/proteins reported	Age groups	N
Chan, KL et al.[26]	2007	Thromboelastography (TEG) [R. K. α, MA, LY30]	< 1 year 1–5 years 6–10 years 11–16 years Adults	n = 24 n = 24 n = 26 n = 26 n = 25
Sosothikul, D et al.[85]	2007	PT, APTT, fibrinogen, TAT, PC:Ac, TF, FVIIa, sTM, vWF (Ag & RCo), D-dimer, tPA, PAI-1, TAFI	1–5 years 6–10 years 11–18 years Adults	n = 19 n = 26 n = 25 n = 26
Mitsiakos, G et al.[86]	2009	INR, PT, APTT, fibrinogen, FII, FV, FVII, FVIII, FIX, FX, FXI, FXII, antithrombin, protein C, protein S, APCr, tPA, PAI-1, vWF	Small-for-growth newborns Appropriate-for-growth newborns	n = 90 n = 98
Newall, F et al.[87]	2008	PF4 and vitronectin	< 1 year 1–5 years 6–10 years 11–16 years Adults	15 per age group
Ries, M et al.[88]	1997	TAT, F1+2, PAP, D-dimer	1–6 years 7–12 years 13–18 years Adults	20 per age group
Boos, J et al.[89]	1989	PIVKA II, FVII, FII, FII:Ag	Day 1, 2, 3 neonates	n = 57 total

Reproduced with permission from *Blood Reviews* 2010;24:63–68 (62).

large part due to the low levels of the contact factors.[2] However, this does not consider the possible roles of qualitative changes in the proteins affecting binding or activation within the assay systems.[7]

Plasma levels of fibrinogen, FV, FVIII, FXIII and vWF are not decreased at birth. Fibrinogen levels increase after birth. Levels of both vWF and high molecular weight multimers are increased at birth and for the first months of life, a fact which makes clinical presentation, or diagnosis of vWD, unlikely during the first 3–4 months of life.[2,33–35]

As stated previously, the vascular endothelium is likely the controller of plasma coagulation protein levels. However, potential mechanisms for exerting that control include influencing both protein translation in the liver or protein clearance. In terms of protein transcription, messenger ribonucleic acid (mRNA) levels have been measured for FVII, FVIII, FIX, and FX, fibrinogen, AT, and protein C in hepatocytes from 5- to 10-week-old human embryos and fetuses and in those from adults. Embryonic–fetal transcripts and adult mRNAs are similar in size; and the nucleotide sequences of mRNA for factors IX and X were identical.[36] However, the expression of mRNA

was variable, with reduced expression of some coagulation proteins in fetuses, and expression equivalent to the adult values for others. The concentrations of prothrombin mRNA in the livers of newborn and adult rabbits do not differ.[36] The mRNA levels of antithrombin (AT) in fetal compared to adult sheep has also been shown to differ.[37] In terms of protein clearance, fibrinogen, whether of fetal or adult origin, is cleared more rapidly in newborn lambs than it is in sheep.[38] Similarly, clearance of fibrinogen is accelerated in premature infants with or without respiratory distress syndrome (RDS). An increased basal metabolic rate in the young may be a factor contributing to the accelerated clearance of proteins.[39]

Thrombin regulation is both delayed and decreased in newborn plasma compared with adult plasma.[40] Thrombin generation in neonates is said to be similar to plasmas from adults receiving therapeutic doses of warfarin or heparin.[40] Thrombin generation in newborn plasma is further decreased in the presence of endothelial cell surfaces, but not to the same extent as adult plasma.[41] Prothrombin concentration directly correlates with the amount of thrombin generated,[40] whereas the concentration of other procoagulants determine the rate of thrombin generation. Thrombin is directly inhibited by antithrombin (AT), heparin cofactor II (HCII) and α_2-macroglobulin (α_2M). In addition, a circulating physiologic anticoagulant in cord blood has properties similar to those of dermatan sulfate.[42] The fetal proteoglycan is present in plasma in concentrations of 0.29 µg/ml, has a molecular weight of 150,000 kd and catalyzes thrombin inhibition by means of the natural inhibitor HCII. The fetal anticoagulant also is present in plasmas from pregnant women and is produced by the placenta.[43] The length of time that the fetal anticoagulant circulates in neonates is not known. Alpha$_2$-macroglobulin (α_2M) is the major inhibitor of thrombin in neonates, being responsible for approximately 60% of thrombin inhibition, compared to only 7% in adults.[44] This increased contribution of α_2M persists throughout childhood, and even during the teenage years α_2M inhibition of thrombin remains twice that observed in adults. Alpha$_2$-macroglobulin compensates, in part, for the low levels of AT in neonates.

Whether the overall activity of the protein C/protein S system varies with age is unknown. However, at birth, plasma concentrations of protein C are very low, and they remain significantly decreased during the first 6 months of life; however, they do not reach adult concentrations until late adolescence.[2,5] Although total amounts of protein S are decreased at birth, functional activity is similar to that in the adult, because protein S is completely present in the free, active form due to the absence of C4 binding protein.[45] Furthermore, the interaction of protein S with activated protein C in newborn plasma may be regulated by the increased levels of α_2M.[46] Plasma concentrations of thrombomodulin are increased in early childhood, decreasing to adult values by the late teenage years; however, whether age influences the endothelial cell expression of thrombomodulin has not been determined.[47–51]

Total tissue factor pathway inhibitor (TFPI) levels in newborn infants are reported as being similar to levels in older children or adults. However, free TFPI is significantly lower in neonates.[52]

The capacity of newborn fibrin clots to bind thrombin has been assessed through the measurement of fibrinopeptide A (FPA) production. Cord plasma clots generate significantly less FPA than do adult plasma clots, because of the decreased plasma concentrations of prothrombin in cord plasma.[53] This observation suggests that thrombi in newborn infants may not have the same propensity to propagate as thrombi in adult patients.

Despite the age-related differences described in the coagulation system, including changes in the concentration of individual coagulation proteins as well as in global tests of coagulation, the hemostatic system in neonates and children does not seem to be "disadvantaged" compared to the "normal" coagulation system of adults. One must consider developmental hemostasis as physiological. There are no data to support either an increased bleeding or thrombotic risk during infancy for any given stimulus and, on the contrary, one could argue that the hemostatic system in neonates protects against bleeding and thrombotic complications compared to adults. It is interesting that when considering individual proteins, many proteins exist at levels during neonatal life that would be associated with disease in adults.[36] Similarly, prolongation of global tests of coagulation, such as the APTT, are not associated with an increase in bleeding, despite the APTT being considerably prolonged compared to that in many adults with clinically relevant vWD.[36] The concentrations of hemostatic proteins as measured by the currently available functional assays are not the key factors in determining clinical phenotype. There is an ongoing requirement for a much better understanding of the relationships between the concentration of hemostatic proteins and functional outcomes of the hemostatic system.

Qualitative changes in plasma protein concentrations

The majority of published research has focused on *quantitative differences* in coagulation proteins based on functional assays.[2,3,5] However, coagulation proteins have complex tertiary structures, as would be expected in proteins that serve multiple functions.[36,54] Post-translational modifications (PTM) to protein structure likely have significant impact on function of hemostatic proteins.[36,54] For example, fibrinogen has been shown to exist in a "fetal" form, in cord blood of term infants.[36] This "fetal" form of fibrinogen has increased sialic acid content compared to adult fibrinogen, a direct result of PTM. Sialic residues of fibrinogen directly bind Ca^{2+}, leading to a decrease in the intermolecular repulsion between fibrinogen chains, and thereby facilitating fibrin polymerization.[55] The phosphorus content of fetal fibrinogen is increased up to four-fold compared to the adult form of this protein.[56,57] Phosphorylation is known to modulate protein structure and function and is involved in the regulation of signaling pathways. Thrombin clotting times are prolonged in newborns, suggesting differences in polymerization of fibrin from "fetal" fibrinogen.[58]

More recently, fibrinogen purified from neonates and children was compared to that from adults. The molecular weight of the Aα fibrinogen chain was consistently higher by up to 1500 Da in neonates and children compared to adults.[59] This trend toward a higher molecular weight of fibrinogen chains in younger age groups was also consistent for the Bβ and γ chains, with differences of up to 400 Da and 500 Da, respectively. These differences in fibrinogen chains could represent multiple additional sialic acid or residues associated with increased glycan branching,[60] in the neonatal and pediatric fibrinogen compared to the adult form of this protein. The same study also demonstrated significant differences in the chromatogram profile (area under the peak and peak height) in neonates and children compared to adults, suggesting differences in the interaction of the fibrinogen molecule from each age group with the chromatography column used, which also implies structural differences for fibrinogen in these age groups.[59]

In addition to fibrinogen, a "neonatal" form of protein C has been detected in the ovine fetus.[61] Compared to the adult two-chain molecule, the "neonatal" protein C has an increased proportion of single-chain molecules. Preliminary reports have also indicated that forms of protein C with increased glycosylation are more prevalent in newborns than in adults. However, there has been very little research examining whether age-related PTMs are relevant in other coagulation proteins, and no reported studies in humans.

Why might developmental hemostasis exist?

As previously discussed, coagulation proteins such as serpins are examples of broadly acting proteins, and many have been shown to also have actions in multiple key biological processes such as inflammation, wound repair and angiogenesis.[17,62] Changing requirements of those systems could equally drive the genetically programmed developmental changes in the hemostatic system, which are therefore seen as

necessary compensations allowing normal hemostatic function. The fundamental question remains as to why the plasma levels of coagulation proteins differ with age.

The absence of tissue factor expression leads to embryonic lethality by days 8.5 to 10.5 in the mouse. Pools of red blood cells can be seen in the yolk sac of these mice embryos.[63] Most interesting was that these embryos lacked the large vitelline vessels that connect the yolk sac and embryonic vasculature, and no blood flow was seen in the yolk sac vessels. Thus, tissue factor is essential for vascular development and integrity during embryonic development. More recent mouse models would suggest this holds true for a number of coagulation proteins.[11] In contrast to tissue factor-null mice, factor VII-deficient mice survived to term, but the majority died in the first 24 hours from intra-abdominal hemorrhage, and the remaining died in the first 3 to 4 weeks of life.[64]

Antithrombin (AT) is a major plasma serine proteinase inhibitor (serpin), the three-dimensional structure of which was determined more than 15 years ago by two independent research groups.[65,66] Antithrombin inhibits thrombin and activated factor X (FXa) generated upon activation of the hemostatic system.[67] Antithrombin inhibits thrombin, and in the presence of unfractionated heparin (UFH), this ability to inhibit thrombin is increased by 1,000-fold.[68] Antithrombin is described as occurring in two distinct isoforms, native AT (NAT) or latent AT (LAT). Recent experiments demonstrate the concentration of the LAT isoform in the healthy population increases significantly with age, such that day 1–3 neonates, have 30% LAT compared to adult levels.[69] In addition to NAT and LAT, AT isolated from adults AT has been shown to circulate as two glycoforms;[70] α-AT has four identical sialylated complex oligosaccharides attached to asparagines, which account for 15% of the 58 kDa total mass; while ß-AT is only glycosylated on three of the potential four asparagine sites.[71] In adults, α-AT constitutes 90–95% of circulating AT, compared to only 5–10% ß-AT, yet ß-AT has higher affinity for UFH and endothelial surfaces, and is a more effective thrombin inhibitor.[71–73] This suggests physiologically and clinically specialized functions for the AT glycoforms, where ß-AT may be vital for controlling thrombogenic events arising from vessel wall injury, while α-AT may be largely responsible for inhibition of fluid-phase thrombin. The location of the carbohydrate side chain at Asn-135 in α-AT (absent in ß-AT) interferes with the binding of UFH due to its proximity to the heparin binding site.[74] As previously discussed, post-translational modifications, including glycosylation or deglycosylation of a single amino acid, particularly in close proximity to the heparin binding site of AT, has significant functional implications for the function of the AT molecule. However, there remains minimal data about the clinical significance of these changes, and in particular variations with age or health state.

Antithrombin has been shown to have potent antiangiogenic properties.[75] Antithrombin downregulates several proangiogenic genes and upregulates a number of antiangiogenic genes. The antiangiogenic forms of AT are known to include heparin binding sites, and heparin is shown to potentiate this effect.[75] This is one of the postulated mechanisms in the positive effect of heparinoids on cancer survival, which is independent of the antithrombotic effect.[76–78] Antithrombin levels are naturally reduced in newborns to less than 50% of the levels observed in adults, and then increase to approach adult levels by approximately 6 months of age.[7] Early evidence supports that there is a difference in the balance of isoforms of AT in newborns compared to adults. One potential explanation for the decreased levels of AT (and the altered balance of isoforms) observed in neonates is related to the role of this protein in angiogenesis.[37] Fetal and early neonatal life is a time of prolific angiogenesis, much more so than any later stage of life, and given the known antiangiogenic properties of AT, then variant forms, or reduced levels of this protein, may well be genetically predetermined at this age as adaptations that improve early survival and healthy development. Such considerations raise the possibility that AT replacement therapy may be detrimental during neonatal life. In the only published randomized trial of AT replacement therapy in newborn infants (as a treatment for lung disease of prematurity), there were seven (11.5%) deaths in the AT-treated group and three (4.9%) deaths in the placebo (no treatment) group.[79] A similar trial (reported only in abstract format) also reported a similar trend in the setting of a clinical trial; however, the mechanism for these findings was never established.[79]

In addition, the low frequency of these events renders a conclusion challenging as to a true difference in outcomes.

Nevertheless, there is a mounting case that age-related changes in the quantity, structure, and/or function of AT and TF are important in normal physiological development, with implications much broader than the coagulation system alone. It is highly possible that other proteins of the coagulation system are similarly important in this way.

Conclusion

The hemostatic system is composed of multiple components which, while often considered separately, are in fact intimately entwined. Each component of the system; vascular endothelium, platelets and the coagulation proteins appear to have significant age-associated changes that are considered physiological. At present we still have much to learn about the age-related changes to each individual component, let alone how their complex interactions change with age. We are hampered by our inability to test these components in physiological systems, and the limitations of currently available in vitro and ex vivo assays. The potential for developmental hemostasis to be a byproduct of developmental changes driven by growth and development within alternative related physiological systems such as angiogenesis is high. Thus we must consider the broader implications of manipulations of the hemostatic system in neonates and children. There remains much research to be performed in this field.

References

1. Bleyer WA, Hakami N, Shepard TH. The development of hemostasis in the human fetus and newborn infant. *J Pediatr*. Nov 1971;**79**(5):838–853.

2. Andrew M, Paes B, Milner R, et al. Development of the human coagulation system in the full-term infant. *Blood*. Jul 1987;**70**(1):165–172.

3. Andrew M, Vegh P, Johnston M, Bowker J, Ofosu F, Mitchell L. Maturation of the hemostatic system during childhood. *Blood*. Oct 1992;**80**(8):1998–2005.

4. Mari D, Mannucci PM, Coppola R, Bottasso B, Bauer KA, Rosenberg RD. Hypercoagulability in centenarians: the paradox of successful aging. *Blood*. Jun 1995;**85**(11):3144–3149.

5. Andrew M, Paes B, Johnston M. Development of the hemostatic system in the neonate and young infant. *Am J Pediatr Hematol/Oncol*. Spring 1990;**12**(1):95–104.

6. Andrew M, Paes B, Milner R, et al. Development of the human coagulation system in the healthy premature infant. *Blood*. Nov 1988;**72**(5):1651–1657.

7. Monagle P, Barnes C, Ignjatovic V, et al. Developmental haemostasis. Impact for clinical haemostasis laboratories. *Thromb Haemost*. Feb 2006;**95**(2):362–372.

8. Kisker CT. The animal models for hemorrhage and thrombosis in the neonate. *Thromb Haemost.* Feb 3 1987;**57**(1):118–122.

9. Goddard J, Lewis RM, Alcala H, Zeller RS. Intraventricular hemorrhage – an animal model. *Biol Neonate.* 1980;**37**(1–2):39–52.

10. Chan A, Jayasuriya K, Berry L, Roth-Kleiner M, Post M, Belik J. Volutrauma activates the clotting cascade in the newborn but not adult rat. *American J Physiol. Lung Cell Mol Physiol.* Apr 2006;**290**(4):L754–760.

11. Kashif M, Isermann B. Role of the coagulation system in development. *Thromb Res.* Jan 2013;**131** Suppl 1:S14–17.

12. Nitschmann E, Berry L, Bridge S, et al. Morphologic and biochemical features affecting the antithrombotic properties of the inferior vena cava of rabbit pups and adult rabbits. *Pediatr Res.* Jan 1998;**43**(1):62–67.

13. Nitschmann E, Berry L, Bridge S, et al. Morphological and biochemical features affecting the antithrombotic properties of the aorta in adult rabbits and rabbit pups. *Thromb Haemost.* May 1998;**79**(5):1034–1040.

14. van Hinsbergh VW. The endothelium: vascular control of haemostasis. *Eur J Obs Gyn, Repro Biol.* 2001;**95**(2):198–201.

15. Lisman T, Platto M, Meijers JC, Haagsma EB, Colledan M, Porte RJ. The hemostatic status of pediatric recipients of adult liver grafts suggests that plasma levels of hemostatic proteins are not regulated by the liver. *Blood.* Nov 10 2011;**117**(6):2070–2072.

16. Monagle P. Who controls the controllers? *Blood.* Feb 10 2011;**117**(6):1778–1779.

17. Taylor FB, Jr., Kinasewitz GT. The diagnosis and management of disseminated intravascular coagulation. *Curr Hematol Rep.* Sep 2002;**1**(1):34–40.

18. Nash MC, Wade AM, Shah V, Dillon MJ. Normal levels of soluble E-selectin, soluble intercellular adhesion molecule-1 (sICAM-1), and soluble vascular cell adhesion molecule-1 (sVCAM-1) decrease with age. *Clin Exp Immunol.* Jan 1996;**103**(1):167–170.

19. Boegehold MA. Endothelium-dependent control of vascular tone during early postnatal and juvenile growth. *Microcirculation (New York, N.Y.: 1994).* Jul 2010;**17**(5):394–406.

20. Allen Graeve JL, de Alarcon PA. Megakaryocytopoiesis in the human fetus. *Arch Dis Child.* Apr 1989;**64**(4 Spec No):481–484.

21. Murray NA, Roberts IA. Circulating megakaryocytes and their progenitors (BFU-MK and CFU-MK) in term and pre-term neonates. *Br J Haematol.* Jan 1995;**89**(1):41–46.

22. Deutsch VR, Olson TA, Nagler A, Slavin S, Levine RF, Eldor A. The response of cord blood megakaryocyte progenitors to IL-3, IL-6 and aplastic canine serum varies with gestational age. *Br J Haematol.* Jan 1995;**89**(1):8–16.

23. Joseph MA, Adams D, Maragos J, Saving KL. Flow cytometry of neonatal platelet RNA. *J Pediatr Hematol/Oncol.* Aug 1996;**18**(3):277–281.

24. Peterec SM, Brennan SA, Rinder HM, Wnek JL, Beardsley DS. Reticulated platelet values in normal and thrombocytopenic neonates. *J Pediatr.* Aug 1996;**129**(2):269–274.

25. Newall F, Barnes C, Ignjatovic V, Monagle P. Heparin-induced thrombocytopenia in children. *J Paediatr Child Health.* May–Jun 2003;**39**(4):289–292.

26. Chan KL, Summerhayes RG, Ignjatovic V, Horton SB, Monagle PT. Reference values for kaolin-activated thromboelastography in healthy children. *Anesth Analg.* Dec 2007;**105**(6):1610–1613, table of contents.

27. Ignjatovic V, Lai C, Summerhayes R, et al. Age-related differences in plasma proteins: how plasma proteins change from neonates to adults. *PLoS One.* 2011;**6**(2):e17213.

28. Reverdiau-Moalic P, Delahousse B, Body G, Bardos P, Leroy J, Gruel Y. Evolution of blood coagulation activators and inhibitors in the healthy human fetus. *Blood.* Aug 1 1996;**88**(3):900–906.

29. Forestier F, Daffos F, Galacteros F, Bardakjian J, Rainaut M, Beuzard Y. Hematological values of 163 normal fetuses between 18 and 30 weeks of gestation. *Pediatr Res.* Apr 1986;**20**(4):342–346.

30. Aballi AJ, De Lamerens S. Coagulation changes in the neonatal period and in early infancy. *Pediatr Clin North Am.* Aug 1962;**9**:785–817.

31. Beverley D, Inwood M, Chance G, Schaus M, O'Keefe B. 'Normal' haemostasis parameters: a study in a well-defined inborn population of preterm infants. *Early Hum Dev.* Apr 1984;**9**(3):249–257.

32. Ignjatovic V, Kenet G, Monagle P. Developmental hemostasis: recommendations for laboratories reporting pediatric samples. *J Thromb Haemost.* Feb 2012;**10**(2):298–300.

33. Katz JA, Moake JL, McPherson PD, et al. Relationship between human development and disappearance of unusually large von Willebrand factor multimers from plasma. *Blood.* May 15 1989;**73**(7):1851–1858.

34. Takahashi Y, Kawaguchi C, Hanesaka Y, et al. Plasma von Willebrand factor-cleaving protease is low in newborns. *Thromb Haemost.* 2001;**86**:285.

35. Weinstein MJ, Blanchard R, Moake JL, Vosburgh E, Moise K. Fetal and neonatal von Willebrand factor (vWF) is unusually large and similar to the vWF in patients with thrombotic thrombocytopenic purpura. *Br J Haematol.* May 1989;**72**(1):68–72.

36. Monagle P, Hagstrom. J. Developmental haemostasis. *Fetal and Neonatal Physiology.* 3rd edn. St. Louis: Elsevier; 2003: pp. 1435–1447.

37. Niessen RW, Lamping RJ, Peters M, Lamers WH, Sturk A. Fetal and neonatal development of antithrombin III plasma activity and liver messenger RNA levels in sheep. *Pediatr Res*. Apr 1996;**39**(4 Pt 1):685–691.

38. Sadowitz PD, Walenga RW, Clark D, Stuart MJ. Decreased plasma arachidonic acid binding capacity in neonates. *Biol Neonate*. 1987;**51**(6):305–311.

39. Schmidt B, Wais U, Pringsheim W, Kunzer W. Plasma elimination of antithrombin III (heparin cofactor activity) is accelerated in term newborn infants. *Eur J Pediatr*. Feb 1984;**141**(4):225–227.

40. Andrew M, Schmidt B, Mitchell L, Paes B, Ofosu F. Thrombin generation in newborn plasma is critically dependent on the concentration of prothrombin. *Thromb Haemost*. Feb 19 1990;**63**(1):27–30.

41. Xu L, Delorme M, Berry L. Thrombin generation in newborn and adult plasma in the presence of an endothelial surface. *Thromb Haemost*. 1991;**65**(6):1230.

42. Andrew M, Mitchell L, Berry L, et al. An anticoagulant dermatan sulfate proteoglycan circulates in the pregnant woman and her fetus. *J Clin Invest*. Jan 1992;**89**(1):321–326.

43. Delorme MA, Xu L, Berry L, Mitchell L, Andrew M. Anticoagulant dermatan sulfate proteoglycan (decorin) in the term human placenta. *Thromb Res*. May 15 1998;**90**(4):147–153.

44. Ignjatovic V, Greenway A, Summerhayes R, Monagle P. Thrombin generation: the functional role of alpha-2-macroglobulin and influence of developmental haemostasis. *Br J Haematol*. Aug 2007;**138**(3):366–368.

45. Moalic P, Gruel Y, Body G, Foloppe P, Delahousse B, Leroy J. Levels and plasma distribution of free and C4b-BP-bound protein S in human fetuses and full-term newborns. *Thromb Res*. Mar 1 1988;**49**(5):471–480.

46. Cvirn G, Gallistl S, Kostenberger M, Leschnik B, Kutschera J, Muntean W. Efficacy of the anticoagulation action of protein S is regulated by the alpha 2 macroglobulin level in cord and adult plasma. *Thromb Haemost*. 2001;Suppl P282 (abstract).

47. Distefano G, Romeo MG, Betta P, Rodono A, Amato M. Thrombomodulin serum levels in ventilated preterm babies with respiratory distress syndrome. *Eur J Pediatr*. Apr 1998;**157**(4):327–330.

48. Knofler R, Hofmann S, Weissbach G, et al. Molecular markers of the endothelium, the coagulation and the fibrinolytic systems in healthy newborns. *Semin Thromb Hemost*. 1998;**24**(5):453–461.

49. Nako Y, Ohki Y, Harigaya A, Tomomasa T, Morikawa A. Plasma thrombomodulin level in very low birthweight infants at birth. *Acta Paediatr*. Oct 1997;**86**(10):1105–1109.

50. Yurdakok M, Yigit S. Plasma thrombomodulin, plasminogen activator and plasminogen activator inhibitor levels in preterm infants with or without respiratory distress syndrome. *Acta Paediatr*. Sep 1997;**86**(9):1022–1023.

51. Yurdakok M, Yigit S, Aliefendioglu D, Dundar S, Kirazli S. Plasma thrombomodulin levels in early respiratory distress syndrome. *Turk J Pediatr*. Jan–Mar 1998;**40**(1):85–88.

52. Suarez CR, Menendez CE, Walenga JM, Fareed J. Neonatal and maternal hemostasis: value of molecular markers in the assessment of hemostatic status. *Semin Thromb Hemost*. Oct 1984;**10**(4):280–284.

53. Patel P, Weitz J, Brooker LA, Paes B, Mitchell L, Andrew M. Decreased thrombin activity of fibrin clots prepared in cord plasma compared with adult plasma. *Pediatr Res*. May 1996;**39**(5):826–830.

54. Bock SRC, et al. Antithrombin III and heparin cofactor II. *Hemostasis and Thrombosis: Basic Principles and Clinical Practice*. 4th edn. Philadelphia: Lippincott Williams and Wilkins; 2001: pp. 321–334.

55. Dang C, Shin C, Bell W, Nagaswami C, Weisel J. Fibrinogen sialic acid residues are low affinity calcium binding sites that influence fibrin assembly. *J Biol Chem*. 1989;**264**(25):15104–15108.

56. Witt I, Muller H. Phosphorus and hexose content of human foetal fibrinogen. *Biochim Biophys Acta*. Nov 1970;**221**(2):402–404.

57. Hamulyak K, Nieuwenhuizen W, Devilee PP, Hemker HC. Re-evaluation of some properties of fibrinogen, purified from cord blood of normal newborns. *Thromb Res*. Nov 1983;**32**(3):301–310.

58. Witt I, Muller H, Kunzer W. Evidence for the existence of foetal fibrinogen. *Thromb Diath Haemorrh*. Aug 1969;**22**(1):101–109.

59. Ignjatovic V, Ilhan A, Monagle P. Evidence for age-related differences in human fibrinogen. *Blood Coagul Fibrinol*. Mar 2011;**22**(2):110–117.

60. Andrew M, Mitchell L, Berry LR, Schmidt B, Hatton MW. Fibrinogen has a rapid turnover in the healthy newborn lamb. *Pediatr Res*. Mar 1988;**23**(3):249–252.

61. Manco-Johnson M, Spedale S, Peters M, et al. Identification of a unique form of protein C in the ovine fetus: developmentally linked transition to the adult form. *Pediatr Res*. 1995;**37**:685–691.

62. Monagle P, Ignjatovic V, Savoia H. Hemostasis in neonates and children: pitfalls and dilemmas. *Blood Rev*. Mar 2010;**24**(2):63–68.

63. Huang ZF, Higuchi D, Lasky N, Broze GJ, Jr. Tissue factor pathway inhibitor gene disruption produces intrauterine lethality in mice. *Blood*. Aug 1997;**90**(3):944–951.

64. Rosen ED, Chan JC, Idusogie E, et al. Mice lacking factor VII develop normally but suffer fatal perinatal bleeding. *Nature*. Nov 1997;**390**(6657):290–294.

65. Carrell RW, Stein PE, Fermi G, Wardell MR. Biological implications of a 3 A structure of dimeric antithrombin. *Structure*. Apr 1994;**2**(4):257–270.

66. Schreuder HA, de Boer B, Dijkema R, et al. The intact and cleaved human antithrombin III complex as a model for serpin–proteinase interactions. *Nat Struct Biol*. Jan 1994;**1**(1):48–54.

67. Olson ST, Bjork I, Shore JD. Kinetic characterization of heparin-catalyzed and uncatalyzed inhibition of blood coagulation proteinases by antithrombin. *Methods Enzymol*. 1993;**222**:525–559.

68. Levi M. All heparins are equal but some are more equal than others. *J Thromb Haemost*. 2003;**1**:884–885.

69. Karlaftis V, Attard C, Monagle P, Ignjatovic V. Latent antithrombin levels in children and adults. *Thromb Res*. Jan 2013;**131**(1):105–106.

70. Chan A, Berry L, Paredes N, Parmar N. Isoform composition of antithrombin in a covalent antithrombin–heparin complex. *Biochem Biophys Res Commun*. 2003;**309**(4):986–991.

71. Picard V, Ersdal-Badju E, Bock S. Partial glycosylation of antithrombin III asparaginase-135 is caused by the serine in the third position of its N-glycosylation consensus sequence and is responsible for production of beta-antithrombin III isoform with enhanced heparin activity. *Biochemistry*. 1995;**34**:8433–8440.

72. Carlson T, Atencio A, Simon T. Comparison of the behaviour in vivo of two molecular forms of antithrombin III. *Biochem J*. 1985;**225**(3):557–564.

73. Witmer MR, Hatton MW. Antithrombin III beta associates more readily than antithrombin III-alpha with uninjured and de-endothelialized aortic wall in vitro and in vivo. *Arterioscler Thromb*. 1991;**11**(3):530–539.

74. Turk B, Brieditis I, Bock SC, Olson ST, Bjork I. The oligosaccharide side chain on Asn-135 of alpha-antithrombin, absent in beta-antithrombin, decreases the heparin affinity of the inhibitor by affecting the heparin-induced conformational change. *Biochemistry*. Jun 1997;**36**(22):6682–6691.

75. Schedin-Weiss S, Richard B, Hjelm R, Olson ST. Antiangiogenic forms of antithrombin specifically bind to the anticoagulant heparin sequence. *Biochemistry*. Dec 2008;**47**(51):13610–13619.

76. Adcock DM, Fink LM, Marlar RA, Cavallo F, Zangari M. The hemostatic system and malignancy. *Clin Lymphoma Myeloma*. Aug 2008;**8**(4):230–236.

77. Akl EA, van Doormaal FF, Barba M, et al. Parenteral anticoagulation for prolonging survival in patients with cancer who have no other indication for anticoagulation. *Cochrane Database Syst Rev*. 2007(3):CD006652.

78. Wojtukiewicz MZ, Sierko E, Rak J. Contribution of the hemostatic system to angiogenesis in cancer. *Semin Thromb Hemost*. Feb 2004;**30**(1):5–20.

79. Schmidt B, Gillie P, Mitchell L, Andrew M, Caco C, Roberts R. A placebo-controlled randomized trial of antithrombin therapy in neonatal respiratory distress syndrome. *Am J Respir Crit Care Med*. Aug 1998;**158**(2):470–476.

80. Perlman M, Dvilansky A. Blood coagulation status of small-for-dates and postmature infants. *Arch Dis Child*. Jun 1975;**50**(6):424–430.

81. Carcao MD, Blanchette VS, Stephens D, et al. Assessment of thrombocytopenic disorders using the Platelet Function Analyzer (PFA-100). *Br J Haematol*. Jun 2002;**117**(4):961–964.

82. Salonvaara M, Riikonen P, Kekomaki R, et al. Effects of gestational age and prenatal and perinatal events on the coagulation status in premature infants. *Arch Dis Child Fetal Neonatal Ed*. Jul 2003;**88**(4):F319–323.

83. Flanders MM, Crist RA, Roberts WL, Rodgers GM. Pediatric reference intervals for seven common coagulation assays. *Clin Chem*. Sep 2005;**51**(9):1738–1742.

84. Flanders MM, Phansalkar AR, Crist RA, Roberts WL, Rodgers GM. Pediatric reference intervals for uncommon bleeding and thrombotic disorders. *J Pediatr*. Aug 2006;**149**(2):275–277.

85. Sosothikul D, Seksarn P, Lusher JM. Pediatric reference values for molecular markers in hemostasis. *J Pediatr Hematol/Oncol*. Jan 2007;**29**(1):19–22.

86. Mitsiakos G, Papaioannou G, Papadakis E, et al. Haemostatic profile of full-term, healthy, small for gestational age neonates. *Thromb Res*. Jul 2009;**124**(3):288–291.

87. Newall F, Johnston L, Ignjatovic V, Summerhayes R, Monagle P. Age-related plasma reference ranges for two heparin binding proteins – vitronectin and platelet factor 4. *Int J Lab Hematol*. 2008;**31**(6):683–687.

88. Ries M, Klinge J, Rauch R. Age-related reference values for activation markers of the coagulation and fibrinolytic systems in children. *Thromb Res*. Feb 15 1997;**85**(4):341–344.

89. Boos J, Pollmann H, Dominick HC. Vitamin K-dependent coagulation parameters during the first six days of life: incidence of PIVKA II in newborns. *Pediatr Hematol Oncol*. 1989;**6**(2):113–119.

Developmental hemostasis II

Marilyn J. Manco-Johnson

Introduction

Early in the study of hemostasis it was discovered that the coagulation system of children, and especially of newborn and young infants, differed remarkably from that of adults in both quantitative and qualitative features, and yet these differences were not pathologic under normal physiologic conditions and represented an ontogeny of hemostasis [1–10]. Maureen Andrew, in particular, made substantial contributions to the field by systematically assessing various coagulation parameters from preterm infants to adolescents [11–14]. Studies in this field have predominantly reported functional assays of the coagulation proteins, presumably due to the fact that these assays are commonly used in clinical practice. Measurements of immunological levels of the coagulation proteins reported to date are fewer, but include: fibrinogen; prothrombin; von Willebrand factor; tissue plasminogen activator; antithrombin; protein C; free and total protein S, soluble thrombomodulin; soluble endothelial protein C receptor; ADAMTS13; and tissue factor pathway inhibitor [15–25]. Antigen levels are concordant with functional activity in the well newborn infant.

Development of many physiologic systems, including coagulation, is a continuous process over the age span. However, perhaps at no other life phase are dynamic changes in coagulation or manifestations of altered coagulation as dramatic as during the adaptation from fetal to neonatal life. Pediatric thrombosis is primarily a disorder of hospitalized children with underlying medical conditions and triggering provocations. Neonatal thrombosis is similarly a disorder of intensively supported newborn infants with various developmental, genetic and acquired conditions. Multiple components of the hemostatic system differ markedly between healthy newborn infants and healthy children and adults. However, healthy newborn infants rarely manifest excessive bleeding or clotting. In contrast, the sick newborn infant has a predilection to bleeding and clotting, with the rate of thrombosis the highest observed during childhood prior to puberty. This discrepancy between physiologically altered ranges of individual and global coagulation assays in all newborn infants, and thrombotic complications limited to sick infants, along with the lack of animal models of many relevant human neonatal disorders, has made it difficult to assess the relationship between the neonatal hemostatic system and thrombotic disorders. In addition, prior to birth, the fetus is subjected to influences of pregnancy, labor and delivery that may be mediated through the maternal or fetal placental circulation, but which are difficult to detect and quantify. This chapter will describe the characteristics of the physiologic hemostatic system during the perinatal period, alterations that can be detected with thrombotic conditions and potential implications for diagnosis and management. Table 9.1 displays reference ranges for various coagulation parameters in preterm and term infants in comparison to healthy adults [15,16]. Figure 9.1 displays the phases of coagulation discussed below.

Primary hemostasis

The primary phase of hemostasis consists of the exposure of collagen and expression of cellular adhesive proteins on damaged and/or activated endothelium resulting in von Willebrand factor (vWF)-dependent and independent platelet adhesion, activation and aggregation. Platelet activation results in structural changes that support a procoagulant platelet surface that accelerates and localizes coagulation protein activations to the site of injury.

Fetal, neonatal and adult thrombopoiesis have been recently reviewed and highlight substantial biologic differences, including that neonates have higher

Pediatric Thrombotic Disorders, ed. Neil A. Goldenberg and Marilyn J. Manco-Johnson. Published by Cambridge University Press. © Cambridge University Press 2015.

Table 9.1 Coagulation screening tests and coagulation factor levels in fetuses, full-term newborns and adults

| Parameter | In utero fetuses (weeks' gestation) | | | Postnatal | |
	19–23 (n = 20)	24–29 (n = 22)	30–38 (n = 22)	Term newborns (n = 60)	Adults (n = 40)
PT (s)	32.5 (19–45)	32.2 (19–44)†	22.6 (16–30) †	16.7 (12.0–23.5) *	13.5 (11.4–14.0)
PT (INR)	6.4 (1.7–11.1)	6.2 (2.1–10.6) †	3.0 (1.5–5.0)*	1.7 (0.9–2.7) *	1.1 (0.8–1.2)
APTT (s)	168.8 (83–250)	154.0 (87–210) †	104.8 (76–128) †	44.3 (35–52) *	33.0 (25–39)
TCT (s)	34.2 (24–44) *	26.2 (24–28)	21.4 (17.0–23.3)	20.4 (15.2–25.0) †	14.0 (12–16)
Factor					
I (g/l, Von Clauss)	0.85 (0.57–1.50)	1.12 (0.65–1.65)	1.35 (1.25–1.65)	1.68 (0.95–2.45) †	3.0 (1.78–4.50)
I Ag (g/l)	1.08 (0.75–1.50)	1.93 (1.56–2.40)	1.94 (1.30–2.40)	2.65 (1.68–3.60) †	3.5 (2.50–5.20)
IIc (%)	16.9 (10–24)	19.9 (11–30) *	27.9 (15–50) †	43.5 (27–64) †	98.7 (70–125)
VIIc (%)	27.4 (17–37)	33.8 (18–48) *	45.9 (31–62)	52.5 (28–78) †	101.3 (68–130)
IXc (%)	10.1 (6–14)	9.9 (5–15)	12.3 (5–24) †	31.8 (15–50) †	104.8 (70–142)
Xc (%)	20.5 (14–29)	24.9 (16–35)	28.0 (16–36) †	39.6 (21–65) †	99.2 (75–125)
Vc (%)	32.1 (21–44)	36.8 (25–50)	48.9 (23–70) †	89.9 (50–140) †	99.8 (65–140)
VIIIc (%)	34.5 (18–50)	35.5 (20–52)	50.1 (27–78) †	94.3 (38–150)	101.8 (55–170)
XIc (%)	13.2 (8–19)	12.1 (6–22)	14.8 (6–26) †	37.2 (13–62) †	100.2 (70–135)
XIIc (%)	14.9 (6–25)	22.7 (6–40)	25.8 (11–50) †	69.8 (25–105) †	101.4 (65–144)
PK (%)	12.8 (8–19)	15.4 (8–26)	18.1 (8–28) †	35.4 (21–53) †	99.8 (65–135)
HMWK (%)	15.4 (10–22)	19.3 (10–26)	23.6 (12–34) †	38.9 (28–53) †	98.8 (68–135)
ATIII (%)	20.2 (12–31) *	30.0 (20–39)	37.1 (24–55) †	59.4 (42–80) †	99.8 (65–130)
HCII (%)	10.3 (6–16)	12.9 (5.5–20)	21.1 (11–33) †	52.1 (19–99) †	101.4 (70–128)
TFPI (ng/ml) ‡	21.0 (16.0–29.2)	20.6 (13.4–33.2)	20.7 (10.4–31.5) †	38.1 (22.7–55.8) †	73.0 (50.9–90.1)
PC Ag (%)	9.5 (6–14)	12.1 (8–16)	15.9 (8–30) †	32.5 (21–47) †	100.8 (68–125)
PC Act (%)	9.6 (7–13)	10.4 (8–13)	14.1 (8–18) *	28.2 (14–42) †	98.8 (68–129)
Total PS (%)	15.1 (11–21)	17.4 (14–25)	21.0 (15–30) †	38.5 (22–55) †	99.6 (72–118)
Free PS (%)	21.7 (13–32)	27.9 (19–40)	27.1 (18–40) †	49.3 (33–67) †	98.7 (72–128)
Ratio of free PS to total PS	0.82 (0.75–0.92)	0.83 (0.76–0.95)	0.79 (0.70–0.89) †	0.64 (0.59–0.98) †	0.41 (0.38–0.43)
C4b-BP (%)	1.8 (0–6)	6.1 (0–12.5)	9.3 (5–14)	18.6 (3–40) †	100.3 (70–124)

Values are the mean, followed in parentheses by the lower and upper boundaries including 95% of the population.
Abbreviations: Ag, antigenic value; Act, activity; c, coagulant activity.
* p < 0.05
† p < 0.01
‡ Twenty samples were assayed for each group, but only ten for 19- to 23-week-old fetuses.

concentrations of thrombopoietin, increased sensitivity to thrombopoietin, increased megakaryocyte proliferation with ability to generate ten-fold more megakaryocyte progenitors, smaller megakaryocyte size with decreased nuclear ploidy, and full cytoplasmic maturation without polyploidization [26]. The molecular mechanisms responsible for enhanced megakaryocyte production include developmentally regulated pathways and transcription factors that promote simultaneous proliferation and cytoplasmic maturation of megakaryocytes [26]. The fetus and neonate respond to thrombocytopenia by increasing the number, but not the size, of megakaryocytes.

Circulating platelets have been determined in 10- to 12-week fetuses [27]. Plasma platelet counts rise early in gestation and have consistently been reported

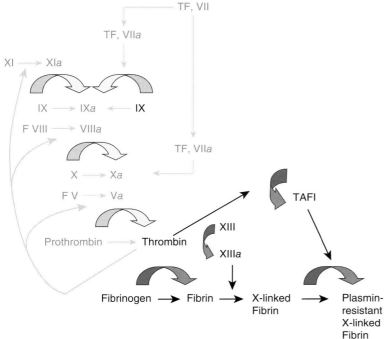

Initiation of coagulation

TF, VII — TF-bearing cell: activated monocyte, exposed sub-endothelial cell

Amplification/propagation of coagulation

Activated platelet surface

Fibrin clot generation

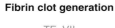

Figure 9.1 Phases of coagulation. Pathways highlighted in black depict the protein activations and products of each phase of coagulation. TF = tissue factor.

Coagulation regulation

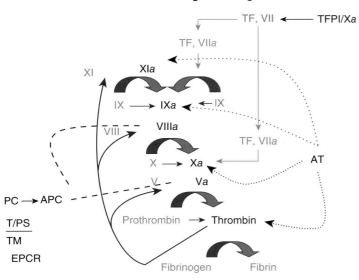

Figure 9.1 (cont.)

within the normal adult reference range of 150–450,000/μl by 20 weeks of fetal life [12,27,28]. However, a recent large study of 47,291 neonates delivered at 22 to 42 weeks' gestation has determined wider ranges of variability, with the 5th percentile being 104,200/μl for infants less than or equal to 32 weeks' gestation, and 123,100/μl for infants 33–42 weeks' gestation; the 95% reached 750,000/μl [29].

Neonatal platelet function has been recently reviewed [26,30,31]. Platelet glycoprotein (GP) receptors Ib and IIb/IIIa as well as the platelet antigen PL^{A1} can be detected on fetal platelets by 16 weeks [32]. The density of fetal platelet receptors varies, with GPIb increased on fetal platelets, the IIb/IIIa complex equal to adult density, and protease activatable receptors, PAR-1 and PAR-4, decreased on fetal platelets [32,33]. In addition, neonatal platelets show decreased aggregation to epinephrine, thrombin, ADP and collagen in conventional lumiaggregometry studies. Platelet function abnormalities have been related to a number of mechanisms, including decreased numbers of alpha-adrenergic receptors in the case of epinephrine, decreased mobilization of normal calcium stores in the case of collagen, decreased PAR receptors in relationship to platelet aggregation to thrombin and decreased downstream signaling from

the thromboxane receptor [33–37]. Differences in the function of platelets from preterm infants mirror those of term infants, but are generally more pronounced [26,34,38]. Platelet function abnormalities differ not only by gestational age, but also by postnatal age, with resolution of most deficiencies by 10–14 days in the report of Bednarek and colleagues but noted to be persistent in healthy children well into childhood by Hézard and others [38,39].

Despite observed decreases in platelet reactivity, platelet function in either the template bleeding time or PFA100 platelet function analyzer is enhanced in stable newborn infants, although a high frequency of thrombocytopenia has been reported in sick preterm infants at risk for intracranial hemorrhage [40–42]. Vascular function in the newborn infant is characterized by increased levels of prostaglandins PGI$_2$ and PGE$_2$, which fall gradually following term birth [43]. Preterm infants are characterized by even higher concentrations of PGI$_2$ and PGE$_2$, as well as increased sensitivity to the vasodilating effects of PGE$_2$ [44]. Neonatal platelet function is most likely enhanced by higher hematocrit and increased plasma concentration of vWF, along with larger vWF multimeric size [11, 12,44,45]. The vWF multimeric size decreases to the adult range by 8 weeks postnatally [44].

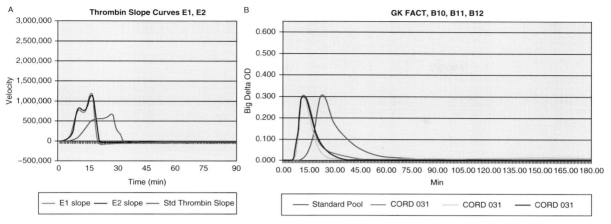

Figure 9.2 Thrombin generation and plasma coagulability in the newborn infant and adult. **A:** First derivative (velocity) of thrombin generation in the newborn infant (yellow/blue) and adult standard pooled plasma (red). **B:** Plasma clot formation and lysis (CloFAL) in the newborn infant (blue/green/yellow) and adult standard pooled plasma (red). (A black and white version of this figure will appear in some formats. For the color version of Figure 9.2, please refer to the plate section.)

The following implications of alterations in primary hemostasis for neonatal thrombosis and antithrombotic therapy can be hypothesized or concluded:

- Increased hematocrit, vWF concentration and vWF multimers support normal to increased primary-phase hemostasis in the term newborn infant.
- In addition to small neonatal arterial caliber, acquired decreases in PGI_2, with elevations in thromboxane TXA_2 associated with hypoxia and sepsis, probably account for the frequent onset of vasospasm with blanched or cyanotic legs following placement of an umbilical or femoral artery catheter in the newborn infant.
- Decreased platelet function and a high frequency of thrombocytopenia in sick preterm infants during their first 2 weeks of life account for the higher risk of bleeding, particularly intracranial hemorrhage, associated with anticoagulant or fibrinolytic therapy in this neonatal population.
- Decreased platelet reactivity and frequent thrombocytopenia in the sick newborn infant render the use of antiplatelet therapy less attractive in this age group.

Secondary hemostasis: Initiation phase of coagulation

Coagulation is initiated by exposure of the cellular transmembrane protein tissue factor (TF) to circulating factor VII in the blood, resulting in rapid autoactivation to activated factor VII (FVIIa) and, via the activation of factor X (FXa), in small amounts of the key procoagulant enzyme thrombin. The TF activity of blood originates from TF-bearing microparticles derived from monocytes or endothelial cells or from a truncated form of the extracellular portion of the TF molecule known as soluble TF.

The TF expression is increased in fetal monocytes and endothelial cells [46,47]. Plasma concentration of soluble TF is increased in the embryo and fetus [48]. Thrombin generation occurs more rapidly in fetal and neonatal plasma, and this has been shown to be due to increased TF activity with decreased tissue factor pathway inhibitor (TFPI), as well as low levels of antithrombin (AT) and protein C (PC) [49–51]. Because the ultimate amount of thrombin generated is dependent upon prothrombin concentration, which is at a mean of 50% adult level at term gestation [11], the newborn infant generates less total thrombin but generates thrombin more rapidly. Enzymatic thrombin generation and plasma clot formation are shown on Figure 9.2, which shows earlier formation of thrombin and clot peaks in the healthy term infant, compared with the healthy child or adult [52,53]. The TF/FVIIa complex additionally activates a small amount of factor IX (FIXa) directly, contributing to increased thrombin generation via activations of FX and prothrombin; plasma concentrations of FIX are very low in preterm and term infants.

The following implications of alterations in the initiation phase of hemostasis for neonatal thrombosis and antithrombotic therapy can be hypothesized or concluded:

• Higher levels of circulating TF activity with lower levels of inhibitors, especially TFPI, may tip the balance of hemostasis in the newborn infant toward hypercoagulability and thrombosis, especially in the frequent clinical settings of sepsis and hypoxia.

• Low levels of AT may heighten and/or prolong the procoagulant activity of early thrombin generation and may limit the efficacy of AT-dependent anticoagulants.

Secondary hemostasis: Amplification and propagation phase of coagulation

In the amplification phase of coagulation, the small amount of the enzyme thrombin generated in the initiation phase of coagulation catalyzes a number of coagulation reactions in a cell-based model that localizes key enzymes and substrates to each other at sites of bleeding [54]. Thrombin activates the procoagulant cofactors, factor V (FV) and factor VIII (FVIII), which increase the rate of thrombin formation 1,000-fold via the tenase and prothrombinase complexes. Thrombin additionally activates the serine proteases, factors XI, IX, X and prothrombin (FII). Activated factor XI (FXIa) increases the amount of factor IXa, generated. Factor IXa anchored to the procoagulant platelet phospholipid surface via FVIIIa, efficiently activates FX to FXa. Factor Xa, similarly anchored to the procoagulant platelet phospholipid surface via FVa, efficiently activates prothrombin to thrombin. The procoagulant polymorphisms factor V Leiden (FVL) and prothrombin 20210 (PTM) prolong the generation of thrombin. The FVL generates a FVa molecule that is resistant to inactivation by a mutation in an activated protein C cleavage site, while the PTM in the promoter region of FII results in a higher concentration of prothrombin, which will result in more active thrombin molecules.

Concentrations of FV and FVIII are within the adult normal range in term infants and near the normal range in preterms [11,12,16,28]. In contrast, concentrations of FXI, FIX, FX and prothrombin are 30% and 50% of normal adult mean in preterm and term infants, respectively [11,12,16,28]. The global screening test, the activated partial thromboplastin time (APTT), is substantially prolonged in the newborn infant, owing to the low levels of procoagulant factors

[11,12,28]. In contrast, the prothrombin time in which activation is driven by tissue factor is only modestly prolonged.

The mechanism(s) for decreased plasma levels of coagulation factors remains unclear. Investigations of hepatic mRNA in humans and animals support active gene translation of coagulation factors in the fetus and neonate in comparison with the adult [55,56]. Studies of protein clearance support rapid clearance of certain coagulation factors, notably fibrinogen, protein C and antithrombin, but not of prothrombin [55,57,58].

Functionality of the coagulation proteins, FII, FVII, FIX, FX, PC, protein S (PS) and protein Z (PZ), is dependent on post-translational vitamin K (VK)-dependent gamma carboxylation. Almost 3% of healthy term infants demonstrate biochemical evidence of VK deficiency with circulation of non-carboxylated prothrombin and other VK-dependent proteins along with more exaggerated decreases in protein clotting function [18]. Under-carboxylated prothrombin and protein C were reported in 7% and 27%, respectively, of cord bloods of healthy term infants and correlated positively with gestational age [59]. There is a steep placental gradient of vitamin K [60,61]. Plasma activities of VK-dependent proteins rise rapidly following VK repletion in deficient newborns, supporting that VK-dependent protein carboxylation and secretion are linked. Other classes of proteins share gamma carboxylation including osteocalcin and matrix Gla proteins, as well as GAS-6, the ligand for tyrosine kinase cell receptors, Tyr, Axl, and Mer. It has been hypothesized that vitamin K-dependent proteins may be critical to embryogenesis, cell proliferation and differentiation, and that vitamin K restriction in utero may be a physiologic protection against mutagenesis during rapid cellular proliferation. The VK-dependent factors increase at a variable rate such that factors VII and X achieve adult levels in the first weeks after birth and free protein S concentration is greater than normal adult levels at 3 months, while levels of prothrombin and protein C do not achieve the adult reference range until puberty, such that the 50th percentile of protein C activity and antigen levels in the child between 6 months and 11 years equals the 10th percentile for normal adult [11,14]. Flanders et al. assayed functional activities of protein C, protein S and AT in 887 healthy children aged 7 to 17 years in comparison to 120 adults [62]. In this large pediatric population, median protein C activity was found to be significantly lower than adult at all ages (7–9, 10–11, 12–13, 14–15 and 16–17 years), with a statistically significant increase in protein C for each year of life of 1.41 U/ml (CI: 0.87–1.94). Neonates are recommended to receive supplemental vitamin K at birth to prevent skin, gastrointestinal and intracranial hemorrhage that is characteristic of vitamin K deficiency.

The following implications of alterations in the amplification phase of hemostasis for neonatal thrombosis and antithrombotic therapy can be hypothesized or concluded:

- Low levels of factors XII, XI and IX result in APTT prolongation by unfractionated heparin (UFH) that is often greater than the anti-Xa activity and not representative of the anticoagulant activity. Therefore, most pediatric hematologists monitor UFH in the newborn infant with anti-Xa activity and increasingly rely on low molecular weight heparin (LMWH) as the subacute anticoagulant for newborn infants with thromboembolic disorders.
- Because of physiologically low levels of vitamin K-dependent proteins, unreliable intake and variable gastrointestinal absorption, it is difficult to achieve safe, stable anticoagulation using warfarin anticoagulation in newborn and young infants.
- The prothrombotic contribution of FVL and PTM as single thrombophilic traits is not known definitively, but these two traits by themselves are probably not strong risk factors for perinatal thrombosis.

Regulation of coagulation

Components of the procoagulant protein system (secondary hemostasis) can be divided into three groups: initiation by TF/FVIIa, serial enzymatic activations by serine proteases (XIa, IXa, Xa and IIa) and amplification by activated cofactors (FVIIIa and FVa). Each of these procoagulant groups has its own regulation. The TF/FVIIa system is regulated by TFPI. The TFPI when complexed with FXa forms a quarternary complex with a complex of TF with FVIIa. The serine proteases are all inactivated by AT and this inactivation is catalyzed by physiologic glycosaminoglycans, such as heparin sulfate and dermatan sulfate, on the endothelial cell surface. The AT acts as a pseudosubstrate, and following cleavage of AT by serine proteases, an irreversible complex is formed which is cleared from the circulation by serpin receptors on Kupfer cells in the liver. Finally, the activated cofactors FVa and FVIIIa

are inactivated via cleavage by activated PC (APC). The PC is activated when bound to the endothelial transmembrane receptor thrombomodulin (TM). The activation of PC and subsequent inactivation of FVa and FVIIIa is augmented by the PC cofactor protein S (PS) as well as the endothelial PC receptor (EPCR) and protein Z (PZ).

Developmental deficiencies in coagulation regulation are among the more striking features of neonatal hemostasis and have been deemed most likely responsible for the peak in thrombosis during the neonatal period. Activity of TF is increased in neonatal plasma, while TFPI is decreased such that the TF pathway plays an important role in the hypercoagulability of the newborn, particularly in settings of TF expression with sepsis or hypoxia. Antithrombin is present at about 50% of adult level in the term infant and shows normal structure and function in the newborn infant [63]. The sick preterm infant is at risk for acquired AT deficiency with consumptive coagulopathy, which conveys a poor prognosis for intracranial hemorrhage and mortality [64,65]. In addition, heparin has an increased volume of distribution and accelerated clearance from newborn plasma [17]. The combination of accelerated heparin clearance with physiologically low and frequently pathologically depressed levels of AT accounts for the considerable difficulty in achieving therapeutic anticoagulation with UFH during the neonatal period. The PC system is least developed in the preterm and term infant, and shows the most delayed postnatal maturation (see secondary hemostasis, above) [11,12,14,16,19,20].

There are likely multiple pathways affecting plasma levels of coagulation proteins. Expression of most coagulation factors in the fetus is regulated at the level of transcription rather than translation [66]. The regulatory mechanisms of plasma and cellular expression for most coagulation proteins during states of health and disease have yet to be determined and could have profound implications for understanding and treating various neonatal disease states. Studies of the fetal and neonatal lamb determined that plasma levels of AT increase linearly throughout gestation and during the neonatal period parallel to similar increases in fetal and neonatal hepatic mRNA for AT [56]. In this model, plasma levels of PS showed rapid plasma increases just prior to and following spontaneous delivery at birth, although hepatic mRNA was dramatically increased to five times the maternal level throughout the third trimester of gestation, suggesting an inhibitory mechanism on mRNA translation or protein synthesis, release or clearance prior to birth [56]. Studies in the ovine (sheep) fetus indicated that plasma levels of PC are expressed early in gestation but persist at a very low level until a gestationally determined maturation, which coincides with signaling of labor and delivery. While hepatic mRNA showed increased expression around term gestation, plasma concentrations of PC actually decreased with very slow postnatal rise [56,67]. The perinatal ovine shifts in fetal hepatic mRNA expression of PC were developmentally linked to physiologic term birth and may be responding to corticosteroids or other hormonal triggers of labor. Models of normal and diabetic pregnancies in the ovine model determined that insulin levels correlated inversely with levels of vitamin K-dependent proteins, PC, PS and FX, in the ewe and lamb, with insulin accounting for 12% of the physiologic regulation of PC; AT levels were not affected by insulin [68]. In contrast, the ovine model of diabetic pregnancy showed modest but significant increases in fibrinogen and factor V, VII and XI associated with elevated insulin levels [69]. The abnormalities were most pronounced in conditions of maternal hyperglycemia and hyperinsulinemia. An increase in procoagulant proteins and decrease in PC may account, in part, for the high rate of thrombosis found in infants of mothers with gestational diabetes.

In addition, there are subtle structural differences between the fetal and adult forms of PC in both the human and the sheep due to developmentally regulated post-translational alterations, which may impact protein kinetics or levels [67,70]. These are similar to described post-translational alterations in fibrinogen forms seen between the newborn infant and the adult [71]. Mean levels of PC are 40% of adult in healthy term infants, but are commonly undetectable (less than 10%) in sick preterm infants; in this setting severe acquired PC deficiency appears to be a risk factor for perinatal thrombosis [19,20]; PC activation may partially compensate for low plasma PC levels. Cellular thrombomodulin is widely distributed in early fetal life; soluble thrombomodulin is more than three times the healthy adult concentration by the end of the second trimester, and then slowly decreases throughout gestation, infancy and childhood to reach adult levels by adolescence [72].

The following implications of alterations in the regulation of coagulation for neonatal thrombosis and antithrombotic therapy can be hypothesized or concluded:

- TF-mediated coagulation activation is dominant in newborn infants. Disorders that express increased amounts of TF, such as sepsis, inflammation and vascular damage by catheters, provide strong prothrombotic signals that easily overwhelm the relatively underdeveloped TF regulation.
- The availability of plasma-derived, viral-inactivated replacement concentrates for AT and PC offers the potential for supportive care of severe genetic or acquired deficiency, particularly in settings where anticoagulation is contraindicated or ineffective.
- Genetic deficiencies of coagulation regulatory proteins, PC, PS and AT, can present with in utero or perinatal stroke and renal vein thrombosis [73–78]. Severe (homozygous and compound heterozygous) deficiencies of PC and PS have presented shortly after birth with disseminated intravascular coagulation and purpura fulminans [76–78]. These disorders require prompt recognition and confirmation, as replacement and anticoagulant treatment is associated with good thrombotic and quality of life outcomes (see also Chapter 13 on severe thrombophilias).
- Although it would be reasonable to hypothesize that sick preterm infants with severe acquired AT deficiency and consumptive coagulopathy would have improved outcomes with AT replacement, such therapy, while safe, has not improved outcomes, including mortality, blood replacement needs or days of mechanical ventilation [79,80]. Furthermore, targeting supraphysiologic levels of AT via replacement therapy has been associated with a non-significant trend toward increased bleeding, suggesting that the therapeutic inhibitor replacement should target physiologic levels in healthy infants [81].

Fibrin clot formation

The pivotal procoagulant enzyme, thrombin, is critical to formation of the stable fibrin clot. Thrombin cleaves the N-terminal region (or E domain) of the Aα chain of fibrinogen to expose a polymerization site located in the Aα and Bβ chains [82]. The polymerization site in the E domain combines non-covalently with a complementary binding pocket on the γ chain in the D domain of an adjacent molecule. These lateral associations between the D and E domains of fibrinogen form the staggered overlapping fibrin double strands.

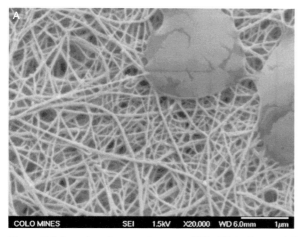 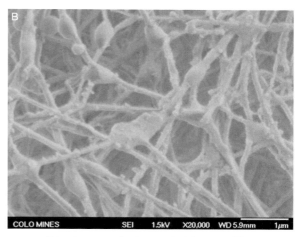

Figure 9.3 Scanning electron microscopy (EM) of fibrin clots made from neonatal blood compared with normal adult. **A**: EM of fibrin clot made from normal pooled adult plasma. **B**: EM of fibrin clot made from normal cord plasma.

Thrombin also activates factor XIII which cross-links lysine and glutamine residues of the Aα and γ chains of fibrin, thus stabilizing the clot [83].

Fibrin clots from neonatal blood are more transparent and have decreased tensile strength [84]. Fibrinogen has been isolated from cord blood and determined to differ from the adult molecule with increased sialic acid and phosphorus, thinner fibrils and decreased N-terminal alanine residues in the Aα chain [84]. Figure 9.3 shows a fibrin clot from cord blood in comparison to normal adult fibrin and discloses differences in fibrin fibril thickness and organization. The thrombin time is slightly prolonged at birth and reaches the adult range by 3 weeks postnatal age. However, data regarding a unique fetal form of fibrinogen are not consistent, and altered function of fibrinogen from cord plasma was not found using careful purification techniques by Hamulyak and colleagues; this group duplicated functional abnormalities by the addition of large molecular weight fibrin degradation fragments [85]. It is likely that such abnormalities in earlier studies could be related to the propensity of the sick newborn infant to coagulation activation and consequent fibrinogen cleavage.

The following implications of fibrin formation for neonatal thrombosis and antithrombotic therapy can be hypothesized or concluded:

- Although there are several indicators of defective clot formation in the newborn infant, these findings probably are of limited clinical significance, as the sick newborn manifests an increased rate of thrombosis relative to older infants and children.

- Despite evidence for defective fibrin clot formation, the stable infant does not bleed excessively.

- The sick preterm infant is also prone to bleeding, especially intracranial hemorrhage, and the question of supporting fibrin clot formation in a manner that is hoped to not appreciably increase thrombotic risk, for example with factor XIII supplementation, has not been addressed.

Fibrin dissolution and fibrinolysis

Fibrin clot lysis with restoration of vascular blood flow is an essential component of hemostasis. Fibrin is the primary regulator of fibrinolysis. Plasminogen, the precursor form of the fibrinolytic serine protease plasmin, binds with high affinity to partially degraded fibrin. Similarly, the activator of plasminogen, tissue plasminogen activator (tPA), binds with high affinity to clot-bound plasminogen. Both tPA and plasminogen bind to lysine-rich residues on fibrin. The tPA, following release from endothelial cells in response to stasis or agonists such as exercise or DDAVP, cleaves fibrin-bound plasminogen to yield plasmin, which in turn cleaves fibrin. Fibrinolysis is inhibited by a number of regulators. The thrombin activatable fibrinolytic inhibitor (TAFI) is activated by thrombin bound to TM [86]. Activated TAFI (TAFIa) removes lysine residues, thus limiting the binding of plasminogen to fibrin and tPA to plasminogen. The TAFI activation, by complexes of thrombin with TM, is dominant in medium and large vessels with low TM concentration, while PC activation predominates in small vessels where TM concentration is high. Thus, clot persistence is promoted in large vessels and fibrinolysis is favored in small vessels. The tPA is regulated by complex formation with its inhibitor, plasminogen activator inhibitor type 1 (PAI-1), such that only free or unbound tPA participates in plasmin activation. The PAI-1 is additionally regulated by binding to APC, whereby APC binding to PAI-1 effectively increases the concentration of free tPA. Plasmin is inhibited by α_2-antiplasmin.

Plasma concentrations of plasminogen are approximately 40% at term [11,15,28]. A fetal form of plasminogen has been reported with reduced activation to plasmin and slower inactivation by antiplasmin in association with increased sialic acid [87,88]. Experiments utilizing both adult and fetal fibrin as well as adult and fetal plasminogen suggest that differences in glycosylation, if any, are minor [89]. The more recent work found that differences in the activation of fetal and adult plasmin are less dramatic than previously reported and primarily result in a prolonged lag phase of enzyme activation for the fetal form, while interactions of both fetal and adult plasmin with fibrin of either fetal or adult origin are similar [89]. Interestingly a similar prolonged lag phase of plasmin activation is determined in plasma of patients with uncontrolled diabetes mellitus that normalizes with glucose control and, to a lesser extent, by in vitro non-enzymatic glycosylation of plasma, supporting that differences in activation of fetal plasminogen are most likely caused by subtle alterations in glycosylation. Plasma concentrations of TAFI have shown a median of 27% of adult levels at birth [90]. In this study, median levels of PAI-1 activity and antigen were also low, although the range was broad. Other studies of cord blood have determined brisk tPA activity with relatively lower PAI-1 activity, although these levels may likely be affected by the process of labor and delivery [91]. As noted above, levels of PC are low in the term and preterm infant, demonstrate subtle differences in molecular form and are vulnerable to consumption. In vitro neonatal fibrinolysis as demonstrated on euglobulin clot lysis time or whole plasma fibrinolysis is brisk [15,28,90]. However, in vitro lysis of newborn clots by therapeutic thrombolytic agents has been reported to be reduced compared with effects on adult clots [92]. Clinically, low levels of plasminogen are often replaced using fresh frozen plasma during neonatal fibrinolytic therapy [93]. Twenty-two neonates in two series treated

with systemic thrombolysis for arterial and atrial thrombi have shown 86% rate of complete lysis with 4.5% major hemorrhage [94,95]. Not unexpectedly, higher rates of bleeding have been reported for preterm infants treated during the first week of life [96].

The following implications of fibrinolysis for neonatal thrombosis and antithrombotic therapy can be hypothesized or concluded:

- Although quantitative and qualitative deficiencies in neonatal fibrinolysis have been reported, physiologic fibrinolysis is probably balanced with thrombus formation in the stable term and preterm infant.
- Newborn infants undergoing low-dose tPA therapy have often responded to somewhat higher dosing compared with older children [93,94].
- Therapeutic thrombolysis can be maximized by replacing low levels of plasminogen in fresh frozen plasma.
- Poor resolution of neonatal renal vein and other perinatal venous thrombi may relate to prenatal onset and clot organization before birth, as well as to delayed thrombus diagnosis and/or institution of therapy.
- Careful consideration should be given to the use of therapeutic thrombolysis in the newborn infant with an expected increased risk of intracranial hemorrhage.

Conclusions and future directions

Despite marked differences in antigen levels, functional activities and plasma half-lives of multiple coagulation components between newborn infants and adults, functional hemostasis is remarkably robust in the newborn infant, and abnormal bleeding or clotting is rare. Experiments conducted in chronically catheterized stable fetal animals support a conclusion that altered plasma protein expression is a function of ontogeny, is developmental and physiologic, and not the result of perinatal immaturity or perturbation of the hemostatic system. Unique features of the newborn hemostatic system likely reflect different functions of coagulation proteins in fetal and neonatal development, as these features are preserved across species.

However, the stressed infant is prone to both bleeding and clotting complications, many of which are life-threatening. The challenge of future neonatal hemostasis research is to define physiologic requirements for optimal hemostasis in the newborn infant and the unique mechanisms by which hemostatic balance is achieved during perinatal life. Increasingly, as new therapies for which evidence is derived in adults and children are applied to thrombotic disorders in the newborn infant, it is imperative to understand the uniquely balanced hemostatic system of the infant, in order to maximize safety and efficacy of new therapeutic products and procedures as applied to this unique age group.

References

1. Aballi AJ, De Lamerens S. Coagulation changes in the neonatal period and early infancy. Pediatr Clin North Am 1962;**9**:785–817.

2. Barnard DR, Simmons MA, Hathaway WE. Coagulation studies in extremely preterm infants. Pediatr Res 1979;**13**:1330–5.

3. Niederhoff H, Künzer W. Physiology of hemostasis in newborn infants. I. Monatsschr Kinderheilkd 1985;**133**:130–6.

4. Robertson BR, Pandolfi M, Nilsson IM. "Fibrinolytic capacity" in healthy volunteers at different ages as studied by standardized venous occlusion of arms and legs. Acta Med Scand 1972;**191**(3):199–202.

5. Bucher U, Robert Y, Riedwyl H. Retention of platelets by glass beads. Variation with the age of the individual. Thromb Diath Haemorrh 1973;**29**(3):671–8.

6. Podolsak B, Mingers AM, Oller J. Thrombocyte functions, thromboelastograms and fibrinogen of healthy children in different age groups. Eur J Pediatr 1977;**127**(1):27–39.

7. Podolsak B, Peter G, Oller J. Correlations between age-dependent protein and lipid concentrations in plasma and platelet functions in children. Eur J Pediatr 1979;**132**(1):21–35.

8. Muntean W. Haemostasis in premature and newborn babies. Padiatr Padol 1980;**15**(2):109–20.

9. Ambrus CM. Ontogeny of fibrinolysin system and its role in pathogenesis of hyaline membrane disease of infants. Fed Proc 1966;**25**:68–72.

10. von Kaulla KN, von Kaulla E, Butterfield J. Fibrinolytic activity, thrombin inhibitor and kinetics of clot formation in premature infants with respiratory distress syndrome. Acta Paediatr Scand 1965 Nov;**54**(6):587–92.

11. Andrew M, Paes B, Milner R, Johnston M, Mitchell L, Tollefsen DM, Powers P. Development of the human coagulation system in the full term infant. Blood 1987;**70**:165–72.

12. Andrew M, Paes B, Milner R, Johnston M, Mitchell L, Tollefsen DM, Castle V, Powers P. Development of the human coagulation system in the healthy premature infant. Blood 1988;**72**:1651–7.

13. Andrew M, Paes B, Johnston M. Development of the hemostatic system in the neonate and young infant. Am J Pediatr Hematol/Oncol 1990;**12**:95–104.

14. Andrew M, Vegh P, Johnston M, Bowker J, Ofosu F, Mitchell L. Maturation of the hemostatic system during childhood. Blood 1992;**80**:1998–2005.

15. Reverdiau-Moalic P, Gruel Y, Delahousse B, Rupin A, Huart MC, Body G, Leroy J. Comparative study of the fibrinolytic system in human fetuses and in pregnant women. Thromb Res 1991;**61**:489–99.

16. Reverdiau-Moalic P, Delahousse B, Body G, Bardos P, Leroy J, Gruel Y. Evolution of coagulation activators and inhibitors in the healthy human fetus. Blood 1996;**88**:900–6.

17. McDonald MM, Jacobson LJ, Hay WW, Jr., Hathaway WE. Heparin clearance in the newborn. Pediatr Res 1981;**15**:1015–18.

18. Shapiro AD, Jacobson LJ, Armon ME, Manco-Johnson MJ, Hulac P, Lane PA, Hathaway WE. Vitamin K deficiency in the newborn infant: prevalence and perinatal risk factors. J Pediatr 1986;**109**:675–80.

19. Manco-Johnson MJ, Marlar RA, Jacobson LJ, Hays T. Severe protein C deficiency in newborn infants. J Pediatr 1988;**113**:359–63.

20. Manco-Johnson MJ, Abshire TC, Jacobson LJ, Marlar RA. Severe neonatal protein C deficiency: prevalence and thrombotic risk. J Pediatr 1991;**119**:793–8.

21. Sthoeger D, Nardi M, Karpatkin M. Protein S in the first year of life. Br J Haematol 1989;**72**:424–8.

22. Sosothikul D, Seksarn P, Lusher JM. Pediatric reference values for molecular markers in hemostasis. J Pediatr Hematol/Oncol 2007;**19**:22.

23. Klarmann D, Eggert C, Geisen C, Becker S, Seifried E, Klingebiel T, Kreuz W. Association of ABO (H) and I blood group system development with von Willebrand factor and factor VIII plasma levels in children and adolescents. Transfusion 2010;**50**:1571–80.

24. Ishii A, Yamada S, Yamada R, Fujibayashi S, Hamada H. t-PA activity and antigen in the newborn and infant. J Perinat Med 1992;**20**:465–9.

25. Nowak-Göttl U, Vielhaber H. Elevated levels of soluble thrombomodulin in plasma from children with Arg 506 to Gln mutation in the factor V gene. Eur J Haematol 1997;**58**:51–5.

26. Sola-Visner M. Platelets in the neonatal period: developmental differences in platelet production, function and hemostasis and the potential impact of therapies. Hematology Am Soc of Hematol Educ Program 2012;**1**:506–11.

27. Bleyer WA, Hakami N, Shepard TH. The development of hemostasis in the human fetus and newborn infant. J Pediatr 1971;**79**:838–53.

28. Hathaway WE, Bonnar J. Hemostatic disorders of the pregnant woman and newborn infant. New York, NY: Elsevier Science Publishing Company; 1987, pp. 57–75.

29. Wiedmeier SE, Henry E, Sola-Visner MC, Christensen RD. Platelet reference ranges for neonates, defined using data from over 47,000 patients in a multihospital healthcare system. J Perinatol 2009;**29**:130–6.

30. Strauss T, Sidlik-Muscatel R, Kenet G. Developmental hemostasis: primary hemostasis and evaluation of platelet function in neonates. Semin Fetal & Neonatal Medicine 2011;**16**:301–4.

31. Ferrer-Marin F, Stanworth S, Josephson C, Sola-Visner M. Distinct differences in platelet production and function between neonates and adults: implications for platelet transfusion practice. Transfusion 2013; epub ahead of print, doi:10.1111/trf.12343. accessed 10/21/2013.

32. Gruel Y, Boizard B, Daffos F, Forestier F, Caen J, Wautier JL. Determination of platelet antigens and glycoproteins in the human fetus. Blood 1986;**68**:488–92.

33. Schlagenhauf A, Schweintzger S, Birner-Gruenberger R, Leschnik B, Muntean W. Newborn platelets: Lower levels of protease-activated receptors cause hypoaggregability to thrombin. Platelets 2010;**21**:641–7.

34. Sitaru AG, Holzhauer S, Speer CP, Singer D, Obergfell A, Walter U, Grossmann R. Neonatal platelets from cord blood and peripheral blood. Platelets 2005;**16**:203–10.

35. Gelman B, Setty BN, Chen D, Amin-Hanjani S, Stuart MJ. Impaired mobilization of intracellular calcium in neonatal platelets. Pediatr Res 1996;**39**:692–6.

36. Israels SJ, Odaibo FS, Robertson C, McMillan EM, McNicol A. Deficient thromboxane synthesis and response to platelets from premature infants. Pediatr Res 1997;**41**:218–23.

37. Corby DG, O'Barr TP. Decreased alpha-adrenergic receptors in newborn platelets: cause of abnormal response to epinephrine. Dev Pharmacol Ther 1981;**2**:215–25.

38. Bednarek FJ, Bean S, Barnard MR, Frelinger AL, Michelson AD. The platelet hyporeactivity of extremely low birth weight neonates is age-dependent. Thromb Res 209;**124**:42–5.

39. Hézard N, Potron G, Schlegel N, Amory C, Leroux B Nguyen P. Unexpected persistence of platelet hyporeactivity beyond the neonatal period: a flow cytometric study in neonates, infants and older children. Thromb Haemost 2003;**90**:116–23.

40. Fuesner JH. Normal and abnormal bleeding times in neonates and young children utilizing a fully standardized template technic. Am J Clin Pathol 1980;**74**:73–7.

41. Israels SJ, Cheang T, McMillarn-Ward EM, Cheang M. Evaluation of primary hemostasis in neonates with a new in vitro platelet function analyzer. J Pediatr 2001;**138**:116–9.

42. McDonald MM, Johnson ML, Rumack CM, Koops BL, Guggenheim MA, Babb C, Hathaway WE. Role of coagulopathy in newborn intracranial hemorrhage. Pediatrics 1984;**74**:26–31.

43. Majed BH, Khalil RA. Molecular mechanisms regulating the vascular prostacyclin pathways and their adaptation during pregnancy and in the newborn. Pharmacol Rev 2012;**64**:540–82.

44. Katz JA, Moake JL, McPherson PD, Weinstein MJ, Moise KJ, Carpenter RJ, Sala DJ. Relationship between human development and disappearance of unusually large von Willebrand factor multimers from plasma. Blood 1989;**73**:1851–8.

45. Weinstein MJ, Blanchard R, Moake JL, Vosburgh E, Moise K. Fetal and neonatal von Willebrand factor (vWF) is unusually large and similar to the vWF in patients with thrombotic thrombocytopenic purpura. Br J Haematol 1989;**72**:68–72.

46. Rivers RP, Hathaway WE. Studies on tissue factor activity and production by leukocytes of human umbilical cord and adult origin. Pediatr Res 1975;**9**:167–71.

47. Grabowski EF, Carter CA, Tsukurov O, Conroy N, Hsu CY, Abbott W, et al. Comparison of human umbilical vein and adult saphenous vein endothelial cells: implications for newborn hemostasis and for models of endothelial cell function. J Pediatr Hematol/Oncol 2000;**22**:266–8.

48. Luther T, Flossel C, Mackman N, Bierhaus A, Kasper M, Albrecht S, et al. Tissue factor expression during human and mouse development. Am J Pathol 1996;**149**:101–3.

49. Streif W, Paes B, Berry L, Andrew M, Andreasen RB, Chan AKC. Influence of exogenous factor VIIa on thrombin generation in cord plasma of full-term and pre-term newborns. Blood Coag Fibrinol 2000;**11**:349–57.

50. Cvirn G, Gallistl S, Leschnik B, Muntean W. Low tissue factor pathway inhibitor (TFPI) together with low antithrombin allows sufficient thrombin generation in neonates. J Thromb Haemost 2003;**1**:263–8.

51. Cvirn G, Callistl S, Muntean W. Effects of antithrombin and protein C on thrombin generation in newborn and adult plasma. Thromb Res 1999;**93**:183–90.

52. Simpson ML, Goldenberg NA, Jacobson LJ, Bombardier CG, Hathaway WE, Manco-Johnson MJ. Simultaneous thrombin and plasmin generation capacities in normal and abnormal states of coagulation and fibrinolysis in children and adults. Thromb Res 2011;**127**:317–23.

53. Goldenberg NA, Hathaway WE, Jacobson L, Manco-Johnson MJ. A new global assay of coagulation and fibrinolysis. Thromb Res 2005;**116**:345–56.

54. Hoffman M, Monroe DM III. A cell-based model of hemostasis. Thromb Haemost 2001;**85**:958–65.

55. Karpatkin M, Lee M, Cohen L, McKinnell J, Nardi M. Synthesis of coagulation proteins in the fetus and neonate. J Pediatr Hematol/Oncol 2000;**22**:276–80.

56. Manco-Johnson MJ, Jacobson LJ, Hacker MR, Townsend SF, Murphy J, Hay WW, Jr. Development of coagulation regulatory proteins in the fetal and neonatal lamb. Pediatr Res 2002;**52**:580–88.

57. Andrew M, Mitchell L, Berry LR, Schmidt B, Hatton MW. Fibrinogen has a rapid turnover in the healthy newborn lamb. Pediatr Res 1988;**23**:249–52.

58. Manco-Johnson MJ, Hacker MR, Jacobson LJ, Hay WW, Jr. Pharmacokinetics of protein C and antithrombin in the fetal lamb: a model to predict human neonatal replacement dosing. Neonatology 2009;**95**:279–85.

59. Bovill EG, Soll RF, Lynch M, Bhushan F, Lancesman M, Frije M, et al. Vitamin K1 metabolism and the production of descarbosy prothrombin and protein C in the term and premature neonate. Blood 1993;**81**:77–83.

60. Shearer MJ, Rahim S, Barkhan P, Stimmler L. Plasma vitamin K1 in mothers and their newborn babies. Lancet 1982;**2**(8296):460–3.

61. Mandelbrot L, Buillaumont M, Leclercq M, Lefrere JJ, Gozin D, Daffos F, Forestier F. Placental transfer of vitamin K1 and its implications in fetal hemostasis. Thromb Haemost 1988;**60**:39–43.

62. Flanders MM, Phansalkar AR, Crist RA, Roberts WL, Rodgers GM. Pediatric reference intervals for uncommon bleeding and thrombotic disorders. J Pediatr 2006;**149**:275–7.

63. McDonald MM, Hathaway WE, Reeve EB, Leonard BD. Biochemical and functional study of antithrombin III in newborn infants. Thromb Haemost 1982;**47**:56–8.

64. McDonald MM, Johnson ML, Rumack CM, Koops BL, Guggenheim MA, Babb C, Hathaway WE. Role of coagulopathy in newborn intracranial hemorrhage. Pediatrics 1984;**74**:26–31.

65. Peters M, Ten Cate JW, Breederveld C, DeLeeuw R, Emeis J, Koppe J. Low antithrombin III levels in neonates with idiopathic respiratory distress syndrome: poor prognosis. Pediatr Res 1984;**18**:273–6.

66. Kawamoto S, Matsumoto Y, Miuno K, Okubo K, Matsubara K. Expression profiles of active genes in human and mouse livers. Gene 1996;**174**:151–8.

67. Manco-Johnson MJ, Spedale S, Peters M, Townsend SF, Jacobson LJ, Christian J, Krugman SD, Hay WW, Jr., Sparks JW. Identification of a unique form of protein C in the ovine fetus: developmentally linked transition to the adult form. Pediatr Res 1995;**37**:365–72.

68. Manco-Johnson MJ, Carver T, Jacobson LJ, Townsend SF, Hay WW, Jr. Hyperglycemia-induced hyperinsulinemia decreases maternal and fetal plasma protein C concentration during ovine gestation. Pediatr Res 1994;**36**:293–9.

69. Kisker CT, Manco-Johnson M. Effect of hyperinsulinemia on the development of blood coagulation in the lamb fetus. Pediatr Res 1995;**38**:169–72.

70. Greffe BS, Marlar RA, Manco-Johnson MJ. Neonatal protein C: molecular composition and distribution in normal term infants. Thromb Res 1989;**56**:91–8.

71. Grieninger G, Lu X, Cao Y, Fu Y, Kudryk BJ, Galanakis DK, Hertzberg KM. Fib 420, the novel fibrinogen subclass: newborn levels are higher than adult. Blood 1997;**90**:2609–14.

72. Menashi S, Aurousseau MH, Gozin D, Daffos F, D'Angelo A, Forestier F, Boffa MC. High levels of circulating thrombomodulin in human foetuses and children. Thromb Haemost 1999;**81**:906–9.

73. Olivieri M, Bidlingmaier C, Schetzeck S, Borggräfe I, Geisen C, Kurnik K. Arterial thrombosis in homozygous antithrombin deficiency. Hämostaseologie 2012;**32**(Suppl 1):S79.

74. Orlando C, Lissens W, Hasaerts D, Jochmans K. Identification of two de novo mutations responsible for type I antithrombin deficiency. Thromb Haemost 2012;**107**:187–8.

75. Kumar R, Moharir M, Yau I, Williams S. A novel mutation in the Serpin C1 gene presenting as unprovoked neonatal cerebral sinus venous thrombosis in a kindred. Pediatr Blood Cancer 2013;**60**:133–6.

76. Hartman K, Manco-Johnson MJ, Rawlings JS, Bowen DR, Marlar RA. Homozygous protein C deficiency: early treatment with warfarin. Amer J Pediatr Hematol/Onc 1989;**11**(4):395–401.

77. Mahasandana C, Suvatte V, Marlar RA, Manco-Johnson MJ, Jacobson L, Hathaway WE. Neonatal purpura fulminans associated with homozygous protein S deficiency. Lancet 1990;**335**:61–2.

78. Goldenberg NA, Manco-Johnson MJ. Protein C deficiency. Haemophilia 2008;**14**:1214–21.

131

79. Niebler RA, Christensen M, Berens R, Wellner H, Mikhailov T, Tweddell JS. Antithrombin replacement during extracorporeal membrane oxygenation. Artif Organs 2011;**35**:1024–8.

80. St. Peter SD, Little DC, Calkins CM, Holcomb GW III, Snyder CL, Ostlie DJ. The initial experience of antithrombin III in the management of neonates with necrotizing enterocolitis. J Pediatr Surg 2007;**42**:704–8.

81. Schmidt B, Gillie P, Mitchell L, Andrew M, Caco C, Roberts R. A placebo-controlled randomized trial of antithrombin therapy in neonatal respiratory distress syndrome. Am J Respir Crit Care Med 1998;**158**:470–6.

82. Mosesson MW, Siebenlist KR, Meh DA. The structure and biologic features of fibrinogen and fibrin. Annals NY Acad Sci 2001;**936**:11–30.

83. Schroeder V, Kohler HP. New developments in the area of factor XIII. J Thromb Haemost 2013;**11**:234–44.

84. Burnstein M, Lewis S, Walter P. Sur l'existence du fibriogène foetal. Sang 1954;**25**:102.

85. Hamulyák K, Nieuwenhuizen W, Devilée PP, Hemker HC. Re-evaluation of some properties of fibrinogen, purified from cord blood of normal newborns. Thromb Res 1983;**32**:301–10.

86. Colucci M, Semeraro N. Thrombin activatable fibrinolytic inhibitor: at the nexus of fibrinolysis and inflammation. Thromb Res 2012;**129**:314–19.

87. Benavent A, Estelles A, Aznar J, Martinez-Sales V, Gilabert J, Fornas E. Dysfunctional plasminogen in full term newborn-study of active site of plasmin. Thromb Haemost 1984;**51**:67–70.

88. Ries M. Molecular and functional properties of fetal plasminogen and its possible influence on clot lysis in the newborn period. Semin Thromb Haemost 1997;**23**:247–52.

89. Ries M, Easton RL, Lonstaff C, Zenkar M, Corran PH, Morris HR, Dell A, Gaffney PJ. Differences between neonates and adults in tissue-type-plasminogen activator (t-PA)-catalyzed plasminogen activation with various effectors and in carbohydrate sequences of fibrinogen chains Thromb Res 2001;**103**:173–84.

90. Smith AA, Jacobson LJ, Miller BI, Hathaway WE, Manco-Johnson MJ. A new euglobulin clot lysis assay for global fibrinolysis. Thromb Res 2003;**112**:3299–37.

91. Åstedt B, Lindoff C. Plasminogen activators and plasminogen activator inhibitors in plasma of preterm and term newborns. Acta Pædiatr 1997;**86**:111–13.

92. Andrew M, Brooker L, Leaker M, Paes B, Weitz J. Fibrin clot lysis by thrombolytic agents is impaired in newborns due to a low plasminogen concentration. Thromb Haemost 1992;**68**:325–30.

93. Manco-Johnson MJ. How I treat venous thrombosis in children. Blood 2006;**107**:1–9.

94. Wang M, Hays T, Balasa V, Bagatell R, Gruppo R, Grabowski EF, Valentino LA, Tsao-Wu G, Manco-Johnson MJ, for the Pediatric Coagulation Consortium. Low-dose tissue plasminogen activator thrombolysis in children. J Pediatr Hematol/Oncol 2003;**25**:379–86.

95. Hartmann J, Hussein A, Trowitzsch E, et al. Treatment of neonatal thrombus formation with recombinant tissue plasminogen activator: six years experience and review of the literature. Arch Dis Child Fetal Neonatal Ed 2001;**85**:F18–22.

96. Zenz W, Arlt F, Sodia S, Berghold A. Intracerebral hemorrhage during fibrinolytic therapy in children: a review of the literature of the last thirty years. Semin Thromb Hemost 1997;**23**:321–32.

Chapter 1

Pediatric thrombophilia evaluation: Considerations for primary and secondary venous thromboembolism prevention

Ulrike Nowak-Göttl, Gili Kenet, and Neil A. Goldenberg

Introduction

Venous thromboembolism (venous TE; VTE) is a rare disease that was increasingly recognized and diagnosed in pediatrics in the past decade, usually as a secondary complication of primary underlying diseases such as sepsis, cancer, congenital heart disease, elevated endogenous testosterone, or after therapeutic interventions such as central venous lines (Table 10.1) [1–13]. Pediatric VTE is a severe disease for which long-term outcomes include lack of thrombus resolution in 50% of cases and the development of post-thrombotic syndrome (PTS) in nearly one-fourth of patients [8–11]. Within the entire childhood population, neonates are at the greatest risk for VTE (5.1/100,000 live births per year in Caucasian children) [1,2,6,14], with a second peak in incidence during puberty and adolescence. The annual incidence of venous events was estimated to be 0.07 to 0.14 per 10,000 children, or 5.3 per 10,000 hospital admissions of children and 24 per 10,000 admissions of neonates to neonatal intensive care units [1,6,12–14].

To date, the results of single studies on the risk of VTE onset and recurrence associated with inherited thrombophilia (IT) are contradictory or inconclusive, mainly due to lack of statistical power. Apart from acquired thrombophilic abnormalities such as antiphospholipid antibodies [15–17], deficiencies of antithrombin, protein C, or protein S and the coagulation factor V (G1691A), and factor II (G20210A) variants have been established as risk factors for incident VTE events in adults [18–23]. The ITs have been described as additional risk factors in populations of children with provoked and unprovoked VTE, with and without underlying disease [24–56].

Follow-up data for VTE recurrence in children are available from a few reports and suggest a recurrence rate of approximately 3% in neonates, 6–11% at 2 years in largely unselected cases (provoked and unprovoked incident VTE), and 21% in children with unprovoked VTE [7,10,12,13,38,48,49,51,54,56].

Role of developmental hemostasis on the risk of VTE in children

The coagulation system of children evolves with age, as evidenced by marked physiological differences in the concentration of the majority of blood clotting proteins, a concept known as "developmental hemostasis" [57,58] (see also Chapters 8 and 9). Evidence suggests that these age-related changes in protein concentration are not isolated to the coagulation system, but are in fact evident across multiple protein systems within the plasma proteome. There are numerous proteins which change in plasma abundance with age [59]. These age-related differences in the plasma proteome may not just be limited to childhood. Studies of centenarians suggest that age-related changes also continue through adult life [60]. In general, the hemostatic system in neonates is a balanced physiologic system despite low concentrations of plasma coagulation proteins with prolonged prothrombin time and partial thromboplastin time. On one hand, apart from the risk periods previously mentioned [1,2,6,14], there is evidence that children are protected from thrombosis. For example, patients with congenital AT, protein C, or protein S deficiencies, or with activated protein C resistance (APCR) [61–65] usually do not present with unprovoked thrombosis until late teenage years or even later, except in severe/moderately severe deficiency states. In addition, VTE secondary to

Pediatric Thrombotic Disorders, ed. Neil A. Goldenberg and Marilyn J. Manco-Johnson. Published by Cambridge University Press. © Cambridge University Press 2015.

Table 10.1 Pooled odds ratios and 95% confidence intervals (in brackets) for genetic traits and persistent antiphospholipid antibodies associated with a first TE onset in children and in pediatric patients with recurrent TE

Inherited* thrombophilia	OR (cerebrovascular occlusion) fixed-effects model (95% CI)	OR (VTE) fixed-effects model (95% CI)
First TE onset		
Protein C deficiency	9.3 [4.8–18.0]	7.7 [4.4–13.4]
Protein S deficiency	3.2 [1.2–8.4]	5.8 [3.0–11.0]
Antithrombin deficiency	7.1 [2.4–22.4]	9.4 [3.3–26.7]
Factor V G1691A	3.3 [2.6–4.1]	3.6 [3.8–4.8]
Factor II G20210A	2.4 [1.7–3.5]	2.6 [1.6–4.4]
Lipoprotein(a)	6.5 [4.5–8.7]	4.5 [3.3–6.2]
LA/aPL*	6.6 [3.5–12.4]	4.9 [2.2–10.9]
≥ Two inherited ITs	11.9 [5.9–23.7]	9.5 [4.9–18.4]
TE recurrence		
Protein C deficiency	–	2.4 [1.2–4.4]
Protein S deficiency	–	3.1 [1.5–6.5]
Antithrombin deficiency	–	3.0 [1.4–6.3]
Factor V G1691A	–	1.4 [0.9–2.0]
Factor II G20210A	4.3 [1.1–16.2]	1.9 [1.01–3.5]
Lipoprotein(a)	–	0.8 [0.5–1.4]
≥ Two inherited ITs	–	4.5 [2.9–6.9]

Abbreviations: OR: odds ratio; IT: inherited thrombophilia; LA/aPL: lupus anticoagulants/antiphospholipid antibodies; TE: thromboembolism; VTE: venous thromboembolism.
*LA/aPL are acquired thrombophilic traits.
(Source: References 73–75.)

acquired risk factors occurs considerably less frequently in children compared to adults. For example, VTE in patients with underlying kidney disease occurs in only 2% of children compared with approximately 20% of adults [66–71]. Furthermore, prepubertal children undergoing abdominal or orthopedic surgery do not standardly receive primary thromboprophylaxis with anticoagulation because secondary thromboses are rare in this age group [72]. Thus, for comparable risk factors, whether inherited or acquired, thrombotic risk is substantially reduced in children compared to adults, which suggests the presence of protective mechanisms [73].

Role of acquired and inherited thrombophilia in incident pediatric TE

The distribution of IT varies in different countries, with respect to the population genetic background and the number of patient/controls investigated.

In three recent systematic reviews and meta-analyses including observational studies in pediatric patients with VTE and arterial ischemic stroke, more than 70% of patients had at least one clinical risk factor [73–75]. The pooled odds ratios (OR) showed statistically significant associations of factor V G1691A, factor II G20210A, deficiencies of protein C, protein S, and antithrombin, elevated lipoprotein(a), and combined IT with incident TE [75]. The presence of acquired lupus anticoagulants/ antiphospholipid antibodies (APA) was also found by meta-analysis to be associated with incident TE [76]. As further detailed in Table 10.1, the pooled OR (single IT) for VTE onset ranged from 2.4 for the factor II G20210A variant (cerebrovascular occlusion) to 9.4 in children with antithrombin deficiency (VTE). In addition, the pooled OR for persistent antiphospholipid antibodies/lupus anticoagulants was 6.6 for children with cerebrovascular occlusion and 4.9 for pediatric cases with VTE [74,75]. However, given the low incidence of VTE in healthy children, the authors do not routinely perform "screening" (i.e., testing in asymptomatic individuals with no prior VTE events) for IT or APA in children who have a negative family history of early VTE (see also later section on role of IT in setting of positive family history of VTE).

Role of IT in pediatric VTE recurrence

Recent meta-analyses have demonstrated statistically significant associations with recurrent VTE for inherited deficiencies of protein C (OR: 2.4), protein S, (OR: 3.1) or antithrombin (OR:3.0); the factor II variant (OR: 2.1) and combined IT [73]. Interestingly, in all three pediatric meta-analyses of observational studies, age at first thromboembolic onset, publication year, or study country were all found to not significantly alter the strength of association between the aforementioned ITs and recurrence risks. Given these meta-analysis findings, as well as individual study findings of a high risk of recurrent VTE in children with unprovoked incident VTE (particularly with combined IT) [38], the authors typically perform IT "diagnostic evaluation" (i.e., testing in affected individuals with VTE) in children with unprovoked VTE. Furthermore, given that VTE recurrence is not rare in children with provoked incident VTE, and given also that the presence of IT other than factor V G1691A and lipoprotein(a) have been found in the aforementioned meta-analyses to increase VTE recurrence risk, the authors also routinely perform this limited IT testing in such children in order to inform patient/parent counseling and evaluation of management considerations based upon associated risks of recurrent VTE. (For further details, please see also section below on Potential implications for treatment.)

Other prognostic biomarkers of coagulation and fibrinolysis in pediatric VTE recurrence

In a single-institution cohort study published in the *New England Journal of Medicine* in 2004 [48], Goldenberg *et al.* evaluated the relationship of plasma factor VIII activity and D-dimer concentration in children with thrombosis (mostly venous, and including both provoked and unprovoked

events) with long-term outcomes. Adverse outcome was defined as a composite endpoint of thrombus persistence upon completion of 3–6 months anticoagulation, recurrence, and/or (among patients with thrombi involving the upper/lower venous systems) the occurrence of PTS. Confirming previous findings in adults with symptomatic VTE, the findings of this study indicated that a plasma factor VIII level of more than 150 IU per deciliter and a plasma D-dimer level of more than 500 ng per milliliter, separately or together, are significant and independent risk factors for a poor composite poor outcome (one or more of the aforementioned outcomes) in children with thrombosis. Elevated factor VIII levels, D-dimer levels, or both early in the course of the disease were highly predictive of a poor outcome, but remained predictive at 3–6 months post-event, with odds ratios ranging from 4.7 to 6.1 for a poor outcome. Further studies are warranted to clarify the role of elevated factor VIII and D-dimer levels in predicting recurrent VTE specifically (and separately in groups of children with provoked and unprovoked incident VTE). In addition, the interaction of these markers of coagulation activation and fibrinolysis with inherited or acquired thrombophilias should be explored among pediatric age groups and various ethnic backgrounds.

Role of acquired and inherited thrombophilia and biomarkers of coagulation and fibrinolysis in pediatric post-thrombotic syndrome (PTS)

A recent systematic review has indicated that PTS occurs in 23% of children following upper/lower extremity deep venous thrombosis [77]. Limited evidence exists regarding prognostic factors for PTS in children. An early study implicated biomarkers of hypercoagulability and/or inflammation (specifically, D-dimer and FVIII) [48], and a small prospective series suggested a protective effect of acute thrombolytic approaches in occlusive proximal limb DVT [78]. Very recently, a bi-institutional cohort study reported preliminary findings that acute presence of the lupus anticoagulant (assessed by dilute Russell viper venom time) is associated with a significantly increased risk of clinically significant PTS [79].

135

Role of IT in asymptomatic children with family histories of early-onset (including pediatric-onset) VTE: Potential implications for risk assessment in primary VTE prevention

In a recent cohort study, 533 first- and second-degree relatives of 206 white pediatric VTE patients were tested for IT (deficiencies of antithrombin, protein C, and protein S; the factor V G1691A and factor II G20210A variants), and the incidence of symptomatic VTE was determined relative to IT status. The risk for VTE was significantly increased among family members with, versus without, IT (hazard ratio [HR] 7.6, 95% confidence interval [CI]: 4.00–14.45; p < 0.001), and was highest among carriers of antithrombin, protein C, or protein S deficiency (HR 25.7, 95% CI: 12.2–54.2; p < 0.001). Annual incidences of VTE were 2.82% (95% CI: 1.63–4.80%) among family members found to be carriers of antithrombin, protein C, or protein S deficiency, 0.42% (95% CI: 0.12–0.53%) for factor II G20210A, 0.25% (95% CI: 0.12–0.53%) for factor V G1691A, and 0.10% (95% CI: 0.06–0.17%) in relatives with no IT [80].

In addition, a single-institution study has found that multiple thrombophilias are common in children with a positive family history of early-onset VTE [81], warranting consideration of IT testing and episodic primary thromboprophylaxis with anticoagulation in these children during future episodes of heightened thrombotic risk (e.g., prolonged immobility; central venous catheterization). Nevertheless, the safety and efficacy of such an approach has not been established, and also awaits further validation of VTE risk models in children.

A particularly difficult and not uncommon clinical question concerns the advisability of IT testing in a child following early extensive or fatal thrombosis (often massive PE) in a first-degree relative. There are no data with which to guide decisions in this setting, although the importance of positive family history in predicting thrombosis risk, irrespective of thrombophilia findings, has been reported [82].

The genome-wide perspective of pediatric VTE

Since approximately 2007 there has been a remarkable advance in our ability to dissect the genetic basis of common traits and complex thrombotic and hemostatic disorders. In other fields, genome-wide association studies (GWAS) have successfully identified numerous novel loci with modest to large effect sizes associated with common disease phenotypes. Venous thromboembolism and arterial ischemic stroke are illustrative of multifactorial diseases, in which multiple heritable and environmental risk factors affect the overall disease risk.

Inherited thrombophilia is known to run within families and a small proportion of familial IT can be attributed to rare but highly penetrant genetic variants, such as in protein C or antithrombin deficiency. However, environmental triggers play an important role in thrombogenesis [83]. Very recently, results were presented from a GWAS using the Illumina 660W Infinium SNP array in a large family-based sample comprising 241 nuclear families with pediatric VTE [84]. Using this family-based approach, four SNPs exceeded the threshold for genome-wide significance using 100,000 bootstrap permutations ($p < 10^{-5}$), interpreted as most likely true associations. Among these, two SNPs residing in a region on chromosome 6q13 comprising the gene for beta-1,3-glucoronyltransferase 2, a member of the human natural killer 1 carbohydrate pathway, were associated with pediatric VTE, with genome-wide significance for the corresponding GA haplotype of this gene. In addition, rs1565242, an SNP residing in the 3'UTR of a hypothetical gene on chromosome 15, was also associated with VTE in white children. Future large-scale pediatric genomic analysis of putative ITs will help to expand the current knowledge of risks for incident and recurrent VTE in children.

Potential implications for treatment

Adult patients with a first episode of VTE will receive oral anticoagulation for at least 3 months, 6 to 12 months in the case of idiopathic VTE, and at least 6 to 12 months following pulmonary embolism [85]. Decisions on extending anticoagulant therapy are individually based on the perceived risks of VTE recurrence and anticoagulant-related bleeding. Whether long-term continuation of anticoagulant treatment should be considered after a first VTE in carriers of a thrombophilic trait is still a matter of debate [86,87].

In children, the presence of mild IT should not generally warrant (in the opinion of the authors and according to recent American College of Chest Physician [ACCP] guidelines) an extended duration of anticoagulation in children, beyond the typically recommended durations of 3–6 months (usually 3 months) for a first VTE occurrence and 6–12 months (usually 6 months) for VTE recurrence. However, such children may warrant episodic, transient secondary thromboprophylaxis with anticoagulation during future times of heightened prothrombotic risk (i.e., re-exposure to VTE provocations). In addition, contrary to ACCP guidelines, the authors often extend duration of anticoagulation beyond a recommendation of 6–12 months in children with a first episode of unprovoked VTE in whom more severe ITs (e.g., presumed or documented homozygous or compound heterozygous anticoagulant deficiencies, homozygous factor V Leiden, or factor II G20210A variants) or multiple ITs (two or more) are disclosed. This practice is based upon findings from the DURAC trial in adult VTE suggesting a substantially increased recurrence risk among patients with homozygous ITs [88], as well as German multicenter prospective cohort study data indicating a greatly increased recurrence risk in children with multiple ITs [38].

In children with a first VTE, definitively powered randomized controlled clinical trials (RCTs) are lacking and treatment guidelines are mainly adapted from adults [89,90]. More than in adults, the prolonged use of anticoagulant treatment in a highly physically active (and often injury-prone) pediatric population must be weighed against the risk of bleeding. In the absence of highest-quality evidence from RCTs, it is hoped that findings of the meta-analyses cited above will help physicians to decide along with parents and patients in which cases prolonged anticoagulant treatment and/or the use of episodic secondary prophylactic anticoagulation may be warranted [73–75]. In addition, future multicenter RCTs should investigate the influence of IT on VTE outcomes, in a setting in which anticoagulant treatment duration is standardized; indeed, this serves as one of the exploratory aims of the ongoing Kids-DOTT trial (NCT00687882).

Conclusions

Recent meta-analyses have shown deficiencies of antithrombin, protein C, and protein S, presence of the factor V G1691A and factor II G20210A variants, elevated lipoprotein(a), and combined IT to be significantly associated with incident VTE and (except for factor V G1691A and lipoprotein(a)) with recurrent VTE as well. Given the low incidence of VTE in healthy children, the authors do not routinely perform

IT screening in asymptomatic children with no prior VTE events and a negative family history of early VTE. However, given the high risk of recurrent VTE in children with unprovoked incident VTE (particularly with combined IT), the authors do typically perform IT diagnostic testing in children with unprovoked VTE. Further, given that VTE recurrence is not rare in children with provoked incident VTE and that the presence of IT other than factor V G1691A and lipoprotein(a) have been found in meta-analyses to increase this risk, the authors also routinely perform this limited IT testing in such children. Nevertheless, given the limitations of meta-analyses of observational studies, future research should evaluate the influence of IT on VTE outcomes within the context of a multicenter RCT in which treatment duration is standardized.

References

1. Andrew M, David M, Adams M, et al. Venous thromboembolic complications (VTE) in children: first analyses of the Canadian Registry of VTE. Blood. 1994;**83**:1251–1257.

2. Schmidt B, Andrew M. Neonatal thrombosis: report of a prospective Canadian and international registry. Pediatrics. 1995;**96**:939–943.

3. Journeycake JM, Buchanan GR. Thrombotic complications of central venous catheters in children. Cur Opin Hematol. 2003;**10**:369–374.

4. Revel-Vilk S. Central venous line-related thrombosis in children. Acta Haematol. 2006;**115**:201–206.

5. Normann S, deVeber G, Fobker M, et al. Role of endogenous testosterone concentration in pediatric stroke. Ann Neurol. 2009;**66**:754–758.

6. Nowak-Göttl U, von Kries R, Göbel U. Neonatal symptomatic thromboembolism in Germany: two year survey. Arch Dis Child Fetal Neonatal Ed. 1997;**76**: F163–167.

7. Revel-Vilk S, Sharathkumar A, Massicotte P, et al. Natural history of arterial and venous thrombosis in children treated with low molecular weight heparin: a longitudinal study by ultrasound. J Thromb Haemost. 2004;**2**:42–46.

8. Goldenberg NA, Donadini MP, Kahn SR, et al. Post-thrombotic syndrome in children: a systematic review of frequency of occurrence, validity of outcome measures, and prognostic factors. Haematologica. 2010;**95**:1952–1959.

9. Journeycake J, Eshelman D, Buchanan GR. Post-thrombotic syndrome is uncommon in childhood cancer survivors. J Pediatr. 2006;**148**:275–277.

10. Goldenberg NA. Long-term outcomes of venous thrombosis in children. Curr Opin Hematol. 2005;**12**: 370–376.

11. Kuhle S, Koloshuk B, Marzinotto V, et al. A cross-sectional study evaluating post-thrombotic syndrome in children. Thromb Res. 2003;**111**:227–233.

12. Massicotte MP, Dix D, Monagle P, et al. Central venous catheter-related thrombosis in children: analysis of the Canadian Registry of Venous Thromboembolic Complications. J Pediatr. 1998;**133**:770–776.

13. Monagle P, Adams M, Mahoney M, et al. Outcome of pediatric thromboembolic disease: a report from the Canadian Childhood Thrombophilia Registry. Pediatr Res. 2000;**47**:763–766.

14. van Ommen CH, Heijboer H, Büller HR, et al. Venous thromboembolism in childhood: a prospective two-year registry in The Netherlands. J Pediatr. 2001;**139**:676–681.

15. Levy DM, Massicotte MP, Harvey E, et al. Thromboembolism in paediatric lupus patients. Lupus. 2003;**12**:741–746.

16. Berkun Y, Padeh S, Barash J, et al. Antiphospholipid syndrome and recurrent thrombosis in children. Arthritis Rheum. 2006;**55**:850–855.

17. Günes AM, Baytan B, Günay U. The influence of risk factors in promoting thrombosis during childhood: the role of acquired factors. Pediatr Hematol Oncol. 2006;**23**:399–410.

18. Salomon O, Steinberg DM, Zivelin A, et al. Single and combined prothrombotic factors in patients with idiopathic venous thromboembolism: prevalence and risk assessment. Arterioscler Thromb Vasc Biol. 1999;**19**:511–518.

19. Ehrenforth S, von Depka Prondsinski M, Aygören-Pürsün E, et al. Study of the prothrombin gene 20201 GA variant in FV: Q 506 carriers in relationship to the presence or absence of juvenile venous thromboembolism. Arterioscler Thromb Vac Biol. 1999;**19**:276–280.

20. Prandoni P, Lensing AW, Cogo A, et al. The long-term clinical course of acute deep venous thrombosis. Ann Intern Med. 1996;**125**:1–7.

21. van den Belt AG, Sanson BJ, Simioni P, et al. Recurrence of venous thromboembolism in patients with familial thrombophilia. Arch Intern Med. 1997;**157**:2227–2232.

22. Simioni P, Sanson BJ, Prandoni P, et al. Incidence of venous thromboembolism in families with inherited thrombophilia. Thromb Haemost. 1999 **81**:198–202.

23. Sofi F, Marcucci R, Abbate R, et al. Lipoprotein(a) and venous thromboembolism in adults: a meta-analysis. Am J Med. 2007;**120**:728–733.

24. Nuss R, Hays T, Manco-Johnson M. Childhood thrombosis. Pediatrics. 1995;**96**:291–294.

25. Nowak-Göttl U, Koch HG, Aschka I, et al. Resistance to activated protein C (APCR) in children with venous or arterial thromboembolism. Br J Haematol. 1996;**92**:992–998.

26. Aschka I, Aumann V, Bergmann F, et al. Prevalence of factor V Leiden in children with thromboembolism. Eur J Pediatr. 1996;**155**:1009–1014.

27. Uttenreuther-Fischer MM, Vetter B, Hellmann C, et al. Paediatric thrombo-embolism: the influence of non-genetic factors and the role of activated protein C resistance and protein C deficiency. Eur J Pediatr. 1997;**156**:277–281.

28. Sifontes MT, Nuss R, Hunger SP, et al. The factor V Leiden mutation in children with cancer and thrombosis. Br J Haematol. 1997;**96**:484–489.

29. Toumi NH, Khaldi F, Ben Becheur S, et al. Thrombosis in congenital deficiencies of AT III, protein C or protein S: a study of 44 children. Hematol Cell Ther. 1997;**39**:295–299.

30. Sifontes MT, Nuss R, Hunger SP, et al. Activated protein C resistance and the factor V Leiden mutation in children with thrombosis. Am J Hematol. 1998;**57**:29–32.

31. Hagstrom JN, Walter J, Bluebond-Langner R, et al. Prevalence of the factor V Leiden mutation in children and neonates with thromboembolic disease. J Pediatr. 1998;**133**:777–781.

32. Ehrenforth S, Junker R, Koch HG, et al. Multicentre evaluation of combined prothrombotic defects associated with thrombophilia in childhood. Childhood Thrombophilia Study Group. Eur J Pediatr. 1999;**158**:S97–104.

33. Schobess R, Junker R, Auberger K, et al. Factor V G1691A and prothrombin G20210A in childhood spontaneous venous thrombosis – evidence of an age-dependent thrombotic onset in carriers of the factor V G1691A and prothrombin G20210A mutation. Eur J Pediatr. 1999;**158**:S105–108.

34. Nowak-Göttl U, Junker R, Hartmeier M, et al. Increased lipoprotein (a) is an important risk factor for venous thromboembolism in childhood. Circulation. 1999;**100**:743–748.

35. Lawson SE, Butler D, Enayat MS, Williams MD. Congenital thrombophilia and thrombosis: a study in a single centre. Arch Dis Child. 1999;**81**:176–178.

36. Junker R, Koch HG, Auberger K, et al. Prothrombin G20210A gene mutation and further prothrombotic risk factors in childhood thrombophilia. Arterioscler Thromb Vasc Biol. 1999;**19**:2568–2572.

37. Kuhle S, Lane DA, Jochmanns K, et al. Homozygous antithrombin deficiency type II (99 Leu to Phe

mutation) and childhood thromboembolism. Thromb Haemost. 2001;**86**:1007–1011.

38. Nowak-Göttl U, Junker R, Kreuz W, et al. Childhood Thrombophilia Study Group. Risk of recurrent venous thrombosis in children with combined prothrombotic risk factors. Blood. 2001;**97**:858–862.

39. deVeber G, Andrew M, Adams C, et al. Cerebral sinovenous thrombosis in children. N Engl J Med. 2001;**345**:417–423.

40. Revel-Vilk S, Chan A, Bauman M, Massicotte P. Prothrombotic conditions in an unselected cohort of children with venous thromboembolic disease. J Thromb Haemost. 2003;**1**:915–921.

41. Bonduel M, Hepner M, Sciuccati G, et al. Factor V Leiden and prothrombin gene G20210A mutation in children with venous thromboembolism. Thromb Haemost. 2002;**87**:972–977.

42. van Ommen CH, Heijboer H, van den Dool EJ, et al. Pediatric venous thromboembolic disease in one single center: congenital prothrombotic disorders and the clinical outcome. J Thromb Haemost. 2003;**1**:2516–2522.

43. Young G, Manco-Johnson M, Gill JC, et al. Clinical manifestations of the prothrombin G20210A mutation in children: a pediatric coagulation consortium study. J Thromb Haemost. 2003;**1**:958–962.

44. Atasay B, Arsan S, Günlemez A, et al. Factor V Leiden and prothrombin gene 20210A variant in neonatal thromboembolism and in healthy neonates and adults: a study in a single center. Pediatr Hematol Oncol. 2003;**20**:627–634.

45. Heller C, Heinecke A, Junker R, et al. Cerebral venous thrombosis in children: a multifactorial origin. Circulation. 2003;**108**:1362–1367.

46. El-Karaksy H, El-Koofy N, El-Hawary M, et al. Prevalence of factor V Leiden mutation and other hereditary thrombophilic factors in Egyptian children with portal vein thrombosis: results of a single-center case-control study. Ann Hematol. 2004;**83**:712–715.

47. Kenet G, Waldman D, Lubetsky A, et al. Paediatric cerebral sinus vein thrombosis. A multi-center, case-controlled study. Thromb Haemost. 2004;**92**:713–718.

48. Goldenberg NA, Knapp-Clevenger R, Manco-Johnson MJ, Mountain States Regional Thrombophilia Group. Elevated plasma factor VIII and D-dimer levels as predictors of poor outcomes of thrombosis in children. New Engl J Med. 2004;**351**:1081–1088.

49. Kosch A, Kuwertz-Bröking E, Heller C, et al. Renal venous thrombosis in neonates: prothrombotic risk factors and long-term follow-up. Blood. 2004;**104**:1356–1360.

50. Rask O, Berntorp E, Ljung R. Risk factors for venous thrombosis in Swedish children and adolescents. Acta Paediatr. 2005;**94**:717–722.

51. Marks SD, Massicotte P, Steele BT, et al. Neonatal renal venous thrombosis: clinical outcomes and prevalence of prothrombotic disorders. J Pediatr. 2005;**146**:811–816.

52. Brandão LR, Williams S, Kahr WH, et al. Exercise-induced deep vein thrombosis of the upper extremity. 2. A case series in children. Acta Haematol. 2006;**115**:214–220.

53. Tavil B, Ozyurek E, Gumruk F, et al. Antiphospholipid antibodies in Turkish children with thrombosis. Blood Coagul Fibrinol. 2007;**18**:347–352.

54. Kreuz W, Stoll M, Junker R, et al. Familial elevated factor VIII in children with symptomatic venous thrombosis and post-thrombotic syndrome: results of a multicenter study. Arterioscler Thromb Vasc Biol. 2006;**26**:1901–1906.

55. Albisetti M, Moeller A, Waldvogel K, et al. Congenital prothrombotic disorders in children with peripheral venous and arterial thromboses. Acta Haematol. 2007;**117**:149–155.

56. Kenet G, Kirkham F, Niederstadt T, et al. Risk factors for recurrent venous thromboembolism in the European collaborative paediatric database on cerebral venous thrombosis: a multicentre cohort study. Lancet Neurol. 2007;**6**:595–603.

57. Andrew M, Paes B, Milner R, et al. Development of the human coagulation system in the full-term infant. Blood. 1987;**70**:165–172.

58. Andrew M, Vegh P, Johnston M, Bowker J, Ofosu F, Mitchell L. Maturation of the hemostatic system during childhood. Blood. 1992;**80**:1998–2005.

59. Ignjatovic V, Lai C, Summerhayes R, et al. Age-related differences in plasma proteins: how plasma proteins change from neonates to adults. PLoS One 2011;**6**(2):e17213.

60. Mari D, Mannucci PM, Coppola R, et al. Hypercoagulability in centenarians: the paradox of successful aging. Blood. 1995;**85**:3144–3149.

61. Bjarke B, Herin P, Blomback M. Neonatal aortic thrombosis. A possible clinical manifestation of congenital antithrombin 3 deficiency. Acta Paediatr Scand. 1974;**63**:297–301.

62. De Stefano V, Leone G, Ferrelli R, et al. Severe deep vein thrombosis in a 2-year-old child with protein S deficiency. Thromb Haemost. 1987;**58**:1089.

63. Israels SJ, Seshia SS. Childhood stroke associated with protein C or S deficiency. J Pediatr. 1987;**111**:562–564.

64. Mannino FL, Trauner DA. Stroke in neonates. J Pediatr. 1983;**102**(4):605–610.

65. Shapiro ME, Rodvien R, Bauer KA, Salzman EW. Acute aortic thrombosis in antithrombin III deficiency. JAMA. 1981;**245**:1759–1761.

66. Andrassy K, Ritz E, Bommer J. Hypercoagulability in the nephrotic syndrome. Klin Wochenschr. 1980;**58**:1029–1036.

67. Kanfer A, Kleinknecht D, Broyer M, Josso F. Coagulation studies in 45 cases of nephrotic syndrome without uremia. Thromb Diath Haemorrh. 1970;**24**:562–571.

68. Kauffmann RH, Veltkamp JJ, Van Tilburg NH, Van Es LA. Acquired antithrombin III deficiency and thrombosis in the nephrotic syndrome. Am J Med 1978;**65**:607–613.

69. Kuhlmann U, Blattler W, Pouliadis G, Siegenthaler W. Complications of nephrotic syndrome with special reference to thromboembolic accidents. Schweiz Med Wochenschr. 1979;**109**:200–209.

70. Schrader J, Kostering H, Zuchner C, al. Antithrombin III-Bestimmung im Schnelltest: Ein Vergleich mit Partigen-Platten undeinem chromogenen Substrat. Lab Med. 1981;**5**:211–218.

71. Thaler E, Balzar E, Kopsa H, Pinggera WF. Acquired antithrombin III deficiency in patients with glomerular proteinuria. Haemostasis. 1978;**7**:257–272.

72. Hanson SJ, Punzalan RC, Greenup RA et al. Incidence and risk factors for venous thromboembolism in critically ill children after trauma. J Trauma. 2010;**68**:52–56.

73. Young G, Albisetti M, Bonduel M, et al. Impact of inherited thrombophilia on venous thromboembolism in children: A systematic review & meta-analysis of observational studies. Circulation. 2008;**118**:1373–1382.

74. Kenet G, Lütkhoff LK, Albisetti M, et al. Impact of inherited thrombophilia on arterial ischemic stroke and cerebral sinovenous thrombosis in children: a systematic review and meta-analysis of observational studies. Circulation. 2010;**121**:1838–1847.

75. Kenet G, Aronis S, Berkun Y, et al. Impact of persistent antiphospholipid antibodies on symptomatic thromboembolism in children: A systematic review & meta-analysis [observational studies]. Semin Thromb Haemost. 2011;**37**:802–809.

76. Avčin T, Cimaz R, Silverman ED, et al. Pediatric antiphospholipid syndrome: clinical and immunologic features of 121 patients in an international registry. Pediatrics. 2008;**122**:e1100–1107.

77. Goldenberg NA, Donadini MP, Kahn SR, Crowther M, Kenet G, Nowak-Göttl U, Manco-Johnson MJ. Post-thrombotic syndrome in children: a systematic review of frequency of occurrence, validity of outcome measures, and prognostic factors. Haematologica. 2010;**95**:1952–1959.

78. Goldenberg NA, Durham JD, Knapp-Clevenger R, Manco-Johnson MJ. A thrombolytic regimen for high-risk deep venous thrombosis may substantially reduce the risk of postthrombotic syndrome in children. Blood. 2007;**110**:45–53.

79. Lyle CA, Gibson E, Lovejoy AE, Goldenberg NA. Acute prognostic factors for post-thrombotic syndrome in children with limb DVT: a bi-institutional cohort study. Thromb Res. 2013;**131**:37–41.

80. Holzhauer S, Goldenberg NA, Junker R, et al. Inherited thrombophilia in children with venous thromboembolism and the familial risk of thromboembolism: An observational study. Blood. 2012;**120**:1510–1515.

81. Calhoon MJ, Ross CN, Pounder E, Cassidy D, Manco-Johnson MJ, Goldenberg NA. High prevalence of thrombophilic traits in children with family history of thromboembolism. J Pediatr. 2010;**157**:485–489.

82. Nowak-Göttl U, Langer C, Bergs S, et al. Genetics of hemostasis: differential effects of heritability and household components influencing lipid concentrations and clotting factor levels in 282 pediatric stroke families. Environ Health Perspect. 2008;**116**:839–843.

83. Arning A, Hiersche M, Bidlingmaier C, et al. A Genome-Wide Association Study Identifies Novel Susceptibility Genes for Pediatric Venous Thrombosis. Blood (ASH Annual Meeting Abstracts). Nov 2011;**118**:3336.

84. Vossen CY, Walker ID, Svensson P, et al. Recurrence rate after first venous thrombosis in patients with familial thrombophilia. Arterioscler Thromb Vasc Biol. 2005;**25**:1992–1997.

85. De Stefano V, Rossi E, Paciaroni K, Leone G. Screening for inherited thrombophilia: indications and therapeutic implications. Haematologica. 2002;**87**:1095–1108.

86. Prandoni P, Noventa F, Ghirarduzzi A, et al. The risk of recurrent venous thromboembolism after discontinuing anticoagulation in patients with acute proximal deep vein thrombosis or pulmonary embolism. A prospective cohort study in 1,626 patients. Haematologica. 2007;**92**:199–205.

87. Lindmarker P, Schulman S, Sten-Linder M, Wiman B, Egberg N, Johnsson H. The risk of recurrent venous thromboembolism in carriers and non-carriers of the G1691A allele in the coagulation factor V gene and the G20210A allele in the prothrombin gene. DURAC Trial Study Group. Duration of Anticoagulation. Thromb Haemost. 1999;**81**:684–9.

88. Büller H, Agnelli G, Hull RD, et al. Antithrombotic therapy for venous thromboembolic disease. The

seventh ACCP conference on antithrombotic and thrombolytic therapy. Chest. 2004;**126**:S401–428.

89. Monagle P, Chan AK, Goldenberg NA et al; American College of Chest Physicians. Antithrombotic Therapy in Neonates and Children: Antithrombotic Therapy and Prevention of Thrombosis, 9th edn: American College of Chest Physicians Evidence-Based Clinical Practice Guidelines. Chest. 2012;**141**(2 Suppl):e737S–801S.

90. Bidlingmaier C, Kenet G, Kurnik K, et al. Safety and efficacy of low molecular weight heparin in children: a systematic review of the literature and meta-analysis of single-arm studies. Semin Thromb Hemost. 2011;**37**:814–25.

Role of global assays in thrombosis and thrombophilia

Meera Chitlur and Mindy L. Simpson

Introduction

Hemostasis is a complex process and is difficult to monitor in its entirety. Many laboratory tests have been developed to discern specific parts of the coagulation process in an attempt to diagnose disorders such as a tendency toward bleeding or clotting abnormally, and/or to predict clinical outcomes in these disorders. Because an in vitro test is simply a model of an in vivo process, it is important to understand what each test is measuring and its limitations. Traditional clotting assays such as the prothrombin time (PT) and activated partial thromboplastin time (APTT) measure the time for initiation of clot formation when, following initiation of coagulation in plasma via differing activators (PT: "thromboplastin," comprised of tissue factor and phospholipid; APTT: "partial thromboplastin," comprised of phospholipid without tissue factor), thrombin mediates the conversion of fibrinogen to fibrin. The endpoint of the PT and APTT occurs when only approximately 5% of thrombin has been produced [1]. PT and APTT also do not provide information regarding the rate and extent of clot formation, nor lytic function. As for other global tests, they are non-specific assays and, for abnormal test results, further testing is generally warranted to evaluate causality. Specific testing may include factor assays to evaluate for a factor deficiency or antibody testing to assess for inhibitory antibodies. The need for improved testing of hemostasis has been long recognized but an accepted standardized test is not yet widely available.

Thrombophilic states and the propensity toward thrombosis are difficult to diagnose/predict with laboratory assays. Testing for thrombophilia can be cumbersome, generally requiring testing for individual abnormalities, and may be difficult with smaller patients due to the amount of blood required for comprehensive testing. There is a need for improved thrombophilia/thrombosis testing and monitoring. Global assays attempt to better define the complete course of clot formation and breakdown through avenues such as the measurement of thrombin generation, fibrin formation, plasmin generation, and clot dissolution. Through a more complete picture of the hemostatic process, global assays may fill the gaps in knowledge regarding hemostatic abnormalities.

The two most commonly employed global assay methodologies in both clinical practice and applied research are thrombin generation assays (TGA) and thromboelastography, which measure thrombin generation and fibrin clot formation over time in a clotting plasma or whole blood sample, respectively. Both assays have been used in the broad evaluation of hemostatic abnormalities, including both bleeding and thrombotic disorders. Despite limitations of methods standardization and result interpretation, these global assays offer an approach to the evaluation of hemostatic balance that may allow for more individualized management.

The use of global assays in the evaluation of pediatric thrombophilia, thrombosis, and thrombotic complications is an ongoing field of study. In addition to TGA and thromboelastography, there are a multitude of additional global assays in use, most commonly in research laboratories and in varying stages of development and practice. In this chapter, we describe the common global assays as well as a few of the less common assays, highlighting how they may contribute to the understanding of the complex process of blood clot formation and breakdown. We also describe the current use of these assays in the field of pediatric thrombosis.

Pediatric Thrombotic Disorders, ed. Neil A. Goldenberg and Marilyn J. Manco-Johnson. Published by Cambridge University Press. © Cambridge University Press 2015.

Assays that measure clot formation and lysis

Thromboelastography

Thromboelastography was first described by Hartert in 1948 as a method to evaluate the coagulation status of soldiers injured on the battle field, using a single sample of whole blood [2]. The original instrument has undergone significant modifications to make it more reliable and user friendly, but the principle remains the same. Current instruments include the TEG® 5000 Thromboelastograph® Hemostasis Analyzer system (TEG) manufactured in the USA by Haemonetics Corporation (Braintree, MA, USA), and a modified instrument using the term rotational thromboelastometry, ROTEM® delta (ROTEM), manufactured by Tem Innovations GmbH (Munich, Germany). Both systems monitor the changes in viscosity and elasticity of a clot formed in a low-shear environment. The blood sample is placed in a sample cup, into which is suspended a pin which is connected to a torsion wire that is monitored for movement. In the TEG, the cup holding the blood sample oscillates through an angle of 4° 45' with each rotation lasting 10 seconds. Once a clot is formed, this links the surface of the cup to the pin, and the rotational torque of the cup is transmitted to the pin. The magnitude of this oscillation depends on the strength of the fibrin–platelet bonds. As the clot retracts and lyses the transfer of motion to the pin diminishes. In the ROTEM, the cup remains stationary while the pin oscillates and the movement of the pin is monitored via an optical detection system instead of mechanically via a torsion wire. The ROTEM is also equipped with an electronic pipetting system. The basic mechanism for both the TEG and ROTEM is shown in Figure 11.1. The graphical representation of changes in elasticity and viscosity during clot formation and lysis is called the thromboelastograph. The blood samples may be activated either extrinsically using tissue factor or intrinsically using a contact activator (kaolin in TEG/rabbit partial thromboplastin in ROTEM). The ROTEM also allows the assessment of quantitative fibrinogen levels using the tissue factor + platelet antagonist and assessment of the fibrinolytic pathway using tissue factor with aprotinin. The TEG on the other hand has r-TEG, or rapid TEG, which uses a combination of 8% kaolin, human recombinant tissue factor, phospholipids, buffers and stabilizers to provide more rapid activation of sample to obtain faster results. Both instruments also provide heparinase to allow assessment of underlying coagulability and lytic function in samples containing heparin (whether for treatment or as a contaminant). The mechanical differences between the two instruments as mentioned above result in differences in reference ranges. Identical parameters are measured by the two instruments, albeit with differences in nomenclature. A typical thromboelastograph tracing is shown in Figure 11.2.

The parameters traditionally measured in both instruments are:

R time (Reaction time, TEG) or clotting time (CT, ROTEM): Time from start of sample run to first significant clot. This is prolonged by anticoagulation and factor deficiencies.

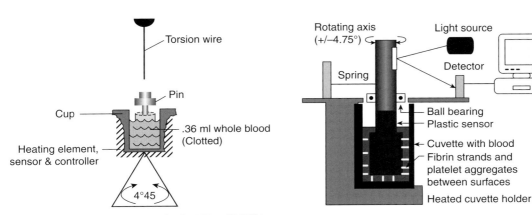

Figure 11.1 The basic mechanism for the TEG and ROTEM.

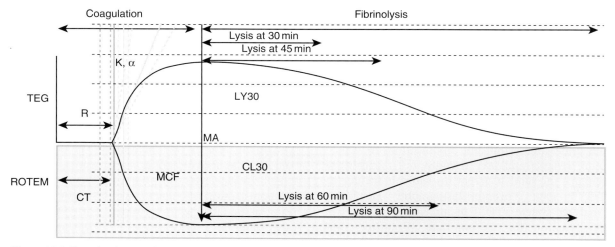

Figure 11.2 Thromboelastograph tracing. (A black and white version of this figure will appear in some formats. For the color version, please refer to the plate section.)

K time (clot formation time, TEG) or rate of clot formation (CFTR, ROTEM): Speed to reach a certain level of clot strength or to generate a clot that measures 2 mm. This is prolonged by low fibrinogen level/platelet dysfunction/anticoagulants.

Angle (α): Rate of clot formation. This reflects function of fibrinogen, increases with improved platelet function.

Maximum amplitude (MA, TEG) or maximum clot firmness (MCF, ROTEM): Measurement of maximum strength or stiffness. This is influenced by platelet function and number.

Clot lysis at fixed time points: Both instruments are able to measure the amount of clot lysis at fixed time points such as 30, 45 and 60 minutes. Ly30, Ly60 on the TEG and CL30, CL60 on the ROTEM.

G (both TEG and ROTEM): Computer-generated measure of clot strength, reflective of the contribution of both the cellular and enzymatic factors in clot formation. This is a calculated measure of clot strength derived from amplitude (A, mm). $G = (5000 \times A)/(100 \times A)$.

Thromboelastography therefore allows the assessment of hemostasis from clot initiation to fibrinolysis. The basic approach of both instruments is based on the presumption that the properties of clot formation such as rate of clot formation, the strength of the clot formed and the stability of the clot are associated with the patient's propensity for either bleeding or thrombosis. The parameters of coagulation are considered to be the R time/CT, K time/CFTR, angle and MA/MCF, while the clot lysis at fixed time points and G are considered measures of fibrinolytic potential. A shortening of the R/CT, K/CFTR, increase in MA/MCF or G and decrease in lysis at 30 minutes are usually considered to be indicators of increased thrombotic potential. The first derivative of the thromboelastographic course can be plotted as a curve and is considered representative of rate of fibrin polymerization. From this curve the maximum rate of clot/fibrin generation (MRTG/MTG) and the time to reach the maximum rate (TMRTG/TMG) can be derived, which have been noted to be increased in patients with increased thrombotic potential [3]. Increased thrombotic potential may also be the result of impaired fibrinolysis. Thromboelastography also models the process downstream of thrombin generation and can reflect the adequacy of platelet activation and fibrin polymerization in the process of clot formation. Therefore in order to facilitate the assessment of fibrinolysis, several researchers have utilized modifications of the assay with addition of fibrinolytic activators like tissue plasminogen activator (tPA). While these methods have proved to be useful in some situations, there is considerable variability related to the use of different initiators of coagulation. Efforts are ongoing to standardize the assay and ensure better reproducibility and reliability [4,5].

Use of thromboelastography in the management of thrombophilia and thrombosis

The incidence of thrombosis, although rising in the pediatric population, is still very small compared to the adult population. Therefore, it is not surprising that relatively few studies have used thromboelastography in the pediatric population for the evaluation of thrombosis. We now briefly review the adult and pediatric literature on this topic in order to provide insight into the potential uses of thromboelastography in the evaluation of hypercoagulability.

Thromboelastography was initially used in the evaluation of the coagulation status of patients with liver disease and transplantation. Since the liver is a vital organ involved in the production of several procoagulant, anticoagulant and fibrinolytic proteins, both hypo- and/or hypercoagulable states have been associated with liver disease. Monitoring coagulation status with thromboelastography during liver transplantation has been an area of great interest [6]. Strong correlations have been found between the platelet count/fibrinogen and MA/MCF, as well as between the INR and R/CT time, as might be expected. However, de Pietri et al. found that, while standard laboratory data obtained during liver resection sometimes revealed a hypocoagulable state, the thromboelastographic tracing revealed normocoagulability. Early identification of a normal coagulation status may be beneficial in preventing interventions that may lead to hypercoagulable complications, such as the use of factor concentrates or antifibrinolytics [7].

Poulsen et al. performed thromboelastography in 76 patients, 2 months after the occurrence of a thrombotic event. A significant decrease in the clotting time and the velocity of clot propagation was noted in patients compared to a control group without history of thrombosis, indicating that patients are hypercoagulable at this time point following a first thrombotic event [8]. In a study by Kupesiz et al., rt-PA was added to whole blood to induce fibrinolysis, along with tissue factor as activator [9]. This facilitated the rapid assessment of the fibrinolytic potential of the sample. This assay was again used to compare the fibrinolysis in patients with non-catheter induced thrombosis to normal pediatric controls and showed a significant difference in TAFI levels and tPA-induced fibrinolysis on thromboelastography in patients with thrombosis when compared to controls [10], while routine measures of thrombotic potential

such as fibrinogen, plasminogen, tPA levels, PAP complexes, PAI and lipoprotein(a) levels were similar in both patients and controls.

Critically ill surgical patients have several derangements of their hemostatic systems, predisposing them to both bleeding and thrombotic complications. There is a significant increase in the risk of thromboembolic events including deep vein thrombosis (DVT) and pulmonary embolism in post-operative adult patients who are critically ill. A study by Kashuk et al. performed r-TEG analysis on 152 critically ill patients in the surgical ICU, comparing groups of patients with and without thromboembolic complications. For each 1 dyne/cm^2 increase in G, there was an associated 25% increase in odds of thromboembolic events [11]. Patients who undergo splenectomy following trauma are also noted to be at an increased risk for thromboembolic events. A 1994 study by Geerts et al. showed that 58% of trauma patients who underwent splenectomy developed thromboembolic complications [12]. This was confirmed in a more recent study by Watters et al., who observed DVT in 7% of patients in the splenectomy group, and none in the non-splenectomy group [13]. An increase in platelet count, decrease in tPA levels and increase in PAI levels were noted post-splenectomy. Evaluation of the residual hypo- or hypercoagulability via thromboelastography following splenectomy showed evidence of increased fibrin cross-linking and increase in the overall clot strength. It is however important to note that comparative studies will be necessary to develop clinically useful reference ranges. Also, since these are adult studies, the relevance to the pediatric population remains to be determined.

Monitoring of anticoagulation is a challenging issue both in children and adults. The advancements in surgical techniques and the increasing use of mechanical circulatory support devices such as cardiopulmonary bypass circuits (CPB), extracorporeal membrane oxygenation (ECMO) and ventricular assist devices (VAD) in children have increased the need for strategies to more accurately monitor the coagulation status. The principal causes of morbidity and mortality with the use of these interventions are bleeding and thrombosis. Thrombotic complications are the result of contact of blood with the extracorporeal circuit resulting in massive inflammatory and clotting response. Therefore, aggressive systemic anticoagulation becomes necessary to prevent activation of cellular and enzymatic pathways of coagulation. This degree of anticoagulation then predisposes to increased risk of bleeding. Accurate monitoring techniques to prevent both thrombosis and bleeding therefore become extremely important. The tests that are commonly used are the platelet count, fibrinogen levels, APTT, the activated clotting time (ACT), measurement of heparin concentrations and the anti-Xa assay. Routine coagulation assays have not correlated with survival and have not been useful in predicting either thrombotic or bleeding complications. The role of thromboelastography in providing an ongoing coagulation profile in patients on ECMO, CPB and VAD is being investigated. In patients on VADs, a combination of anticoagulants and antiplatelet agents are used. Thromboelastography has been found to be useful in providing information on the combined effect of these multiple agents on the coagulation system [14]. While it may not replace the current testing methods, it has been suggested to be an aide in monitoring these patients [15,16].

The role of thromboelastography in assessment of coagulopathy in patients with extensive trauma is being actively investigated in adults. In a large study by Halcomb et al. in 1974 consecutive trauma patients were studied with both conventional coagulation tests and r-TEG on admission. The authors found the TEG results to be more timely and quite informative in predicting both bleeding and hyperfibrinolysis. While bleeding was the major cause of death in trauma patients, stabilized trauma patients were noted to be more hypercoagulable than controls [12,17]. Hypothermia is noted to be common after trauma and the effect of hypothermia on coagulation was studied by Differding et al. in 46 patients using thromboelastography at different temperatures. Clot strength was noted to be unaffected by hypothermia and clotting factor function was more affected by hypothermia than platelet function, contributing to the hypercoagulability [18]. This ability to assess the interaction between platelets and clotting factors and evaluate clot strength and lysis gives thromboelastography several potential diagnostic implications.

The major advantage of a point of care monitoring device such as TEG or ROTEM is the fast turnaround time and the ability to assess coagulation in whole blood, allowing for the interactions between the enzymatic and cellular coagulation factors. The ability to measure the clot formation in real time provides the unique opportunity to assess the different phases of coagulation and fibrinolysis with one sample of blood. The major drawback of this system is its lack of

standardization. A working group through the International Society on Thrombosis and Haemostasis is striving to standardize these tests and ensure reliable results. Continued efforts in this arena would ensure that the studies become more comparable and allow the tests to move from the research to clinical laboratories.

Use of Clot Formation and Lysis (CloFAL) and Overall Hemostasis Potential (OHP) assays in management of thrombosis/thrombophilia

Fibrin clot formation and breakdown can be evaluated by turbidity measurements where an increase in turbidity reflects the aggregation of fibrin fibers. The Clot Formation and lysis assay (CloFAL) [19] and the Overall Hemostasis Potential assay (OHP) [20–22] are two global assays of hemostasis based on turbidimetric fibrin measurement.

The CloFAL assay is performed on platelet poor plasma (PPP) where coagulation is initiated with calcium, 5 pM tissue factor and phospholipid, while fibrinolysis is enhanced with the addition of 450 ng/ml tissue plasminogen activator (tPA). Kinetic blanked dual-wavelength (405 and 605 nm) absorbance measurements are obtained in a spectrophotometer over 3 hours. A waveform describing clot formation and lysis is generated with data on the following parameters: time to maximum amplitude, maximum amplitude (MA), coagulation index (CI – area under the curve through 30 minutes), area under the curve (AUC, cumulative for the entire assay), and a fibrinolytic index (FI_2) [19,23,24] as depicted in Figure 11.3. The CloFAL assay has been utilized in both adults and children to evaluate both bleeding and clotting disorders [19,23–25].

In a 2012 publication, CloFAL was used to monitor hypercoagulability and hypofibrinolysis in 50 children following an acute venous thromboembolism (VTE) [23]. The CloFAL AUC parameter was analytically sensitive to hypercoagulable states and the modified fibrinolytic index (FI_2) was sensitive to both hyper- and hypofibrinolytic states. Additionally, the AUC was significantly increased in the acute phase post-event, denoting hypercoagulability, whereas the FI_2 was significantly decreased, denoting hypofibrinolysis. These findings offer a novel approach to studying and understanding the contribution that plasma coagulative and fibrinolytic changes (including the strong influence of fibrinogen) make around thrombotic events in

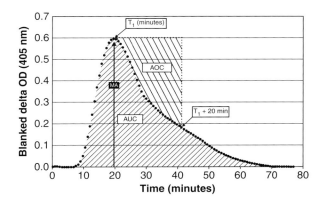

Figure 11.3 CloFAL assay waveform in pooled normal adult plasma, demonstrating AUC and FI$_2$ calculated parameters. FI$_2$ is calculated based on AUC. *Reprinted with permission from Elsevier (Thromb Res 2012;130:343–349).*

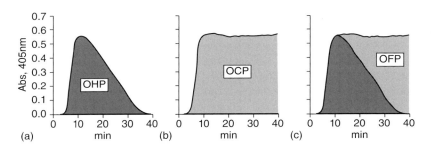

Figure 11.4 (a) Overall hemostasis potential (OHP). (b) Overall coagulation potential (OCP). (c) Overall fibrinolytic potential (OFP) assayed in normal pooled plasma samples. Abs, absorbance. *Reprinted with permission from Antovic (Semin Thromb Hemost 2010;36:772–779).*

children. Further studies to assess the utility in possible VTE outcome prediction are ongoing [26].

The OHP assay is performed on PPP containing a low concentration of exogenous thrombin (0.04 IU/ ml), calcium, phospholipids, and 330 ng/ml tPA. Fibrin formation and breakdown is monitored spectrophotometrically at a wavelength of 405 nm over 40 minutes. Area under the curve (AUC) is the determined parameter, and the assay develops two fibrin aggregation curves (and therefore 2 AUC calculations) for each sample where the assay is run with and without the addition of tPA. The overall hemostasis potential (OHP) is the AUC with tPA added, whereas the overall coagulation potential (OCP) is the AUC without tPA. The overall fibrinolysis potential (OFP) is the difference between the OHP and the OCP, as shown in Figure 11.4. The clot lysis time (CLT) can be determined as an additional parameter [20–22,27].

The OHP assay has been studied in hypercoagulable conditions where increased coagulation and impaired fibrinolysis were detected in subjects with acquired arterial thrombotic events [28], pre-eclampsia [29], coronary heart disease in elderly females [21], patients < 45 years of age with previous stroke or transient ischemic

attack [30] and elderly patients with stroke [31]. Thrombophilic conditions have also been evaluated with OHP. When 88 women with previous VTE were evaluated, the OHP was most significantly increased in those with factor V Leiden mutation [32]. A modified OHP assay known as the coagulation inhibitor potential (CIP) assay has been shown to detect major thrombophilias when the reagents include Protac (a protein C activator) and heparin pentasaccharide (activator of antithrombin) [33–35]. Finally, the OHP has been tested in monitoring anticoagulant therapy including low molecular weight heparin (dalteparin), where there were immediate changes in hemostatic balance after the medication injection and overall the OHP values were inversely related to anti-Xa activity [36]. There are no studies utilizing OHP technology in pediatrics; therefore, the utility in assessing pediatric thrombosis and thrombophilia is yet to be determined.

Assays that measure fibrinolysis alone

The importance of fibrinolysis in the maintenance of hemostatic balance is often under-recognized. Conditions of hypofibrinolysis may predispose to

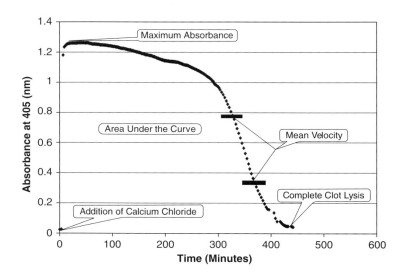

Figure 11.5 Spectrophotometric tracing of euglobulin clot formation and lysis. A representative standard pool curve is shown here with the four measured parameters labeled. *Reprinted with permission from Elsevier (Thromb Res 2003;112:329–337).*

thrombosis, but frequently are not evaluated for due to lack of available testing. There are few tests that focus on measuring fibrinolysis alone, but two examples include the euglobulin clot lysis time (ELT), which has been modified to the automated euglobulin clot lysis assay (ECLA), and the global fibrinolytic capacity (GFC) [37,38].

Euglobulin clot lysis assay (ECLA) and global fibrinolytic capacity (GFC)

The euglobulin clot lysis time (ELT) was first described in 1959 [39] and subsequently modernized using a computerized kinetic spectrophotometer in 2003, known as the ECLA [37]. The euglobulin fraction of plasma is composed of several proteins, including fibrinogen, plasminogen, tPA, plasminogen activator inhibitor (PAI-1), factor VIII, and TAFI. In the ECLA, a euglobulin fraction is prepared by adding citrated plasma to acetic acid in a glass tube, which is then placed on ice for 10 minutes and subsequently centrifuged at 2000 × g at 25°C for 5 minutes. The euglobulin fraction is resuspended in a solution of sodium chloride and sodium borate, stirred with a glass rod, placed in a 37°C water bath for 90 seconds, restirred, and finally placed back into the water bath for an additional 90 seconds. The sample is then transferred to a 96-well microtiter plate where calcium is added, and the absorbance is measured at 405 nm in a spectrophotometer for 720 minutes. Maximum absorbance is the peak absorbance at 405 nm. Other parameters measured include the lysis time, AUC, and mean velocity, as shown in Figure 11.5. The ECLA has

been evaluated in neonates, children, adults, and pregnant females. Abnormal fibrinolysis has been studied via ELT or ECLA technology in multiple hypercoagulable states and conditions. Hypofibrinolysis (prolongation of ELT) has been found in studies of idiopathic, secondary, and recurrent VTE [40–43].

The GFC is based on the measurement of clot lysis via fibrin degradation product (FnDP) generation during a 3-hour in vitro incubation at 37°C of clotted whole blood [38]. Whole blood is collected in tubes containing sodium chloride, bovine serum albumin (BSA), and thrombin with or without aprotinin. The tubes are mixed and then incubated at 37°C for 3 hours. Clots are released from the tube wall and then centrifuged at 2000 × g for 20 minutes at 4°C. The FnDP are determined by ELISA. The GFC (in mcg/ml) is the difference between the FnDP level from the sample with aprotinin and the FnDP level from the sample without aprotinin. The GFC has been used to study patients with coronary artery disease [38] and patients with liver cirrhosis [44]. There are few studies of thrombosis/thrombophilia with GFC, but impaired fibrinolytic capacity was found in patients with Cushing's disease when evaluated for hypercoagulability [45]. Future studies are needed to determine the utility of GFC in children and in hypercoagulable states.

Assays that measure thrombin generation alone

Thrombin generation is required for the final conversion of fibrinogen to fibrin in the formation of a fibrin clot, and therefore determines the extent of a thrombotic process. Thrombin is considered to be the key enzyme of the coagulation process. Thrombin generation assays (TGA) measure the ability of plasma to generate thrombin in vitro when coagulation is activated by a trigger, such as tissue factor. Monitoring of thrombin generation over time in plasma affords a broad assessment of coagulation including: (1) initiation, where small amounts of thrombin instigate clot formation; (2) propagation, via a thrombin burst; and (3) termination, where thrombin activity ceases. These processes incorporate pro- and anticoagulant factors that regulate thrombin generation, giving an improved overall picture of an individual's clot formation capacity and therefore acting as a "global" assay of coagulation [46]. A potential and debated limitation is the degree to which changes in quantity and function of fibrinogen are measurable via thrombin generation assay.

Thrombin generation testing was first introduced in 1953 by means of subsampling activated plasma to quantify thrombin by measuring the ability to clot fibrinogen [47]. Over the past 60 years, the technology has evolved to using chromogenic or fluorescent thrombin substrates added to plasma and continuous measurement of thrombin activity via the substrates. A variety of thrombin generation assays have been developed over the years including those that utilize fluorogenic substrates such as the Calibrated Automated Thrombogram (CAT, Thrombinoscope BV, Maastricht, The Netherlands) and Technothrombin TGA (Technoclone, Vienna, Austria), and those that utilize chromogenic substrates such as the Endogenous Thrombin Potential Assay (Siemens Healthcare Diagnostic Inc., Deerfield, IL, USA) and Pefakit Thrombin Dynamics Test (Pentapharm, Basel, Switzerland). The CAT assay as developed by Hemker is the best known [48–50].

The CAT assay uses a low-affinity fluorogenic thrombin substrate (Z-Gly-Gly-Arg-AMC) to continuously monitor thrombin generation in a plasma sample where coagulation is triggered by the addition of tissue factor and phospholipids. The reaction occurs in a microtiter plate with measurement wells and calibrator wells. In the measurement wells, tissue factor, phospholipids, and calcium are added to the sample plasma, which induces thrombin formation. Conversely, in the calibrator wells, "thrombin calibrator" consisting of thrombin bound to α_2-macroglobulin, which cannot be inhibited by plasma protease inhibitors, is added to the sample plasma along with calcium and the

fluorogenic substrate, where the fluorogenic substrate is converted at a constant rate, thereby providing known thrombin activity. The developing fluorescence is recorded over time. The tracing from the calibrator wells provides the calibration factor needed to determine the actual thrombin concentration (in nM) from the resultant tracing of generated thrombin in the measurement wells. The final thrombin generation curve (thrombogram) is calculated by taking the first derivative of the corrected fluorescent tracing and is characterized by the following progression: lag phase (coagulation initiation), thrombin burst (propagation), and dissolution (termination). Parameters reported include the lag time, peak time, peak height, and area under the curve (i.e., the endogenous thrombin potential, ETP), as shown in Figure 11.6. The lag time frequently correlates with plasma clotting times and the ETP represents the total enzymatic work done by thrombin during the recorded time. In general, hypocoagulable states are suggested by long lag times and decreased ETP or peak heights, whereas hypercoagulable states are suggested by short lag times and increased ETP or peak heights. It is hypothesized that the ETP is the most predictive CAT parameter for bleeding/thrombotic risks [46].

The TGAs can be run under a variety of experimental conditions to suit specific study questions. Most often, the trigger for coagulation initiation is tissue factor, but the concentration can be altered to modify the extent that the intrinsic pathway contributes to thrombin generation. In the presence of low tissue factor concentration, it has been shown that all of the coagulation factors, except factor XI, influenced the TGA, whereas high tissue factor concentration allowed only the extrinsic pathway to influence TGA results [51]. Additionally, soluble thrombomodulin or activated protein C can be added to make the assay more sensitive to the protein C anticoagulant pathway. The fluorescent technology for the current TGA allows thrombin generation to be measured in platelet-rich plasma (PRP) as well as PPP. When evaluating tissue factor-triggered PRP, the platelet function contributes to the assay results, notably the onset and rate of thrombin generation, whereas the coagulant activity determines the total amount of thrombin generated, or ETP [52]. Finally, there is large interindividual variation in thrombin generation, which can be attributed to naturally variable plasma levels of assay determinants such as coagulation factors, as well as biological variables such as age, gender, body mass index, genetic conditions, pregnancy, and medications, such as hormonal therapy

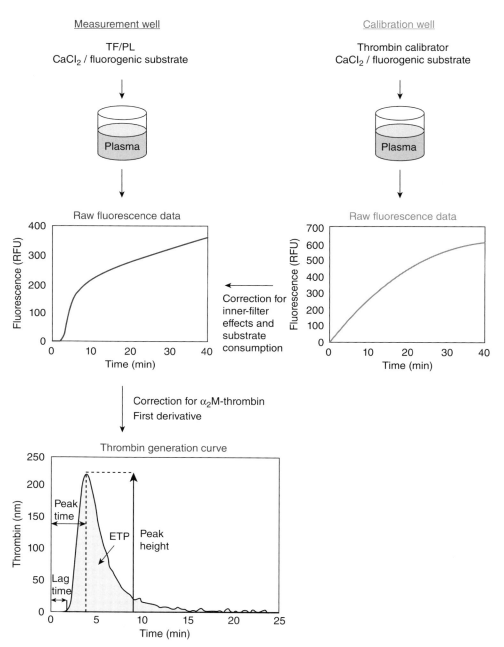

Figure 11.6 CAT assay principle and parameters of the thrombin generation curve. The CAT assay requires two fluorescence measurements in the same plasma. In the measurement well, coagulation is triggered with tissue factor (TF), phospholipids (PL), and CaCl₂; in the calibration well, only the thrombin calibrator (i.e., a known amount of a₂M-thrombin) and CaCl₂ are added to plasma. Thrombin activity in both wells is monitored continuously via conversion of a low-affinity fluorogenic substrate added to plasma. The thrombin generation curve is obtained by taking the first derivative that the fluorescence recorded in the measurement well after: (i) correction for inner-filter effects and substrate consumption (based on the fluorescence measured in the calibration well); and (ii) subtraction of the fluorescence signal deriving from a₂M-thrombin (based on a mathematical algorithm). The thrombin generation curve can be described in terms of lag time, peak time, peak height, and area under the curve (endogenous thrombin potential, ETP). *Reprinted with permission from Elsevier (Thromb Res 2011;127(Suppl 3):S21–S25).*

[53–58]. The highly variable assay conditions make this technology difficult to standardize for widespread clinical use.

Use of TGA for pediatric thrombophilia/ thrombosis evaluation

Few studies in the pediatric population utilize TGAs to predict thrombophilia or evaluate thrombosis. However, TGA has been used in this capacity in adult cohorts. It has been evaluated in congenital thrombophilic states such as antithrombin, protein C, and protein S deficiencies as well as factor V Leiden and prothrombin gene mutations. Additionally, TGA parameters have been studied to determine if they may be predictive of venous thromboembolism (VTE) or recurrent VTE. Representative studies are presented below where TGA has been overall predictive in the populations studied when performed under appropriate assay conditions.

In a study of children with active vs. inactive Crohn's disease, TGA ETP and peak height were significantly higher during times of active disease, attributed to the inflammatory state. This may represent a high-risk time for thrombotic potential and a high index of suspicion should be heeded [59]. This study highlights the need for further studies in this area.

The TGA has been studied in its relationship to inherited thrombophilic genetic mutations including factor V Leiden and prothrombin G20210A mutations. In a pilot study of first-degree relatives of patients with VTE and factor V Leiden, abnormal thrombin generation was associated with having factor V Leiden and/or other prothrombotic states. Here, TGA was performed in the presence and absence of thrombomodulin (TM), where TM makes the assay more sensitive to the protein C pathway, and the factor V Leiden mutation is relevant causing activated protein C resistance [60]. Similarly, in a study published in 2010, the ETP was higher in patients with the prothrombin gene mutation when compared to normal controls. Additionally, ETP was significantly higher in patients with the prothrombin gene mutation and a history of VTE than those asymptomatic with the gene mutation [61]. A similar study in 2007 compared thrombin generation between carriers and non-carriers for the prothrombin G20210A gene mutation and found that there was a "dose-dependent" effect of the PT 20210A allele on virtually all thrombin generation parameters. The lag time was shortest in normal controls and progressively prolonged in heterozygotes and homozygotes for the prothrombin gene mutation. Peak height and ETP progressively increased from normal to heterozygous and ultimately homozygous subjects [62].

The TGA has been shown sensitive to deficiencies of natural anticoagulants including antithrombin, protein C, and protein S under appropriate assay conditions. A study of antithrombin deficiency and TGA demonstrated an increased mean ETP for mutations most associated with thrombotic risk, including type 1 or type IIRS/ PE. Type IIHBS heterozygosity of antithrombin deficiency is associated with a low VTE risk and there was no increased ETP in these subjects. These findings illustrate the importance of phenotypic as well as genotypic differences, but note that TGA did not fully discriminate between subjects with thrombogenic defects and other defects [63]. Protein S is an anticoagulant protein that stimulates activated protein C and tissue factor pathway inhibitor. Protein S deficiency is a thrombotic risk factor and thrombin generation assays sensitive to activated protein C and tissue factor pathway inhibitor activities confirmed that these are hypercoagulable states with elevated thrombin generation [64].

The CAT assay has been evaluated in recognizing prothrombotic phenotypes. In a 2006 retrospective study, adult patients with a history of VTE were compared to normal controls. Thrombin generation with soluble thrombomodulin showed a higher ETP in subjects with oral contraceptives, a history of VTE with an identified prothrombotic risk factor, and a history of VTE without an identified prothrombotic risk factor when compared to normal controls. The group with a history of thrombosis and an identified prothrombotic risk factor had higher ETP values than the group with a history of thrombosis but no identified risk factors. Therefore under these conditions, the CAT assay was able to detect a prothrombotic phenotype with a sensitivity of 0.93 [65].

The TGA results may impact the risk assessment for first-time and recurrent thrombotic events. Thrombin generation was significantly higher in patients after an acute DVT compared to a normal healthy population. Notably, thrombin generation varied over time in patients with thrombosis, whereas thrombin generation in the reference population remained stable over time [66]. In a study where 360 patients and 404 control subjects underwent thrombin generation testing, ETP results above the 90th percentile had a 1.5-fold increased risk of first DVT. In this study though, ETP was not predictive of

151

recurrent thrombotic events [67]. In contrast, in 2008, Tripodi evaluated the utility of TGA (as measured 1 month after cessation of anticoagulant therapy) in assessing risk of recurrent DVT in 254 patients followed after a first episode of unprovoked VTE. Thrombin generation was measured in the presence and absence of thrombomodulin. The ETP and peak height results in the presence of thrombomodulin revealed that an ETP of > 960 nm/min or peak height of > 193 nm were associated with hazard ratios of VTE recurrence of 3.41 (1.34–8.68, 95% CI) or 4.57 (1.70–12.2, 95% CI), respectively when compared to those with ETP < 563 nm/min or peak < 115 nm [68]. Additionally, in a prospective cohort study published in 2008, TGA was done on 188 patients with first-time unprovoked VTE or provoked by a non-surgical trigger. Subjects with high ETP had a significantly higher rate of unprovoked recurrent thrombosis compared to those with low ETP. [69]. In a different approach, thrombin generation has been shown to identify patients at low risk of recurrent VTE. A study from Austria presented 914 subjects with a history of first spontaneous VTE who were followed prospectively for recurrence, which occurred in 100 (11%) of subjects. Peak thrombin generation was measured at a median of 13 months (3 weeks to 94 months) after discontinuation of anticoagulation. Those subjects without recurrence had lower thrombin generation than those with recurrence. After 4 years, the patients with thrombin generation less than 400 nM had a recurrence probability of 6.5%, whereas those with more than 400 nM thrombin generation had a 20% recurrence risk [70].

Although TGA appears to be a potential tool to evaluate thrombophilic states and the risk of recurrent VTE in adults, studies utilizing TGA in pediatric thrombosis and thrombophilia are lacking. This is an important area for future research.

Assays that measure both thrombin generation and plasmin generation

Hemostatic balance is maintained by the coagulation and fibrinolytic systems. Thrombin and plasmin are considered to be the key enzymes in coagulation and fibrinolysis, respectively. Recently, two assays have been developed that measure thrombin and plasmin generation directly: the simultaneous thrombin and plasmin generation assay (STP) and the novel hemostasis assay

(NHA) [71,72]. Both the STP and NHA utilize similar techniques to TGAs where the enzyme of interest is tracked through measurement of specific fluorogenic substrates. Although neither of these assays has been used to date to evaluate thrombotic risk or thrombophilias, the potential of such assays for generating novel information regarding an individual's hemostatic balance is important.

Simultaneous thrombin and plasmin generation assay (STP) and novel hemostasis assay (NHA)

The STP utilizes thrombin- and plasmin-specific fluorogenic substrates that track the generation of each (thrombin substrate: Boc-Val-Pro-Arg-MCA; plasmin substrate: Boc-Glu-Lys-Lys-MCA). Coagulation is initiated with tissue factor (5 pM), phospholipid, and calcium in PPP, while fibrinolysis is accelerated with tPA (450 ng/ml). The generation of thrombin and plasmin are measured in separate wells but simultaneously. The data are then aggregated for analysis. Profound impairments in thrombin generation were seen in extrinsic and common pathway factor deficiencies (with the notable exception of fibrinogen), and also in factor VIII and IX deficiencies. Plasmin generation was sensitive to fibrinogen, plasminogen, exogenous tPA, and alpha-2 antiplasmin. An advantage of the STP assay over TGA is that plasmin generation in STP was found to be sensitive to altered levels of fibrinogen. The protein C pathway has not yet been evaluated with STP. Similar to other TGAs, this assay should be able to evaluate PRP as well as whole blood given the fluorogenic assay condition [71]. The STP reference ranges have been established in pediatric and adult normal subjects.

The STP parameters from the raw curves of thrombin and plasmin generation as well as the first derivative curves are assessed, including the lag time (time to clot initiation), maximal velocity (Vmax), maximum amplitude (MA), time to Vmax, time to MA, and area under the curve, as shown in Figure 11.7. Precise amounts of thrombin and plasmin are not recorded, but results are reported as relative changes as compared to a normal standard.

The NHA monitors thrombin and plasmin generation simultaneously via fluorescent substrates in a sample from a single well (thrombin substrate: Bz-beta-Ala-Gly-Arg-AMC; plasmin substrate: bis-(CBZ-

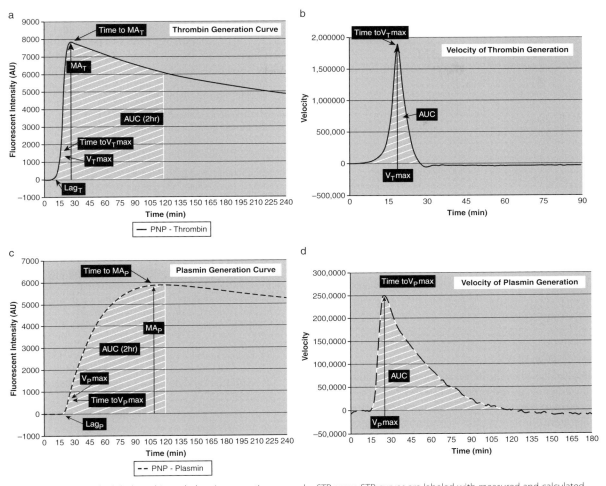

Figure 11.7 Normal adult thrombin and plasmin generation curves by STP assay. STP curves are labeled with measured and calculated parameters. a. Thrombin generation; b. Velocity of thrombin generation; c. Plasmin generation; d. Velocity of plasmin generation. Parameters include: LagT = thrombin lag time (time to start of thrombin generation), VTmax = maximum velocity of thrombin generation, time to VTmax = time to the maximum velocity of thrombin generation, MAT = maximum amplitude of thrombin generation, time to MAT = time to MA of thrombin generation, LagP = plasmin lag time (time to start of plasmin generation), VPmax = maximum velocity of plasmin generation, time to VPmax = time to the maximum velocity of plasmin generation, MAP = maximum amplitude of plasmin generation, time to MAP = time to MA of plasmin generation, AUC (2hr) = area under the curve over the first 2 hours, AUC (1st derivative [velocity] curves) = area under the velocity curve. *Reprinted with permission from Elsevier (Thromb Res 2011;127:317–323).*

L-Phe-L-Arg)-rhodamine. Similar to the STP, coagulation is initiated with tissue factor (0.28 pM), calcium, and phospholipid, while fibrinolysis is accelerated through the addition of tPA (193 IU/ml) [72]. The tPA concentration was specifically chosen to make the plasmin generation sensitive to thrombin activatable fibrinolysis inhibitor (TAFI) activation [73]. The initial work on the NHA has only evaluated adult subjects.

The NHA parameters are defined from the first derivative of the fluorescence signal. Thrombin generation parameters include: (1) lag time (from

initiation to thrombin generation), (2) peak time (time to reach the maximal rate), (3) peak height (maximal velocity of production), and (4) area under the curve (total amount of thrombin generated). Plasmin generation parameters include: (1) plasmin peak (representing the point of clot lysis by plasmin), (2) fibrin lysis time (FLT), and (3) plasmin potential (area under the plasmin curve during FLT). These parameters are depicted in Figure 11.8.

Further research is necessary to determine the utility of the NHA and STP assays in pediatric thrombosis and thrombophilia states.

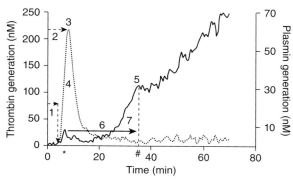

Figure 11.8 Novel hemostasis assay. Simultaneous thrombin and plasmin generation. First derivative of TG (–) and PG (– – –) experiment derived from a measurement in a single well. Thrombin generation signal was divided in four parameters: [1] lag time (minute), [2] thrombin peak time (minute), [3] thrombin peak height (nM), [4] area under the curve (AUC) (nM/minute). Plasmin generation yielded three parameters: [5] the plasmin peak (nM), [6] the fibrin lysis time (FLT) (minute), [7] plasmin potential (nM/minute). Surrogate peak time is marked by * and plasmin peak time is marked by #. *Reprinted with permission from Elsevier (Thromb Res 2012;129(6):681–687).*

Summary

Global assays of coagulation and fibrinolysis add to the knowledge of an individual's hemostatic balance and may help in the evaluation of thrombotic or thrombophilic conditions. While thromboelastography and TGA have been used most widely in clinical practice in non-thrombotic conditions and in clinical research settings of thrombosis/thrombotic risk, additional global assays applied in pediatric thrombosis research have included CloFAL, OHP, and ECLA. Further work dedicated to pediatric thrombosis is needed for all modalities discussed here in order to realize the full potential for global assays to contribute to the understanding of thrombosis/thrombophilia and its optimal management.

References

1. Brummel KE, Paradis SG, Butenas S, Mann KG. Thrombin functions during tissue factor-induced blood coagulation. *Blood.* 2002 Jul 1;**100**(1):148–52.

2. Hartert H. [Not Available]. *Klin Wochenschr.* 1948 Oct 1;**26**(37–38):577–83.

3. Park MS, Martini WZ, Dubick MA, Salinas J, Butenas S, Kheirabadi BS, et al. Thromboelastography as a better indicator of hypercoagulable state after injury than prothrombin time or activated partial thromboplastin time. *J Trauma.* 2009 Aug;**67**(2):266–75;discussion 75–6.

4. Chitlur M, Lusher J. Standardization of thromboelastography: values and challenges. *Semin Thromb Hemost.* 2010 Oct;**36**(7):707–11.

5. Chitlur M, Sorensen B, Rivard GE, Young G, Ingerslev J, Othman M, et al. Standardization of thromboelastography: a report from the TEG-ROTEM working group. *Haemophilia.* 2011 May;**17**(3):532–7.

6. Herbstreit F, Winter EM, Peters J, Hartmann M. Monitoring of haemostasis in liver transplantation: comparison of laboratory based and point of care tests. *Anaesthesia.* 2010 Jan;**65**(1):44–9.

7. De Pietri L, Montalti R, Begliomini B, Scaglioni G, Marconi G, Reggiani A, et al. Thromboelastographic changes in liver and pancreatic cancer surgery: hypercoagulability, hypocoagulability or normocoagulability? *Eur J Anaesthesiol.* 2010 Jul;**27**(7):608–16.

8. Hvitfeldt Poulsen L, Christiansen K, Sorensen B, Ingerslev J. Whole blood thrombelastographic coagulation profiles using minimal tissue factor activation can display hypercoagulation in thrombosis-prone patients. *Scand J Clin Lab Invest.* 2006;**66**(4):329–36.

9. Kupesiz A, Rajpurkar M, Warrier I, Hollon W, Tosun O, Lusher J, et al. Tissue plasminogen activator induced fibrinolysis: standardization of method using thromboelastography. *Blood Coagul Fibrinolysis.* 2010 Jun;**21**(4):320–4.

10. Kupesiz OA, Chitlur MB, Hollon W, Tosun O, Thomas R, Warrier I, et al. Fibrinolytic parameters in children with noncatheter thrombosis: a pilot study. *Blood Coagul Fibrinolysis.* 2010 Jun;**21**(4):313–19.

11. Kashuk JL, Moore EE. The emerging role of rapid thromboelastography in trauma care. *J Trauma.* 2009 Aug;**67**(2):417–18.

12. Geerts WH, Code KI, Jay RM, Chen E, Szalai JP. A prospective study of venous thromboembolism after major trauma. *N Engl J Med.* 1994 Dec;**331**(24):1601–6.

13. Watters JM, Sambasivan CN, Zink K, Kremenevskiy I, Englehart MS, Underwood SJ, et al. Splenectomy leads to a persistent hypercoagulable state after trauma. *Am J Surg.* May 2010;**199**(5):646–51.

14. Copeland H, Nolan PE, Covington D, Gustafson M, Smith R, Copeland JG. A method for anticoagulation of children on mechanical circulatory support. *Artif Organs.* 2011 Nov;**35**(11):1018–23.

15. Andreasen JB, Hvas AM, Christiansen K, Ravn HB. Can RoTEM(R) analysis be applied for haemostatic monitoring in paediatric congenital heart surgery? *Cardiol Young.* 2011 Dec;**21**(6):684–91.

16. Moganasundram S, Hunt BJ, Sykes K, Holton F, Parmar K, Durward A, et al. The relationship among

thromboelastography, hemostatic variables, and bleeding after cardiopulmonary bypass surgery in children. *Anesth Analg.* 2010 Apr;**110**(4):995–1002.

17. Holcomb JB, Minei KM, Scerbo ML, Radwan ZA, Wade CE, Kozar RA, et al. Admission rapid thrombelastography can replace conventional coagulation tests in the emergency department: experience with 1974 consecutive trauma patients. *Ann Surg.* Sep;**256**(3):476–86.

18. Differding JA, Underwood SJ, Van PY, Khaki RA, Spoerke NJ, Schreiber MA. Trauma induces a hypercoagulable state that is resistant to hypothermia as measured by thromboelastogram. *Am J Surg.* May;**201**(5):587–91.

19. Goldenberg NA, Hathaway WE, Jacobson L, Manco-Johnson MJ. A new global assay of coagulation and fibrinolysis. *Thromb Res.* 2005;**116**(4):345–56.

20. Antovic A. The overall hemostasis potential: a laboratory tool for the investigation of global hemostasis. *Semin Thromb Hemost.* 2010 Oct;**36**(7):772–9.

21. He S, Bremme K, Blomback M. A laboratory method for determination of overall haemostatic potential in plasma. I. Method design and preliminary results. *Thromb Res.* 1999 Oct;**96**(2):145–56.

22. He S, Antovic A, Blomback M. A simple and rapid laboratory method for determination of haemostasis potential in plasma. II. Modifications for use in routine laboratories and research work. *Thromb Res.* 2001 Sep;**103**(5):355–61.

23. Bombardier C, Villalobos-Menuey E, Ruegg K, Hathaway WE, Manco-Johnson MJ, Goldenberg NA. Monitoring hypercoagulability and hypofibrinolysis following acute venous thromboembolism in children: application of the CloFAL assay in a prospective inception cohort study. *Thromb Res.* 2012 Sep;**130**(3):343–9.

24. Goldenberg NA, Hathaway WE, Jacobson L, McFarland K, Manco-Johnson MJ. Influence of factor VIII on overall coagulability and fibrinolytic potential of haemophilic plasma as measured by global assay: monitoring in haemophilia A. *Haemophilia.* 2006 Nov;**12**(6):605–14.

25. Goldenberg NA, Bombardier C, Hathaway WE, McFarland K, Jacobson L, Manco-Johnson MJ. Influence of factor IX on overall plasma coagulability and fibrinolytic potential as measured by global assay: monitoring in haemophilia B. *Haemophilia.* 2008 Jan;**14**(1):68–77.

26. University of Colorado Denver. Evaluation of the Duration of Therapy for Thrombosis in Children (Kids-DOTT). Available from: ClinicalTrials.gov

(Internet). Bethesda (MD): National Library of Medicine (US). 2000- [cited 2014 Apr 7]. Available from: http://clinicaltrials.gov/show/NCT00687882 NLM Identifier: NCT00687882.

27. Antovic A, Blomback M, Sten-Linder M, Petrini P, Holmstrom M, He S. Identifying hypocoagulable states with a modified global assay of overall haemostasis potential in plasma. *Blood Coagul Fibrinolysis.* 2005 Nov;**16**(8):585–96.

28. Antovic JP, Yngen M, Ostenson CG, Antovic A, Wallen HN, Jorneskog G, et al. Thrombin activatable fibrinolysis inhibitor and hemostatic changes in patients with type I diabetes mellitus with and without microvascular complications. *Blood Coagul Fibrinolysis.* 2003 Sep;**14**(6):551–6.

29. Antovic JP, Rafik Hamad R, Antovic A, Blomback M, Bremme K. Does thrombin activatable fibrinolysis inhibitor (TAFI) contribute to impairment of fibrinolysis in patients with preeclampsia and/or intrauterine fetal growth retardation? *Thromb Haemost.* 2002 Oct;**88**(4):644–7.

30. Anzej S, Bozic M, Antovic A, Peternel P, Gaspersic N, Rot U, et al. Evidence of hypercoagulability and inflammation in young patients long after acute cerebral ischaemia. *Thromb Res.* 2007;**120**(1):39–46.

31. Rooth E, Wallen H, Antovic A, von Arbin M, Kaponides G, Wahlgren N, et al. Thrombin activatable fibrinolysis inhibitor and its relationship to fibrinolysis and inflammation during the acute and convalescent phase of ischemic stroke. *Blood Coagul Fibrinolysis.* 2007 Jun;**18**(4):365–70.

32. Antovic A, Blomback M, Bremme K, Van Rooijen M, He S. Increased hemostasis potential persists in women with previous thromboembolism with or without APC resistance. *J Thromb Haemost.* 2003 Dec;**1**(12):2531–5.

33. Andresen MS, Abildgaard U. Coagulation inhibitor potential: a study of assay variables. *Thromb Res.* 2005;**115**(6):519–26.

34. Andresen MS, Abildgaard U, Liestol S, Sandset PM, Mowinckel MC, Odegaard OR, et al. The ability of three global plasma assays to recognize thrombophilia. *Thromb Res.* 2004;**113**(6):411–17.

35. Andresen MS, Iversen N, Abildgaard U. Overall haemostasis potential assays performed in thrombophilic plasma: the effect of preactivating protein C and antithrombin. *Thromb Res.* 2002 Dec;**108**(5–6):323–8.

36. Antovic A, Blomback M, Bremme K, He S. The assay of overall haemostasis potential used to monitor the low molecular mass (weight) heparin, dalteparin, and treatment in pregnant women with previous thromboembolism. *Blood Coagul Fibrinolysis.* 2002 Apr;**13**(3):181–6.

37. Smith AA, Jacobson LJ, Miller BI, Hathaway WE, Manco-Johnson MJ. A new euglobulin clot lysis assay for global fibrinolysis. *Thromb Res.* 2003;**112**(5–6): 329–37.

38. Rijken DC, Hoegee-de Nobel E, Jie AF, Atsma DE, Schalij MJ, Nieuwenhuizen W. Development of a new test for the global fibrinolytic capacity in whole blood. *J Thromb Haemost.* 2008 Jan;**6**(1):151–7.

39. Kowalski E, Kopec M, Niewiarowski. An evaluation of the euglobulin method for the determination of fibrinolysis. *J Clin Pathol.* 1959 May;**12**(3):215–18.

40. Swiatkiewicz A, Jurkowski P, Kotschy M, Ciecierski M, Jawien A. Level of antithrombin III, protein C, protein S and other selected parameters of coagulation and fibrinolysis in the blood of the patients with recurrent deep venous thrombosis. *Med Sci Monit.* 2002 Apr;**8**(4): CR263–8.

41. Doig RG, O'Malley CJ, Dauer R, McGrath KM. An evaluation of 200 consecutive patients with spontaneous or recurrent thrombosis for primary hypercoagulable states. *Am J Clin Pathol.* 1994 Dec;**102** (6):797–801.

42. Harbourne T, O'Brien D, Nicolaides AN. Fibrinolytic activity in patients with idiopathic and secondary deep venous thrombosis. *Thromb Res.* 1991 Dec 1;**64**(5):543–50.

43. Sloan IG, Firkin BG. Impaired fibrinolysis in patients with thrombotic or haemostatic defects. *Thromb Res.* 1989 Sep;**55**(5):559–67.

44. Rijken DC, Kock EL, Guimaraes AH, Talens S, Murad SD, Janssen HL, et al. Evidence for an enhanced fibrinolytic capacity in cirrhosis as measured with two different global fibrinolysis tests. *J Thromb Haemost.* 2012 Oct;**10**(10):2116–22.

45. van der Pas R, de Bruin C, Leebeek FW, de Maat MP, Rijken DC, Pereira AM, et al. The hypercoagulable state in Cushing's disease is associated with increased levels of procoagulant factors and impaired fibrinolysis, but is not reversible after short-term biochemical remission induced by medical therapy. *J Clin Endocrinol Metab.* 2012 Apr;**97**(4):1303–10.

46. Castoldi E, Rosing J. Thrombin generation tests. *Thromb Res.* 2011 Feb;**127**(Suppl 3):S21–5.

47. Macfarlane RG, Biggs R. A thrombin generation test: the application in haemophilia and thrombocytopenia. *J Clin Pathol.* 1953 Feb;**6**(1):3–8.

48. Hemker HC, Giesen P, AlDieri R, Regnault V, de Smed E, Wagenvoord R, et al. The calibrated automated thrombogram (CAT): a universal routine test for hyper- and hypocoagulability. *Pathophysiol Haemost Thromb.* 2002 Sep–Dec;**32**(5–6):249–53.

49. Hemker HC, Al Dieri R, De Smedt E, Beguin S. Thrombin generation, a function test of the haemostatic-thrombotic system. *Thromb Haemost.* 2006 Nov;**96**(5):553–61.

50. Baglin T. Using the laboratory to predict recurrent venous thrombosis. *Int J Lab Hematol.* 2011 Aug;**33**(4):333–42.

51. Duchemin J, Pan-Petesch B, Arnaud B, Blouch MT, Abgrall JF. Influence of coagulation factors and tissue factor concentration on the thrombin generation test in plasma. *Thromb Haemost.* 2008 Apr;**99**(4):767–73.

52. Vanschoonbeek K, Feijge MA, Van Kampen RJ, Kenis H, Hemker HC, Giesen PL, et al. Initiating and potentiating role of platelets in tissue factor-induced thrombin generation in the presence of plasma: subject-dependent variation in thrombogram characteristics. *J Thromb Haemost.* 2004 Mar;**2**(3):476–84.

53. Dielis AW, Castoldi E, Spronk HM, van Oerle R, Hamulyak K, Ten Cate H, et al. Coagulation factors and the protein C system as determinants of thrombin generation in a normal population. *J Thromb Haemost.* 2008 Jan;**6**(1):125–31.

54. Haidl H, Cimenti C, Leschnik B, Zach D, Muntean W. Age-dependency of thrombin generation measured by means of calibrated automated thrombography (CAT). *Thromb Haemost.* 2006 May;**95**(5):772–5.

55. Fritsch P, Kleber M, Rosenkranz A, Fritsch M, Muntean W, Mangge H, et al. Haemostatic alterations in overweight children: associations between metabolic syndrome, thrombin generation, and fibrinogen levels. *Atherosclerosis.* 2010 Oct;**212**(2):650–5.

56. Segers O, van Oerle R, Ten Cate H, Rosing J, Castoldi E. Thrombin generation as an intermediate phenotype for venous thrombosis. *Thromb Haemost.* 2010 Jan;**103** (1):114–22.

57. Rosenkranz A, Hiden M, Leschnik B, Weiss EC, Schlembach D, Lang U, et al. Calibrated automated thrombin generation in normal uncomplicated pregnancy. *Thromb Haemost.* 2008 Feb;**99**(2):331–7.

58. Tchaikovski SN, van Vliet HA, Thomassen MC, Bertina RM, Rosendaal FR, Sandset PM, et al. Effect of oral contraceptives on thrombin generation measured via calibrated automated thrombography. *Thromb Haemost.* 2007 Dec;**98**(6):1350–6.

59. Bernhard H, Deutschmann A, Leschnik B, Schweintzger S, Novak M, Hauer A, et al. Thrombin generation in pediatric patients with Crohn's disease. *Inflamm Bowel Dis.* 2011 Nov;**17**(11):2333–9.

60. Couturaud F, Duchemin J, Leroyer C, Delahousse B, Abgrall JF, Mottier D. Thrombin generation in first-degree relatives of patients with venous thromboembolism who have factor V Leiden. A pilot study. *Thromb Haemost.* 2008 Jan;**99**(1):223–8.

61. Lavigne-Lissalde G, Sanchez C, Castelli C, Alonso S, Mazoyer E, Bal Dit Sollier C, et al. Prothrombin

G20210A carriers: the genetic mutation and a history of venous thrombosis contributes to thrombin generation independently of factor II plasma levels. *J Thromb Haemost*. 2010 May;**8**(5):942–9.

62. Castoldi E, Simioni P, Tormene D, Thomassen MC, Spiezia L, Gavasso S, et al. Differential effects of high prothrombin levels on thrombin generation depending on the cause of the hyperprothrombinemia. *J Thromb Haemost*. 2007 May;**5**(5):971–9.

63. Alhenc-Gelas M, Canonico M, Picard V. Influence of natural SERPINC1 mutations on ex vivo thrombin generation. *J Thromb Haemost*. 2010 Apr;**8**(4):845–8.

64. Castoldi E, Maurissen LF, Tormene D, Spiezia L, Gavasso S, Radu C, et al. Similar hypercoagulable state and thrombosis risk in type I and type III protein S-deficient individuals from families with mixed type I/III protein S deficiency. *Haematologica*. 2010 Sep;**95**(9):1563–71.

65. Dargaud Y, Trzeciak MC, Bordet JC, Ninet J, Negrier C. Use of calibrated automated thrombinography +/- thrombomodulin to recognise the prothrombotic phenotype. *Thromb Haemost*. 2006 Nov;**96**(5):562–7.

66. Ten Cate-Hoek AJ, Dielis AW, Spronk HM, van Oerle R, Hamulyak K, Prins MH, et al. Thrombin generation in patients after acute deep-vein thrombosis. *Thromb Haemost*. 2008 Aug;**100**(2):240–5.

67. van Hylckama Vlieg A, Christiansen SC, Luddington R, Cannegieter SC, Rosendaal FR, Baglin TP. Elevated endogenous thrombin potential is associated with an increased risk of a first deep venous thrombosis but not with the risk of recurrence. *Br J Haematol*. 2007 Sep;**138**(6):769–74.

68. Tripodi A, Legnani C, Chantarangkul V, Cosmi B, Palareti G, Mannucci PM. High thrombin generation measured in the presence of thrombomodulin is associated with an increased risk of recurrent venous thromboembolism. *J Thromb Haemost*. 2008 Aug;**6**(8):1327–33.

69. Besser M, Baglin C, Luddington R, van Hylckama Vlieg A, Baglin T. High rate of unprovoked recurrent venous thrombosis is associated with high thrombin-generating potential in a prospective cohort study. *J Thromb Haemost*. 2008 Oct;**6**(10):1720–5.

70. Hron G, Kollars M, Binder BR, Eichinger S, Kyrle PA. Identification of patients at low risk for recurrent venous thromboembolism by measuring thrombin generation. *JAMA*. 2006 Jul 26;**296**(4):397–402.

71. Simpson ML, Goldenberg NA, Jacobson LJ, Bombardier CG, Hathaway WE, Manco-Johnson MJ. Simultaneous thrombin and plasmin generation capacities in normal and abnormal states of coagulation and fibrinolysis in children and adults. *Thromb Res*. 2011 Apr;**127**(4):317–23.

72. van Geffen M, Loof A, Lap P, Boezeman J, Laros-van Gorkom BA, Brons P, et al. A novel hemostasis assay for the simultaneous measurement of coagulation and fibrinolysis. *Hematology*. 2011 Nov;**16**(6):327–36.

73. van Geffen M, van Heerde WL. Global haemostasis assays, from bench to bedside. *Thromb Res*. 2012 Jun;**129**(6):681–7.

Chapter 12

Heparin-induced thrombocytopenia and thrombosis syndrome in children

Courtney D. Thornburg

Historical perspective

Heparin-induced thrombocytopenia (HIT) and heparin-induced thrombocytopenia and thrombosis syndrome (HITTS) are well-described phenomena, particularly in the adult population. These conditions were first described several decades ago [1,2]. At first, these syndromes were under-recognized, leading to limb and life-threatening thrombosis. Recently, due to increased recognition, testing, availability of novel anticoagulants and high concern for missing a case, the trend has shifted to over-diagnosis.

Pathophysiology

The HIT/HITTS condition requires the interaction between heparin, platelet factor 4 (PF4), immunoglobulin G (IgG) and an Fc receptor on the platelet. This interaction results in procoagulant activity of the platelets and a prothrombotic state. These complexes are most likely to be formed under proinflammatory conditions such as surgery, described by Warkentin as "point immunization" [3]. There is a high rate of thrombosis even once heparin is discontinued. This is because the HIT antibody can bind to heparin-PF4 complexes on the surface of endothelial cells, monocytes and polymorphonuclear (PMN) cells, and lead to vessel injury and inflammation, PMN activation and exposure of tissue factor on monocytes.

Special considerations in children

The pathophysiology of HIT/HITTS likely differs between adults and children. This may be related to differences in PF4 levels and immune response, which contribute to immune complex formation as well as platelet reactivity and underlying prothrombotic risk, which contribute to the incidence of thrombosis in the presence of HIT antibodies [4].

Diagnosis

Clinical symptoms

The primary manifestation of HITTS is thrombosis. Venous thrombosis occurs more often than arterial thrombosis. Thrombosis most often occurs within 5–10 days of initial heparin exposure, and if heparin has been given within the past 100 days, within 24 hours of repeat heparin exposure (rapid HITTS). Thrombosis may also occur weeks after heparin exposure (delayed HITTS). Other manifestations include heparin-induced skin necrosis and acute systemic reaction coincident with heparin infusion. Even in the presence of significant thrombocytopenia, bleeding is rare. In fact, bleeding with thrombocytopenia should decrease the suspicion of HIT.

Scoring system

The prevalence of positive HIT antibodies is much higher than the incidence of HIT/HITTS in both adults and children [5]. Therefore, laboratory testing for HIT should only be done when there is an intermediate to high pretest probability. Otherwise, clinicians may feel compelled to initiate an anticoagulant or switch to a non-heparin anticoagulant when the HIT antibody is non-pathogenic.

Due to the complexity of recognizing and diagnosing HIT/HITTS, most clinicians depend on a pretest probability clinical scoring system to guide testing, diagnosis and management [6–8]. A HIT clinical scoring system was first developed by Warkentin and was designed to estimate the probability of HIT based on the four T's, including the degree of thrombocytopenia, the time of platelet count fall, presence of thrombosis or other sequelae described above, and the absence of other causes of thrombocytopenia. The highest pretest

Pediatric Thrombotic Disorders, ed. Neil A. Goldenberg and Marilyn J. Manco-Johnson. Published by Cambridge University Press. © Cambridge University Press 2015.

Table 12.1 Etiology and mechanism of *acute* thrombocytopenia in hospitalized neonates,* children and adolescents at risk for HIT/HITTS

Etiology	Mechanism
Infection	Immune-mediated, increased destruction or decreased production
Drugs	Immune-(including hapten-)mediated or decreased production
Post-transfusion purpura	Immune-mediated
Disseminated intravascular coagulation (DIC)	Increased destruction
Hypersplenism	Consumption of platelets and increased destruction
Thrombosis	Increased destruction
Hemophagocytic lymphohistiocytosis syndrome (HLH)	Increased destruction
Thrombocytopenic purpura (TTP)	Increased destruction

* In neonates where baseline platelet count is not known, consider inherited thrombocytopenia, maternal immune thrombocytopenia purpura (ITP), or neonatal alloimmune thrombocytopenia (NAT).

Table 12.2 Etiology of thrombocytopenia in children with acquired and congenital heart disease

	Etiology
Cardiac	Cyanotic congenital heart disease Prosthetic valves; "Waring blender" effect Repair of intracardiac defects ECMO Cardiopulmonary bypass* Ventricular assist device (VAD) Heart failure leading to hepatosplenomegaly
Non-cardiac	Infection Drugs Disseminated intravascular coagulation (DIC) Post-transfusion purpura Thrombosis

* Thrombocytopenia lasting longer than 4–5 days post-CPB, or recovery of thrombocytopenia after CBP, followed by recurrent thrombocytopenia 5–14 post-operatively is suspicious for HIT/HITTS.

probability is in patients with a platelet count decline of > 50% but without severe thrombocytopenia, i.e., platelet nadir $\geq 20 \times 10^9$/l; clear onset of thrombocytopenia between days 5–10 after heparin exposure or $\leq$ 1 day if prior heparin exposure within 30 days; new confirmed thrombosis, skin necrosis at sites of subcutaneous heparin injection, and/or acute systemic reaction within 30 minutes after intravenous heparin bolus; and no other apparent causes for thrombocytopenia. Cuker *et al.* recently proposed the HIT expert probability (HEP) score, which has expanded clinical criteria based on expert opinion [8].

Predictive scoring systems have not been validated in children. When utilizing the available scoring systems in children, clinicians should consider the broad differential diagnosis of thrombocytopenia in neonates, children and adolescents. Thrombocytopenia occurs fairly frequently in hospitalized neonates, children and adolescents, who also represent the primary risk group for pediatric HIT/HITTS. Reasons for acute thrombocytopenia in these pediatric patients at risk for HIT/HITTS are shown in Table 12.1. Children with congenital heart disease (CHD) as well as acquired heart disease have a particularly high prevalence of thrombocytopenia. Children who undergo extracorporeal membrane oxygenation (ECMO) and cardiopulmonary bypass are exposed to high concentrations of unfractionated heparin (UFH). They are also frequently thrombocytopenic due to cardiac and non-cardiac factors (Table 12.2). Therefore, discerning whether a HIT antibody is pathogenic is especially challenging in these children.

Laboratory testing

There are two primary types of laboratory tests for the diagnosis of HIT: immunologic and functional.

The immunologic assays are enzyme-linked immunosorbent assays (ELISA), which detect antibodies against the complex of PF4 with heparin. These assays are > 95% sensitive. However, since the assay detects both pathogenic and non-pathogenic antibodies, they are only 50–89% specific. The ELISA measures optical density (OD). The standard cut-off for a positive value is 0.4 and high levels are associated with a higher probability of clinical HIT in the adult population. The functional assays include the ^{14}C-serotonin release assay (SRA), the heparin-induced platelet activation assay (HIPA) and the platelet aggregation test. These assays measure antibody-mediated, heparin-dependent platelet activation and are > 90% sensitive and specific. The higher specificity is attributed to only detecting antibodies capable of activating platelets. In clinical practice a combination of the pretest probability, determined by a scoring system, and results of the ELISA assay guide management. Since the SRAs are not readily available at most institutions, results are not available for real-time clinical decision making.

Epidemiology

Heparin-induced thrombocytopenia occurs in a minority of individuals exposed to heparin [9]. HIT/HITTS is very rare in individuals less than 40 years of age, especially neonates and children. Published rates in children range from 0% to 2–3% [10,11]. Risk factors for HIT/HITTS include drug-related factors and patient-related factors. Risk is higher with UFH compared to low molecular weight heparin (LMWH), bovine compared to porcine heparin, and with duration of heparin exposure greater than or equal to, versus less than 6 days. Patient-related risk factors include surgery, older age and female gender.

Special considerations for children

There are several case reports and case series of children with HIT/HITTS [11–21]. Most cases are in children with complex CHD and/or in the intensive care unit setting. The reported frequency of HIT/HITTS in children depends on the patient population and the laboratory tests used to make the diagnosis. The epidemiology of HIT/HITTS is expected to differ from adults based on potential differences in pathophysiology and differences in heparin utilization [4].

Reasons for heparin prescription in children include treatment of venous and arterial thromboembolism (VTE and ATE, respectively). Although the incidence of VTE is lower in children than in adults, the incidence in children is increasing [22–24]. Low-dose UFH may be used to prevent line occlusion in children with central venous access devices. Low molecular weight heparin is most often used for pharmacologic thromboprophylaxis, but UFH may occasionally be used as an alternative. Pharmacologic thromboprophylaxis is now recognized as an important consideration in the care of the hospitalized child [25], albeit lacking high-quality evidence of safety and efficacy for most "indications." High-dose UFH exposures are encountered more and more frequently in children with congenital and acquired heart disease; UFH is used for children on extracorporeal membrane oxygenation (ECMO), undergoing cardiac surgery with cardiopulmonary bypass (CPB), and undergoing cardiac catheterization. In addition, children with ventricular assist devices (VAD), including the Berlin Heart EXCOR pediatric VAD, are anticoagulated with UFH [26]. Children who undergo surgery for CHD or solid organ transplant are anticoagulated with UFH during the post-operative period [27].

Management

If HIT/HITTS is suspected with intermediate or high clinical probability, the first step is to remove all heparin exposure including flushes and catheters [28]. Four-extremity Doppler ultrasound should be performed to investigate for VTE. Due to the high risk of thrombosis in the setting of HIT a non-heparin anticoagulant should be initiated. Blood for immunologic assay of antibodies against heparin complexed with PF4 should then be sent. Subsequent management depends on test results and clinical probability of HIT/HITTS. If the immunologic assay is positive, a functional assay may be done for confirmation. If the immunologic assay is negative but the clinical probability is high, patients may still be managed as if they have HIT/HITTS. If the immunologic assay is negative and there is low or intermediate clinical probability, HIT is unlikely and heparin may be restarted. Since bleeding is a rare complication of HIT/HITTS and there are limited data regarding the safety of platelet transfusions in HIT/HITTS, adult guidelines recommend against platelet transfusion [29].

Non-heparin anticoagulation

Direct thrombin inhibitors (DTIs) are the non-heparin anticoagulant of choice, because they have not been associated with HIT/HITTS. Direct thrombin inhibitors bind thrombin directly and do not require antithrombin to function. Argatroban and bivalirudin are parenteral DTIs that have been prescribed to children with HIT/HITTS [30]. Argatroban is a synthetic DTI administered by continuous intravenous (IV) infusion. The half-life is approximately 40 minutes and clearance is both weight-dependent and decreased in children compared with adults [31]. It should be used with caution in children with hepatic disease due to dependence on the liver for clearance [31]. Bivalirudin is administered by continuous IV infusion. A bolus may be given prior to the infusion. The half-life is approximately 25 minutes and clearance is decreased with renal insufficiency. Both agents are monitored using the APTT with a goal of 1.5–3 times baseline. Neither DTI has an established antidote for reversal, which complicates management in children at high risk for bleeding. Novel strategies such as bypassing agents may be necessary; there are limited ex vivo data suggesting that rVIIa overcomes the anticoagulant effect of non-heparin anticoagulants including bivalirudin and argatroban as measured by thromboelastography [32].

There is limited pediatric experience with bivalirudin for thrombosis [33], cardiac transplantation [16], CPB [21,34] and percutaneous coronary interventions [35]. Young *et al.* conducted a pilot study of bivalirudin in infants < 6 months of age with thrombosis [33]. Forbes *et al.* conducted a study of bivalirudin in infants and children undergoing percutaneous coronary interventions [35]. In both cases, dose response was similar to that of adults. The US Food and Drug Administration (FDA) has not approved specific pediatric dosing, but the adult dosing recommendations include a 0.75 mg/kg bolus, followed by an infusion of 1.75 mg/kg/h. Dose reduction to 1 mg/kg/h is recommended for adult patients with renal clearance < 30 ml/kg/h, and to 0.25 mg/kg/h for adults on hemodialysis. There is additional pediatric experience with argatroban for ECMO, cardiac catheterization, CPB, hemodialysis and VTE [21,31,36,37]. Young *et al.* published a prospective safey, efficacy and pharmacokinetic (PK) study of argatroban in children ≤ 16 years of age who were suspected of having HIT or were at risk for HIT and required anticoagulation for thrombosis, cardiac catheterization, cardiac surgery, ECMO or hemodialysis. [31,38]. Thirteen of 18 subjects received argatroban by continuous IV infusion. Although argatroban is not formally FDA-approved for use in children, the data from this study are included in the pediatric labeling information for argatroban, with a recommended starting dose of 0.75 micrograms/kg/minute in critically ill children; in the setting of hepatic insufficiency a starting dose of 0.2 micrograms/kg/min is recommended [39].

Transition to warfarin

In most cases, patients with HIT/HITTS will be transitioned from a parenteral DTI to warfarin. Individuals with HIT/HITTS are at risk for limb gangrene if warfarin is started too early in the course. Based on adult guidelines, warfarin should be started once the platelet count is $\geq 150 \times 10^9$/l and should be given concomitantly with a non-heparin anticoagulant for at least 5 days. Recommended starting dose is ≤ 5 mg/day. If transitioning from argatroban to warfarin, clinicians must recognize that argatroban raises the INR in addition to the APTT. Therefore, a patient on argatroban will likely not be therapeutic on warfarin until the INR is > 4, which equates to a warfarin-only effect on INR of 2–3 [40]; a chromogenic plasma factor X activity of < 45% may also be used as an adjunct to the INR to determine when a therapeutic warfarin effect has been achieved. There are adult guidelines for transitioning to warfarin [41].

If anticoagulation with warfarin is not feasible, fondaparinux may be used as an alternative. Fondaparinux is a synthetic pentasaccharide that is administered subcutaneously (SC) once per day; HIT/HITTS associated with fondaparinux has rarely been reported [42]. Young *et al.* conducted a prospective study of the PK and safety of fondaparinux in children ages 1–18 years with VTE and/or a diagnosis of HIT [43]. Based on this study, dosing recommendations are 0.1 mg/kg SC daily; the dose is titrated to achieve a goal anti-factor Xa level (using a fondaparinux standard) of 0.5–1.0 U/ml.

Duration of anticoagulation

The duration of anticoagulation in HIT/HITTS depends on whether there is concomitant thrombosis (i.e., HIT vs. HITTS). As described above, individuals with pathogenic HIT antibodies have a high likelihood of developing thrombosis if no anticoagulation is given. Therefore, adult recommendations suggest anticoagulation for 1–3 months in the absence of thrombosis [41]. If thrombosis is present, children may be anticoagulated based on standard guidelines for management of thrombosis, typically 3–6 months [44].

Heparin re-exposure

Children with HIT/HITTS, particularly those with underlying CHD, may require anticoagulation in the future. The approach to anticoagulation depends on the clinical setting, the timing of a procedure relative to the episode of HIT/HITTS, the current laboratory test results and the type of procedure. If emergent cardiac surgery is required in the setting of acute HIT/HITTS with positive immunologic and functional assays, surgery may be done with a DTI. If there is a remote history of HIT/HITTS and negative immunologic and functional assays, UFH may possibly be used at the time of surgery with very close clinical and hematologic laboratory (i.e., platelet count) monitoring, or else a more cautious approach may be adopted of using an IV DTI in lieu of UFH. For cardiac catheterization, the risk of a bleeding complication with a DTI is low; adult guidelines recommend non-heparin anticoagulation regardless of timing from acute HIT/HITTS and current laboratory profile. In all cases, surgery should be done with close collaboration among hematology, cardiology, surgery and anesthesia.

Future approaches to preventing HIT/HITS

By avoiding heparin exposure, HIT/HITTS may be prevented. However, it is unlikely that utilization of heparin will decline dramatically in the near future. Therefore, alternative strategies to prevent the "point immunization" may be required. Sachais *et al.* proposed the development of small molecules to block PF4 such that the causative immune complex can be disrupted [45]. An alternative strategy may be to prophylactically give 2–0, 3–0 desulfated heparin (ODSH) at the time of heparin infusion; ODSH disrupts PF4 heparin interactions and thereby is suggested to block the formation of complexes and associated antibodies [46].

Table 12.3 Non-heparin anticoagulants* used in pediatric HIT/HITTs

Drug	Type	Mode of administration	Approved indications [47]	Pediatric label information
Argatroban	DTI	IV	Prophylaxis or treatment of thrombosis in adult patients with heparin-induced thrombocytopenia (HIT); in patients with, or at risk for, HIT undergoing percutaneous coronary intervention (PCI)	Yes; note regarding study of seriously ill children, particularly those with hepatic impairment
Bivalirudin	DTI	IV	In adult patients with unstable angina undergoing percutaneous transluminal coronary angioplasty (PTCA); with provisional use of glycoprotein IIb/IIIa inhibitor (GPI) in adult patients undergoing percutaneous coronary intervention (PCI); for adult patients with, or at risk of, HIT or HITTS undergoing PCI	No
Fondaparinux	LMWH	SC	Treatment of DVT/PE in adults when administered in conjunction with warfarin sodium; DVT/PE thromboprophylaxis in adults with: knee replacement surgery, hip replacement surgery, hip fracture surgery or abdominal surgery	Yes [48]; note regarding increased risk of bleeding for individuals < 50 kg, including those in the pediatric population [47]

* There is no standard antidote for any of these non-heparin anticoagulants

Summary

In summary, HIT/HITTS is an adverse drug reaction with often severe, and potentially fatal, consequences. There are few clinical data about HIT/HITTS in children and recommendations for evaluation and management of pediatric HIT/HITTS are primarily extrapolated from adult studies. Clinicians who manage children with anticoagulants must maintain familiarity with risk factors for HIT/HITTS, when and how to test, and how to manage those with suspected and confirmed HIT/HITTS.

References

1. Rhodes GR, Dixon RH, Silver D. Heparin-induced thrombocytopenia with thrombotic and hemorrhagic manifestations. Surg Gynecol Obstet. 1973;**136**(3):409–16.

2. Weismann RE, Tobin RW. Arterial embolism occurring during systemic heparin therapy. AMA Arch Surg. 1958;**76**(2):219–25; discussion 25–7.

3. Warkentin TE. HIT paradigms and paradoxes. J Thromb Haemost. 2011;9(Suppl 1):105–17.

4. Takemoto CM, Streiff MB. Heparin-induced thrombocytopenia screening and management in pediatric patients. Hematology/the Education Program of the American Society of Hematology. 2011;**2011**:162–9.

5. Mullen MP, Wessel DL, Thomas KC, Gauvreau K, Neufeld EJ, McGowan FX, Jr., et al. The incidence and implications of anti-heparin-platelet factor 4 antibody formation in a pediatric cardiac surgical population. Anesth Analg. 2008;**107**(2):371–8.

6. Warkentin TE. New approaches to the diagnosis of heparin-induced thrombocytopenia. Chest. 2005;**127**(2 Suppl):35S–45S.

7. Lo GK, Juhl D, Warkentin TE, Sigouin CS, Eichler P, Greinacher A. Evaluation of pretest clinical score (4 T's) for the diagnosis of heparin-induced thrombocytopenia in two clinical settings. J Thromb Haemost. 2006;**4**(4):759–65.

8. Cuker A, Arepally G, Crowther MA, Rice L, Datko F, Hook K, et al. The HIT Expert Probability (HEP) Score: a novel pre-test probability model for heparin-induced thrombocytopenia based on broad expert opinion. J Thromb Haemost. 2010;**8**(12):2642–50.

9. Cuker A. Update in the diagnosis and management of heparin-induced thrombocytopenia. Clin Adv Hematol Oncol. 2012;**10**(7):453–5.

10. Newall F, Barnes C, Ignjatovic V, Monagle P. Heparin-induced thrombocytopenia in children. J Paediatr Child Health. 2003;**39**(4):289–92.

11. Schmugge M, Risch L, Huber AR, Benn A, Fischer JE. Heparin-induced thrombocytopenia-associated thrombosis in pediatric intensive care patients. Pediatrics. 2002;**109**(1):E10.

12. Ranze O, Ranze P, Magnani HN, Greinacher A. Heparin-induced thrombocytopenia in paediatric patients – a review of the literature and a new case treated with danaparoid sodium. Eur J Pediatr. 1999;**158**(Suppl 3):S130–3.

13. Klenner AF, Lubenow N, Raschke R, Greinacher A. Heparin-induced thrombocytopenia in children: 12 new cases and review of the literature. Thromb Haemost. 2004;**91**(4):719–24.

14. Murdoch IA, Beattie RM, Silver DM. Heparin-induced thrombocytopenia in children. Acta Paediatr. 1993;**82**(5):495–7.

15. Potter KE, Raj A, Sullivan JE. Argatroban for anticoagulation in pediatric patients with heparin-induced thrombocytopenia requiring extracorporeal life support. J Pediatr Hematol/Oncol. 2007;**29**(4):265–8.

16. Almond CS, Harrington J, Thiagarajan R, Duncan CN, LaPierre R, Halwick D, et al. Successful use of bivalirudin for cardiac transplantation in a child with heparin-induced thrombocytopenia. J Heart Lung Transplant. 2006;**25**(11):1376–9.

17. Risch L, Huber AR, Schmugge M. Diagnosis and treatment of heparin-induced thrombocytopenia in neonates and children. Thromb Res. 2006;**118**(1):123–35.

18. Spadone D, Clark F, James E, Laster J, Hoch J, Silver D. Heparin-induced thrombocytopenia in the newborn. J Vasc Surg. 1992;**15**(2):306–11; discussion 11–12.

19. Severin T, Sutor AH. Heparin-induced thrombocytopenia in pediatrics. Semin Thromb Hemost. 2001;**27**(3):293–9.

20. Alsoufi B, Boshkov LK, Kirby A, Ibsen L, Dower N, Shen I, et al. Heparin-induced thrombocytopenia (HIT) in pediatric cardiac surgery: an emerging cause of morbidity and mortality. Semin Thorac Cardiovasc Surg Pediatr Card Surg Annu. 2004;**7**:155–71.

21. Argueta-Morales IR, Olsen MC, DeCampli WM, Munro HM, Felix DE. Alternative anticoagulation during cardiovascular procedures in pediatric patients with heparin-induced thrombocytopenia. J Extra Corpor Technol. 2012;**44**(2):69–74.

22. Raffini L, Huang YS, Witmer C, Feudtner C. Dramatic increase in venous thromboembolism in children's hospitals in the United States from 2001 to 2007. Pediatrics. 2009;**124**(4):1001–8.

23. Setty BA, O'Brien SH, Kerlin BA. Pediatric venous thromboembolism in the United States: a tertiary care complication of chronic diseases. Pediatr Blood Cancer. 2012;**59**(2):258–64.

24. Boulet SL, Grosse SD, Thornburg CD, Yusuf H, Tsai J, Hooper WC. Trends in venous thromboembolism-related hospitalizations, 1994–2009. Pediatrics. 2012;**130**(4):e812–20.

25. Raffini L, Trimarchi T, Beliveau J, Davis D. Thromboprophylaxis in a pediatric hospital: a patient-safety and quality-improvement initiative. Pediatrics. 2011;**127**(5):e1326–32.

26. Fraser CD, Jr., Jaquiss RD, Rosenthal DN, Humpl T, Canter CE, Blackstone EH, et al. Prospective trial of a pediatric ventricular assist device. N Engl J Med. 2012;**367**(6):532–41.

27. Hardikar W, Poddar U, Chamberlain J, Teo S, Bhat R, Jones B, et al. Evaluation of a post-operative thrombin inhibitor replacement protocol to reduce haemorrhagic and thrombotic complications after paediatric liver transplantation. Thromb Res. 2010;**126**(3):191–4.

28. Arepally GM, Ortel TL. Clinical practice. Heparin-induced thrombocytopenia. N Engl J Med. 2006;**355**(8):809–17.

29. Cuker A, Cines DB. How I treat heparin-induced thrombocytopenia. Blood. 2012;**119**(10):2209–18.

30. Young G. New anticoagulants in children: a review of recent studies and a look to the future. Thromb Res. 2011;**127**(2):70–4.

31. Young G, Boshkov LK, Sullivan JE, Raffini LJ, Cox DS, Boyle DA, et al. Argatroban therapy in pediatric patients requiring nonheparin anticoagulation: an open-label, safety, efficacy, and pharmacokinetic study. Pediatr Blood Cancer. 2011;**56**(7):1103–9.

32. Young G, Yonekawa KE, Nakagawa PA, Blain RC, Lovejoy AE, Nugent DJ. Recombinant activated factor VII effectively reverses the anticoagulant effects of heparin, enoxaparin, fondaparinux, argatroban, and bivalirudin ex vivo as measured using thromboelastography. Blood Coagul Fibrinolysis. 2007;**18**(6):547–53.

33. Young G, Tarantino MD, Wohrley J, Weber LC, Belvedere M, Nugent DJ. Pilot dose-finding and safety study of bivalirudin in infants < 6 months of age with thrombosis. J Thromb Haemost. 2007;**5**(8):1654–9.

34. Gates R, Yost P, Parker B. The use of bivalirudin for cardiopulmonary bypass anticoagulation in pediatric heparin-induced thrombocytopenia patients. Artif Organs. 2010;**34**(8):667–9.

35. Forbes TJ, Hijazi ZM, Young G, Ringewald JM, Aquino PM, Vincent RN, et al. Pediatric catheterization laboratory anticoagulation with bivalirudin. Catheter Cardiovasc Interv. 2011;**77**(5):671–9.

36. Wright JM, Watts RG. Venous thromboembolism in pediatric patients: epidemiologic data from a pediatric tertiary care center in Alabama. J Pediatr Hematol/Oncol. 2011;**33**(4):261–4.

37. Hursting MJ, Dubb J, Verme-Gibboney CN. Argatroban anticoagulation in pediatric patients: a literature analysis. J Pediatr Hematol/Oncol. 2006;**28**(1):4–10.

38. Madabushi R, Cox DS, Hossain M, Boyle DA, Patel BR, Young G, et al. Pharmacokinetic and pharmacodynamic basis for effective argatroban dosing in pediatrics. J Clin Pharmacol. 2011;**51**(1):19–28.

39. Argatroban prescribing information 2008 [cited 2012 September 24]. Available from: http://www.access data.fda.gov/drugsatfda_docs/label/2008/020883s014 lbl.pdf

40. Hursting MJ, Lewis BE, Macfarlane DE. Transitioning from argatroban to warfarin therapy in patients with heparin-induced thrombocytopenia. Clin Appl Thromb Hemost. 2005;**11**(3):279–87.

41. Cuker A, Crowther M. 2009 clinical practice guidelines on the evaluation and management of heparin-induced thromboctyopenia (HIT 2009) (cited 2012 September 17). Available from: hematology.org/Practice/Guidelines/4678.aspx

42. Chong BH, Chong JJ. Heparin-induced thrombocytopenia associated with fondaparinux. Clin Adv Hematol Oncol. 2010;**8**(1):63–5.

43. Young G, Yee DL, O'Brien SH, Khanna R, Barbour A, Nugent DJ. FondaKIDS: a prospective pharmacokinetic and safety study of fondaparinux in children between 1 and 18 years of age. Pediatr Blood Cancer. 2011;**57**(6):1049–54.

44. Monagle P, Chan AK, Goldenberg NA, Ichord RN, Journeycake JM, Nowak-Gottl U, et al. Antithrombotic therapy in neonates and children: Antithrombotic Therapy and Prevention of Thrombosis, 9th edn: American College of Chest Physicians Evidence-Based Clinical Practice Guidelines. Chest. 2012;**141**(2 Suppl):e737S–801S.

45. Sachais BS, Rux AH, Cines DB, Yarovoi SV, Garner LI, Watson SP, et al. Rational design and characterization of platelet factor 4 antagonists for the study of heparin-induced thrombocytopenia. Blood. 2012;**119**(25):5955–62.

46. Joglekar MV, Quintana Diez PM, Marcus S, Qi R, Espinasse B, Wiesner MR, et al. Disruption of PF4/H multimolecular complex formation with a minimally anticoagulant heparin (ODSH). Thromb Haemost. 2012;**107**(4):717–25.

47. Donoghue M, Suh KR, Facilitating Development of Anticoagulant Drugs for Use in Pediatric Patients. FDA Presentation to Pediatric Subcommittee of the Oncologic Drugs Advisory Committee. Food and Drugs Administration, 2011.

48. Food and Drugs Administration. Arixtra (fondaparinux sodium) prescribing information, September, 2013: www.accessdata.fda.gov/drugsatfda_docs/label/2013/021345s030lbl.pdf Reference ID: 3372362.

Severe thrombophilias

Cameron C. Trenor III and Marilyn J. Manco-Johnson

Introduction

Thrombophilia denotes a constitutional predisposition to thrombosis; thrombophilic traits may be genetic or acquired. It has not been standard practice to grade thrombophilia by severity, but such a grading could have practical clinical import. Grading of thrombophilia may be performed in a number of ways. The severity of thrombophilia may be regarded as the magnitude of the risk for first (incident) thrombosis, risk for thrombus recurrence or risk for poor thrombotic outcomes such as death or post-thrombotic syndrome. Severity of thrombophilia may also denote the clinical severity of the thrombotic episode, such as thrombotic storm or purpura fulminans. "Thrombophilia," if extended to the larger context of prothrombotic risk beyond blood-based predisposing factors, can also be anatomic, such as external venous compression (e.g., Paget–Schroetter, May–Thurner); however, we will focus in this chapter on hematologic thrombophilia. This includes enhanced procoagulants, diminished anticoagulants and diminished fibrinolysis as mechanisms leading to increased thrombosis.

Genetic thrombophilic traits judged to be more potent often present at an earlier age or manifest recurrence soon after discontinuation of anticoagulation for a previous event. Patients with severe thrombophilia may spontaneously initiate a thrombotic event, while most experience a provoking trigger, tipping the balance in favor of thrombosis. However, the severe thrombophilias may require only a slight trigger (i.e., a mild upper respiratory infection), which may result in sustained activation of coagulation and progressive thrombosis even despite conventional antithrombotic drugs at typical target anticoagulant activity and duration. In this chapter we attempt to describe the subset of pediatric thrombotic syndromes

that are clinically very severe and require a high index of suspicion, prompt diagnosis and immediate institution of appropriate therapy for a favorable outcome.

Severe genetic thrombophilic syndromes

Most severe genetic thrombophilias occur as non-conserved mutations (i.e., not founder effects such as factor V Leiden). Autosomal genetic syndromes are generally characterized as homozygous (an identical mutation on each chromosomal allele, commonly found in settings of consanguinity), compound heterozygous (both alleles affected but by different mutations) or simple heterozygous (a single allele mutation). Type I deficiencies denote a quantitative defect while type II deficiencies are qualitative. Most severe defects are compound heterozygous and quantitative.

Severe/moderately severe protein C deficiency

The prototype of the most severe genetic thrombophilia determined in human thrombotic disease is homozygous or compound heterozygous protein C (PC) deficiency [1]. This genetic disorder is generally related to one or two different null mutations resulting in undetectable circulating plasma PC activity or antigen; by definition PC plasma concentration in severe/moderately severe (hereinafter referred to simply as "severe") PC deficiency is less than than 20 U/dl. Severe PC deficiency most often presents within hours or days of birth with purpura fulminans (PF), a thrombotic disorder of the capillaries and post-capillary venules in soft tissues, particularly the subcutaneous fat. Purpura fulminans manifests as exquisitely painful red lesions caused by small vessel thrombosis with extravasation

Pediatric Thrombotic Disorders, ed. Neil A. Goldenberg and Marilyn J. Manco-Johnson. Published by Cambridge University Press. © Cambridge University Press 2015.

of red blood cells into the skin that quickly become indurated and necrotic resulting in eschars. The skin lesions are accompanied by systemic evidence of disseminated intravascular coagulation (DIC) with thrombocytopenia, hypofibrinogenemia, prolonged PT and APTT, and elevated D-dimer. Once initiated, PF and DIC do not respond to conventional anticoagulation alone and require PC replacement. Infants with severe genetic PC deficiency may also present with large-vessel thrombosis such as renal vein thrombosis, deep vein thrombosis (DVT) or arterial ischemic stroke (AIS). Evidence of prenatal thrombosis may be present and most commonly affects the eyes, the brain and the renal veins. Infants with severe PC deficiency are often born blind from in utero thrombosis of the developing retinal veins [2]. Most affected newborn infants require indefinite anticoagulation or PC replacement to prevent recurrent DIC, while a small minority resolves spontaneous activation of coagulation after resolution of an active lesion. Currently available PC concentrates are produced from pooled human plasma and are subjected to standard viral inactivation procedures (Ceprotin®, Baxter BioScience, Marburg, GE). The volume of distribution of PC is similar to that of other vitamin K-dependent factors or approximately twice the plasma volume, and the half-life is approximately 6–8 hours. Protein C can be replaced during acute episodes of PF with 100 IU/kg bolus and maintenance with 50 IU/kg every 6–8 hours initially, decreasing to every 12 to 48 hours as PF or DIC resolves. The trough plasma PC activity should be maintained above 20 U/dl. Protein C can be replaced in the neonate using fresh frozen plasma (FFP), although volume overload may limit the potential for maintenance of protein C replacement. Addition of anticoagulation generally allows resolution of PF and DIC with lower trough levels of PC. Recurrent episodes of PF and DIC are often triggered by childhood viral infections that affect the endothelium, such as adenovirus; recurrent episodes often first manifest at the site of first neonatal lesions. Many affected children, adolescents and young adults are maintained on continuous PC replacement by either the intravenous or subcutaneous route [3,4]. Doses as low as 50 U/kg given three times weekly have been sufficient to prevent recurrent episodes of PF, DIC and thrombosis. Concomitant use of warfarin with an INR of 1.5–2.0 or 2.0–3.0 has allowed less frequent dosing with PC concentrate.

Following a severe neonatal presentation, infants and children with severe PC deficiency can sometimes be managed with anticoagulation, with stable courses punctuated by episodes of triggered DIC and PF, separated by several months to a year or more. Coagulation activation in affected individuals increases progressively during and after puberty, such that recurrent episodes of PF and DIC are difficult to prevent or control without PC replacement. Anticoagulation can be used concomitantly and can limit the amount of protein concentrate required. Interestingly, a few patients with endogenous PC activity levels of 2% to 7% have not presented with thrombosis until puberty or later [5]. A male with compound heterozygous PC mutations, 7% plasma PC activity and concomitant heterozygous factor V Leiden first presented with a trauma-related DVT at age 15 years. Within 10 years he suffered chronic persistent DIC and recurrent DVT requiring long-term PC replacement and anticoagulation, but did not develop lesions of PF [5]. The phenotype may vary even between affected siblings [6]. Individuals with genetic severe PC deficiency, who are promptly recognized, diagnosed and appropriately supported, can survive to adulthood with good quality of life [1]. Currently, the number of individuals known to be surviving with severe PC deficiency and receiving PC concentrate replacement in North America and Western Europe (approximately 30) is far fewer than that expected based on gene frequency (1/360,000) [7,8]. The small number of individuals supported suggests that most affected individuals die in utero, at birth or during infancy without a diagnosis. An international registry is currently collecting data on the natural history of severe PC deficiency, as well as documenting the safety of replacement and anticoagulant therapy. For information, please access clinicaltrials.gov, Ceprotin Treatment Registry, NCT 01127529. An international database for PC mutations is maintained by the International Society for Thrombosis and Haemostasis, Scientific and Standardization Committee, Subcommittee on Plasma Coagulation Inhibitors [9].

Protein C deficiency can be acquired through multiple mechanisms. Severe PC deficiency can be acquired with multiple bacterial infections, the most common being meningococcemia, resulting in severe DIC and PF, with organ and limb infarction [1]. The mechanism of acquired PC deficiency in sepsis is PC consumption and decreased synthesis. This acquired PF differs somewhat from the genetic syndrome, with purpura more concentrated on the limbs rather than the trunk. While primary treatment is focused on antimicrobial therapy and general supportive care, PC replacement and anticoagulation are sometimes administered to decrease the extent of tissue necrosis and organ infarction. Probable acquired PC deficiency and severe recurrent thrombosis have been described in a teenage girl with ulcerative colitis and antiphospholipid antibodies (APA) [10]. In contrast, genetic PC deficiency complicated by an acquired primary antiphospholipid antibody syndrome (APS) was proposed as a cause of recurrent episodes of AIS in a child [11]. Valproic acid therapy has been implicated as a cause of PC deficiency in patients with seizures and has been associated with AIS in one reported child [12]. Acquired PC deficiency and a clinically severe prothrombotic phenotype have also been reported in a child with acute myelogenous leukemia undergoing chemotherapy [13]. It is often difficult to determine whether PC deficiency determined in the setting of complicated underlying illness is genetic or acquired.

Acquired PC deficiency is most commonly seen in severe bacterial sepsis. A trial consisting of a continuous infusion of recombinant activated PC (APC) was conducted based on the hypothesis that APC is critical to down-regulate inflammation in severe sepsis, to reverse the systemic inflammatory response and consequently to decrease the mortality of sepsis. This therapy has not been proven to be effective in adequately powered clinical trials and, furthermore, was associated with an excess of bleeding, particularly intracranial hemorrhage, in infants less than 60 days of age [14,15]. Recombinant APC was also reported in the therapy of PF caused by severe genetic PC; in this setting APC was partially effective but less effective than zymogen PC replacement [16]. Therefore, APC should not be considered as standard therapy for genetic or acquired PC deficiency.

Severe/moderately severe protein S deficiency

A few case reports have documented severe genetic protein S (PS) deficiency, usually in newborn infants, with a phenotype similar to severe genetic PC deficiency with neonatal PF [17,18]. Congenital blindness may also present in infants with severe genetic PS deficiency [19]. Similar to PC, reported affected babies have usually had compound heterozygosity for two different null mutations and required long-term PS replacement [18,20]. Currently, there is no purified

PS concentrate and PS can be replaced in FFP or some concentrates of vitamin K-dependent proteins. It is necessary to contact the manufacturer regarding the relative concentration of PS in prothrombin complex concentrates. Anticoagulant therapy is important to maintain for thrombotic events in which PS is replaced via these plasma derivates. Compound heterozygosity resulting in both PC and PS deficiency can present with a severe phenotype, including PF [21]. A database of PS mutations is kept by the International Society of Thrombosis and Haemostasis, Scientific and Standardization Committee, Subcommittee on Plasma Coagulation Inhibitors [22].

Severe PS deficiency can also be acquired and associated with a severe clinical phenotype. The prototype of acquired PS deficiency presents following varicella infection and is usually accompanied by APA. Affected children have suffered severe thromboses with myocardial infarction, AIS, PF and limb loss [23]. In one study, molecular mimicry between PS and varicella antigens with cross-reacting antibodies was proposed based on laboratory investigations [24]. Another possible explanation is inhibition of laboratory testing of PS function by lupus anticoagulant.

Severe/moderately severe antithrombin deficiency

Complete deficiency of antithrombin (AT) appears to be incompatible with life, as no live-born infant has been determined to have undetectable plasma levels of antithrombin. Heterozygous antithrombin deficiency is associated with a more severe phenotype than that reported for PC or PS [25,26]. To date, all described cases of homozygous antithrombin mutations are type II and affect the active site, which physiologically reacts with several serine proteases, the heparin binding site or are near the active site loop [27–30]. Antithrombin deficiency has been recently reviewed [30]. A database of AT mutations is maintained by the International Society of Thrombosis and Haemostasis, Scientific and Standardization Committee, Subcommittee on Plasma Coagulation Inhibitors [31]. Antithrombin deficiency can be acquired by a multitude of mechanisms including urinary loss in nephrotic syndrome, gastrointestinal losses in protein-losing enteropathies, decreased synthesis with severe liver disease, the use of L-asparaginase chemotherapy or consumption during sepsis, or on extracorporeal circuits, including extracorporeal membrane oxygenators (ECMO) [32]. A case of acquired AT deficiency in a newborn infant caused by maternal transfer of APA has been reported in association with severe aortic thrombosis [33].

Recombinant human AT purified from transgenic goat milk (Atryn®, GTC Biotherapeutics, Framingham, MA, USA) as well as a human plasma-derived, viral-inactivated lyophilized concentrate (Thrombate®, Grifols, Barcelona, Spain) are available for replacement of severe genetic or acquired deficiencies for prevention or treatment of thrombosis. A severe deficiency may be defined as AT activity less than 30 U/dl beyond the age of 6 months, and less than 20 U/dl in the newborn infant. Plasma AT activity increases by 2% for each U/kg infused [34]. The terminal half-life (beyond 24 hours) of AT in plasma is approximately 60 hours. Antithrombin can be replaced for a severely deficient patient in steady state conditions in doses of 50 U/kg of plasma-derived antithrombin given every other day. The use of AT replacement in pediatric patients has been recently reviewed and 97% of utilization in tertiary care children's hospitals is for acquired deficiencies [35]. Anticoagulation is important to maintain for thrombotic episodes in which AT is being replaced.

Congenital fibrinogen deficiencies and dysfunctions

Congenital fibrinogen deficiencies, including both afibrinogenemia and dysfibrinogenemia, have been associated with severe thrombotic phenotypes. The former association appears, at first, to be counterintuitive, given that afibrinogenemia is a congenital disorder manifesting initially with moderate to severe bleeding. Until recently reports of spontaneous and triggered thrombosis in patients with afibrinogenemia were considered to be rare events and to occur as adverse events related to fibrinogen replacement therapy. A recent review of reported cases of afibrinogenemia support that severe thrombotic events, including AIS and arterial thromboembolism, occur in many patients with afibrinogenemia distant from replacement therapy, and are particularly frequent in the context of surgery [36]. Of note, the presentation of AIS was clinically indistinguishable from hemorrhagic stroke with acute-onset focal neurologic signs in this review; appropriate imaging was required for proper

diagnosis. The pathophysiology of thrombosis in patients with afibrinogenemia has not been fully elucidated. Fibrin functions as a sink for free thrombin and was originally designated as "antithrombin I" [37]. The absence of fibrinogen could result in an excess of free thrombin available to activate platelets and endothelial cells; this theory is supported by a mouse knock-out model of afibrinogenemia [38]. Alternatively, a histological study in one patient with afibrinogenemia and recurrent embolic lesions from the iliac artery demonstrated an intramural hematoma in the arterial medial wall. Excess thrombin generated locally was hypothesized in this case to form poorly organized clots that disengaged and embolized from the site of the hematoma [39]. Patients with afibrinogenemia and recurrent thrombotic events have benefited clinically from routine replacement infusions of fibrinogen [36]. Implantation during early pregnancy is particularly disabled in afibrinogenemia. Essentially all women with afibrinogenemia require fibrinogen replacement prior to or within a few weeks of conception to prevent predictable spontaneous abortion, which occurs around 7 weeks after fertilization [36].

Abnormal fibrinogen function – dysfibrinogenemia – can manifest with either bleeding or thrombotic phenotypes. Certain dysfibrinogenemias have displayed an association with recurrent thrombosis. Studies of purified or expressed dysfunctional protein have suggested that thromboses may occur either as a consequence of decreased thrombin binding to abnormal fibrinogen, resulting in an excess of unregulated thrombin, or by decreased binding of plasminogen and/or tissue plasminogen activator (tPA) to fibrin, causing impairment of activation of fibrinolysis, or by mutations limiting the action of plasmin on the abnormal fibrin [40–42]. Patients with dysfibrinogenemia have been treated with antithrombotic agents more commonly than protein replacement. Women with dysfibrinogenemia have been described with implantation failures very similar to women with afibrinogenemia, and pregnancy in affected women has been similarly facilitated by fibrinogen replacement [36].

Severe tissue factor pathway inhibitor deficiency

Severe deficiency of the tissue factor pathway inhibitor (TFPI) has not been described in a human and is most likely incompatible with life. The knock-out mouse model results in embryonic loss at 10.5 days' gestation, with histologic evidence of consumptive coagulopathy and diffuse fibrin deposition [43]. A chromosomal deletion including one allele of TFPI has been associated with a post-operative deep vein thrombosis in an adolescent, though plasma levels of TFPI were normal [44].

Metabolic disorders

Homocysteinuria

With severe congenital deficiency of cystathionine beta synthase, resultant homocysteiniuria is associated with pediatric presentation of arterial and venous thrombosis in 25% of affected individuals, of which AIS occurs in one-third and peripheral venous thrombosis occurs in half [45]. The exact mechanism of thrombosis in homocysteinuria is unknown, but extremely elevated levels of plasma homocysteine (> 200 μmol/l) in this syndrome are believed to mediate thrombosis through endothelial damage [46].

Congenital disorders of glycosylation

A rare cause of congenital deficiency of antithrombin, protein C and protein S along with other coagulation proteins is a genetic defect in glycosylation (CDG) [47]. Children affected with CDG manifest other signs including dysmorphic features, developmental delay, gastrointestinal, endocrine and central nervous system involvement. This syndrome is comprised of mutations in a number of different genes, but the most common disorder, PMM2-CDG, has been associated with a thrombosis rate of 14%, equally distributed between arterial and venous events, with a mean age of occurrence of 4.6 years [47]. Because procoagulant proteins are also glycosylated, affected children can manifest prolongations of the APTT and PT, with decreased protein activities most commonly of factors XI and IX, as well as bleeding symptoms. However, the thrombotic tendency is not altered by prolongations of global screening tests or decreased activities of procoagulant proteins. Management of anticoagulation therapy is challenging in children with CDG and prolonged baseline APTT and/or PT; use of anti-Xa activity to monitor LMWH or measurements of activities of specific vitamin K-dependent proteins to monitor warfarin is often necessary.

Congenital deficiencies causing hemolytic uremic syndrome/thrombotic thrombocytopenia purpura (HUS/TTP) syndromes: Genetic deficiency of H protein, ADAMTS13, prostacyclin

The HUS/TTP syndromes are characterized by hemolytic anemia and small vessel thrombosis affecting multiple vascular beds. Although sharing many similar clinical features, HUS is a disorder of capillary fibrin deposition and progressive fibrin sclerosis, whereas TTP is characterized histologically by the deposition of platelets and von Willebrand factor (vWF) in the terminal arterioles, while fibrin is conspicuously absent [48–50].

Congenital relapsing hemolytic uremic syndrome (HUS)

Congenital relapsing hemolytic uremic syndrome is a clinical disorder of recurrent episodes of acute capillary fibrin deposition in multiple vascular beds, most notably the kidney glomeruli, leading to complete capillary obstruction, acute renal failure, chronic fibrinosis and obliteration of the glomeruli, and ultimately chronic renal failure. These disorders are characterized by thrombocytopenia, Coomb's negative microangiopathic hemolytic anemia and renal failure. The congenital types are suspected by the early age of presentation, often in the first few months of life, temporal relationship to minor infections and relapsing course [51]. Congenital HUS is caused by genetic mutations in the complement system, and episodes are usually triggered by an acute episode such as infection [51,52]. The complement system is a cascade of enzymatic activities initiated by recognition of antigen–antibody complexes with the goal of killing invading microbes. The complement system is activated by one of three pathways: the classical, lectin and alternative systems. Genetic deficiencies in proteins key to these three pathways are responsible for the familial HUS syndromes. The factor H protein (also known as beta1H globulin) is the main regulator of the complement alternative pathway [53]. The factor H protein binds via multiple sites to the complement component C3b, and via one binding site to sialic acid and cell surfaces. Factor H and membrane cofactor protein (MCP) serve as cofactors to the C3b inactivating enzyme, complement factor I convertase [54]. Factor H protein is essential for the opsonization and cell-killing functions of the alternative pathway. Factor H protein can be replaced with infusions of fresh frozen plasma while the MCP is tissue-associated and reconstituted by renal transplantation. In one child with atypical HUS who was unresponsive to FFP, a good clinical response was achieved with eculizumab (Solaris®, Alexion Pharmaceutics Inc., Cheshire, CT, USA), a humanized monoclonal antibody against terminal complement protein C5 [51].

Congenital TTP

Congenital relapsing TTP is a genetic disorder caused by mutations in the ADAMTS13 molecule, a plasma metalloproteinase required to cleave the vWF after release from the platelet or endothelial cell [49,54–56]. Infants and children affected with congenital TTP manifest recurring episodes of thrombocytopenia, hemolytic anemia and small vessel thrombi that consist primarily of platelets and vWF. The diagnosis of congenital TTP is made by laboratory confirmation of undetectable or very low levels of ADAMTS13 and absence of antibodies to ADAMTS13, which characterize acquired TTP. Some variants of congenital ADAMTS13 deficiency result in more prominent renal disease [57]. The treatment of congenital TTP is replacement of ADAMTS13 with FFP; ADAMTS13 has a relatively long half-life in plasma (2.6 days) and low levels are sufficient to prevent relapsing TTP episodes. One report chronicles a child who was supported with as little as 3.6 ml/kg FFP infused every 2 to 3 weeks for 10 years with satisfactory results [58].

Combined thrombophilias

Most thrombophilic traits, including deficiencies of the more potent coagulation regulatory proteins such as antithrombin, protein C and protein S, result in moderate thrombotic phenotypes that respond as expected to conventional antithrombotic therapy. The syndromes above describe severe thrombotic phenotypes resulting from mutations in single proteins (except for CDG). The last category of thrombophilia results from combined defects in unrelated genes. Substantially more severe thrombotic syndromes can result from defects in two or more regulatory proteins, such as combined deficiencies of protein C and protein S, or protein C and antithrombin [5,21,59–62]. Alternatively, combined thrombophilia may involve two or more mutations in genes each causing a mild to moderate thrombotic phenotype. Salomon and colleagues estimated the relative risk for thrombosis to be greater than 50 in carriers of both the factor V Leiden and prothrombin 20210 mutations [64]. Combined thrombophilias should be suspected in a child with thrombosis when the presentation is early, severe and lacking strong prothrombotic provocation, or recurrent without strong provocation.

Table 13.1 displays a proposed scoring system for thrombophilias with differing weights given to specific thrombophilic traits. Thrombophilia testing should be considered for presentations of severe or very severe clinical thrombotic disorders, as test results have the potential to offer tailored, specific therapies that improve outcomes. Clinical indicators of the severe and combined thrombophilias are shown on Table 13.2.

Special considerations for neonatal presentations of thrombosis and thrombophilia

Prenatal and perinatal presentations with severe thrombosis present a special challenge to the pediatric hematologist. Thrombosis within the pediatric population is common during the neonatal period, particularly AIS. Most cases of neonatal AIS are interpreted as emboli from the placenta through the umbilical vein and across the patent foramen ovale. It is difficult to identify the infant with inherited severe thrombophilia from the background of acquired disorders. To date, there are no established predictors of genetic thrombophilia, except for spontaneous neonatal purpura fulminans, which is characteristic of severe deficiencies of protein C and/or protein S. Some general guidelines are shown in Table 13.2. The neonatal equivalent of spontaneous thrombosis includes thrombosis documented in the absence of any detected maternal or fetal risk factors during pregnancy, labor and delivery. While guidelines do not support routine thrombophilia testing in neonates with thrombosis, it is reasonable to assay protein C, protein S and antithrombin in infants fulfilling one or more risk factors for severe genetic thrombophilia and to test the mother for APA. Protein concentrate replacements exist for protein C and antithrombin and these can be considered for the treatment of newborn infants with thrombosis and less than 30% antithrombin or 20% protein C in the term infant, and less than 15% antithrombin or 10% protein C in the preterm. Consideration can be given to therapy with IVIG and/or steroids for infants with transplacental transfer of high-titer APA.

Table 13.1 Severity of thrombophilia

Trivial/mild; relative risk < 1.5:

Acquired	• Lifestyle, fasting homocysteine < 20 μmol/l • Elevated PAI-1 • Single low-titer APA
Genetic	• Metabolic, fasting homocysteine < 20 μmol/l • Polymorphisms: PAI-1 4G/5G; factor XIII V34D

Mild/moderate; relative risk > 1.5 but rare spontaneous thrombosis:

Acquired *Genetic*	• Persistent elevated FVIII • Factor V Leiden deficiency • Prothrombin mutation heterozygote • Protein C heterozygote (> 40%) • Protein S heterozygote (> 40%) • Antithrombin heterozygote (> 60%) • Hypo-/dysfibrinogenemia • Elevated FVIII • 2 trivial/mild traits

Moderate/severe; provoked or spontaneous thrombosis or with underlying risk factor:

Acquired	• Persistent single high-titer APLA (ISTH definition) • L-asparaginase chemotherapy • Nephrotic syndrome • Inflammatory bowel disease with active colitis
Genetic	• Factor V Leiden homozygote • Prothrombin mutation homozygote • Protein C deficiency 20–40% • Protein S deficiency 20–40% • Antithrombin deficiency 30–60% • ≥ 3 mild/moderate thrombophilic traits

Severe/very severe; spontaneous thrombosis, DIC and/or purpura fulminans:

Acquired	• Heparin-induced thrombocytopenia/thrombosis • Catastrophic antiphospholipid syndrome • Thrombotic storm • Paroxysmal nocturnal hemoglobinuria • Persistent multiple high-titer APA
Genetic	• Severe protein C deficiency (< 20%) • Severe protein S deficiency (< 20%) • Severe antithrombin deficiency (< 30%) • A-/dysfibrinogenemia with arterial and venous thrombosis • Cystathionine B synthase deficiency (homocysteinuria) • Congenital glycosylation defect • Severe deficiency of factor H protein, membrane cofactor protein or ADAMTS13 causing recurrent HUS/TTP syndromes • ≥ 2 moderate/severe or ≥ 4 mild/moderate thrombotic traits

Severe acquired thrombophilic syndromes

Severe acquired thrombophilias are characterized by rapid onset and progression of thrombosis, generally in a previously well child following a triggering factor such as mild trauma or infection. Some features found to a greater or lesser frequency and degree include thrombotic involvement of unusual sites and organs, DIC, thrombocytopenia, hemolytic anemia, autoantibodies and a high mortality rate. Genetic thrombophilic traits may be detected, but are not judged to be sufficient to explain the severe thrombotic event. Table 13.3 lists the relative frequency of various clinical and laboratory findings distinguishing the severe acquired thrombophilias. Note the frequency of overlapping findings, underscoring the difficulty in making a precise diagnosis.

Catastrophic antiphospholipid syndrome

Catastrophic antiphospholipid syndrome (CAPS) is a fulminant form of the antiphospholipid syndrome (APS), which affects 1% of APS patients. Catastrophic antiphospholipid syndrome, which was first described in 1987 and called Asherson syndrome after one of its authors, is a fulminant disorder of rapidly evolving coagulopathy often causing overt DIC and microvascular thrombosis that results in multiple organ dysfunction and a high mortality rate [64]. Massive cytokine release is common, causing the

systemic inflammatory response syndrome (SIRS) with acute respiratory distress syndrome (ARDS), cerebral edema, DIC and microvascular thrombosis; C-reactive protein and erythrocyte sedimentation rate may be greatly elevated. Large-vessel thrombosis can occur but is found in only one-third of patients [65]. Criteria for the diagnosis of CAPS include evidence of involvement of three or more organs, systems or tissues; rapid development of manifestations simultaneously or within a week; histopathologic confirmation of small vessel occlusion in at least one organ or tissue; and laboratory confirmation of APA (moderate to high-titer lupus anticoagulant [LA], anticardiolipin antibody [ACA]) and/or antibodies directed against β_2 glycoprotein [antiβ_2GP1 antibodies])[66]. Children have rarely undergone tissue biopsy and histological diagnosis. Mortality has been reduced from 50 to 30% with combination therapy using anticoagulation, corticosteroids and plasma exchange with or without intravenous immunoglobulin (IVIG) [66]. Approximately half of affected patients have primary APA while the remainder have systemic lupus erythematosis (SLE). Patients with SLE have also benefited from treatment with cyclophosphamide [66]. Rituximab and prostacyclin have also been used, but response rates have not yet been determined. Long-term survivors generally do not experience a recurrent CAPS episode, although further APA-related events have been reported in 19% of patients after an average

Table 13.2 Clinical factors suspicious for severe thrombophilia

- Strongly positive family history and/or consanguinity
- In utero, neonatal or early childhood onset
- Presence of DIC or purpura fulminans
- Life-, limb- or organ-threatening thrombosis
- Multifocal non-contiguous sites of thrombosis
- Rapid progression of thrombosis in spite of appropriate antithrombotic therapy
- Spontaneous thrombosis or thrombus recurrence

Table 13.3 Comparative features of severe acquired thrombophilia

	CAPS [64]	TS	HUS	TTP
Female gender	72%	Equal	Equal	70%
Triggering factor	53%	Usual	Usual	Often
Pulmonary symptoms (ARDS)	64%	No	No	No
Renal dysfunction	71%	No	100%	90%
Central nervous system abnormalities	62%	With CSVT	25%	Frequent
Cardiac abnormalities	51%	Not characteristic	No	No
Skin: livido reticularis, purpura, skin necrosis	50%	Occasionally	No	No
Thrombotic microangiopathy	70%	No	100%	100%
Thrombocytopenia	46%	Frequent	100%	100%
Hemolytic anemia	33%	Not characteristic	100%	100%
DIC	15%	Occasionally	No	Rare
APA	Nearly all	Often	No	Rarely
Schistocytes on red cell smear	+	Not characteristic	100%	100%
Inflammatory markers (SED, CRP)	High	High	Moderately elevated	Moderately elevated

of 67 months of follow-up [67]. Catastrophic anti-phospholipid syndrome is primarily an adult disorder, but has been reported in children as young as infancy [68]. When APA titers are low to moderate, it is difficult to determine their contribution to the fulminant thrombotic course, and the syndrome overlaps that of thrombotic storm (see below) [69].

Thrombotic storm

Thrombotic storm (TS) is characterized by a rapidly progressive, severe prothrombotic phenotype affecting multiple vascular beds (two or more non-contiguous vessels) in the arterial, venous and/or microvascular circulations. Patients with TS tend to be younger, on average, than those with CAPS, with a negative personal and family history for thrombosis [70]. Macrovascular thrombosis is more prominent than small vessel, predominantly DVT and PE, although unusual locations such as abdominal veins or cerebral sinuses may be affected. Arterial lesions occur and, rarely, thrombotic microangiopathy may involve solid organs or skin. Episodes are characteristically preceded by an event such as pregnancy, minor trauma or a mild infection; APA and even heparin-induced thrombocytopenia and thrombosis (HITT) antibodies may be present. Inflammatory markers, including fibrinogen, factor VIII, C-reactive protein and erythrocyte sedimentation rate, tend to be very high in most but not all children. Anticoagulation is the mainstay of therapy. Thrombotic storm is distinguished from the other severe acquired thrombophilias in that it is often rapidly progressive in spite of apparently appropriate standard anticoagulation [71]. Patients have been treated similarly to those with CAPS using high-dose steroids, IVIG, plasmapheresis, cyclophosphamide and rituximab in addition to anticoagulant and fibrinolytic therapies. Direct thrombin inhibitors and fondaparinux have been used due to apparent inefficacy of heparins with fulminant progression and positivity of the heparin-PF4 and serotonin release assays for HITT [71]. There is a high rate of thrombus progression or recurrence when anticoagulation is subtherapeutic, even weeks or months following therapeutic initiation. Late thrombus recurrence has been described [70,71]. Warfarin has been an effective agent for long-term anticoagulation.

Acquired HUS/TTP syndromes

Acquired HUS and TTP were previously considered separate syndromes based upon the differences in etiology (infection in typical HUS and autoantibodies in TTP), as well as differences in pathophysiology with primary deposition of fibrin and red cells in HUS and platelets and vWF in TTP. However, more recent data regarding the dysregulation of complement in many patients with typical HUS have blurred the two boundaries between the two disorders [48,49,54].

Acquired hemolytic uremic syndrome

Acute HUS is an acquired syndrome of acute thrombotic microangiopathy with fibrin aggregates affecting primarily the preglomerular arterioles and extending up to glomerular capillaries [72,73]. Fibrin deposition is triggered by infection, most frequently the shiga toxin associated with E. coli (in the USA and Europe, most frequently O157:H7) and Shigella dysenteriae type 1 (in South America) [72]. Thrombotic acute HUS most frequently affects young children. The renal bed is most frequently involved and 5% of children with acute renal failure caused by HUS will develop chronic renal failure, requiring long-term dialysis and renal transplant. Other vascular beds including the central nervous system and the liver can be involved. Acute HUS is rarely recurrent.

Acquired thrombotic thrombocytopenic purpura

Acquired TTP is an autoimmune disorder mediated by autoantibodies against the plasma metalloproteinase, ADAMTS13 [74,75]. Acquired TTP is a recurrent, relapsing condition of hemolytic anemia, thrombocytopenia and small vessel occlusion involving the central nervous system (CNS) and liver more prominently than in HUS. Seizures are common and AIS can occur. Renal involvement can occur but is less prominent than in HUS. Acquired TTP in pediatrics is diagnosed more frequently in adolescent females during or following pregnancy [75]. The treatment of acquired TTP is plasmapheresis with plasma replacement.

Paroxysmal nocturnal hemoglobinuria

Paroxysmal nocturnal hemoglobinuria (PNH) is a syndrome of disordered complement regulation resulting in intravascular hemolysis and platelet activation. In PNH the complement and coagulation systems intersect with mutual activation. The pathophysiology, molecular mechanisms and management have recently been reviewed [76]. Paroxysmal nocturnal hemoglobinuria is a non-malignant clonal disorder caused by a somatic mutation of the phosphatidylinositol glycan A (PIG-A) gene located on the X chromosome in bone marrow stem cells, resulting in a deficiency of glycosylphosphatidylinositol (GPI) and, consequently, of all GPI-anchored proteins on the cell membrane. The proteins CD55 (which limits cell surface activation of complement) and CD59 (which blocks formation of the membrane attack complex [MAC] consisting of complement proteins C5b, C6, C7, C8 and multiple molecules of C9) are two such GPI-anchored complement regulatory proteins that are absent in PNH cells. The diagnosis of PNH is made by high-sensitivity flow cytometry of peripheral red cells or neutrophils for CD55 and CD59. In PNH, complement is activated resulting in platelet and coagulation activation, red cell hemolysis, depletion of nitric oxide, vascular inflammation and free hemoglobin.

Thrombosis, which can precede other signs of the disorder, constitutes a frequent morbidity of PNH and the primary cause of death in affected patients. Thromboses occur in any site, but abdominal and cerebrosinovenous thromboses are characteristic. Patients with Budd–Chiari syndrome, arising from thrombosis of the hepatic vein, should be carefully considered for PNH testing. Conventional anticoagulation has been only partially effective in preventing thrombosis progression and recurrence. Eculizumab (Solaris®, Alexion Pharmaceutics Inc., Cheshire, CT, USA), a humanized monoclonal antibody that prevents activation of C5 to C5a by the alternative pathway of complement, has dramatically changed the course of PNH [77]. Eculizumab prevents platelet activation, thrombus formation and complement-mediated intravascular hemolysis. Patients with PNH treated with eculizumab require fewer transfusions and are sometimes able to discontinue long-term anticoagulation. There is an associative, but not causal, relationship between PNH and aplastic anemia. Because of an apparent survival advantage of PNH clones, approximately half of patients with aplastic anemia and 15–20% of patients with low-risk myelodysplasia syndromes test positive for PNH when high-resolution flow cytometry is used [77]. Treatment with eculizumab does not affect clonal expansion either positively or negatively.

In the pediatric population, PNH presents most commonly during adolescence. Guidelines for PNH testing include patients with the following: (1) intravascular hemolysis, especially when accompanied by iron deficiency, abdominal pain, thrombosis or cytopenias; (2) other acquired Coombs negative, non-schistocytic, non-infectious hemolytic anemia; (3) thrombosis involving hepatic veins, other abdominal veins, cerebral veins or dermal veins with hemolytic anemia and/or unexplained cytopenias; and (4) evidence of bone marrow failure or cytopenias of unknown etiology [78].

Summary

Consensus guidelines regarding the role of thrombophilia and thrombophilia testing on the incidence, clinical course and management of thrombosis in infants and children are based upon adult thrombotic disease and routine pediatric cases. These guidelines have not accounted for the severity of the thrombophilic tendency or the severity of the thrombotic event, given the limited evidence basis in such subpopulations. However, severe genetic disorders are more likely to manifest early in life. Similarly, infants and children suffer many severe acquired thrombotic disorders. Hence, the pediatric hematologist is at times faced with a catastrophic case of thrombophilia in an infant or child. The pathophysiology of many of these disorders has been elucidated and happily, effective treatments exist for many of them. For these reasons, it is incumbent upon the clinician to be able to recognize signs of severe thrombophilia, perform a targeted evaluation and institute life-saving appropriate therapy expeditiously.

References

1. Goldenberg NA, Manco-Johnson MJ. Protein C deficiency. Haemophilia 2008;**14**:1214–21.

2. Douglas AGL, Rafferty H, Hodgkins P, Nagra A, Foulds NC, Morgan M, Temple IK. Persistent fetal vasculature and severe protein C deficiency. Mol Syndromol 2010;**1**:82–6.

3. Manco-Johnson MJ, Knoebl P, Shapiro AD, Finnerty M, Leman Y, Gelmont D. Registry of patients treated with protein C concentrate (human) in the United States and Europe: Interim results. Annual Meeting of the American Society of Hematology, 12/7/2013, Abst #1146.

4. Dreyfus M, Masterson M, David M, Rivard GE, Müller FM, Kreuz W, et al. Replacement therapy with a

monoclonal antibody purified protein C concentrate in newborns with severe congenital protein C deficiency. Semin Thromb Hemost 1995;21:371–81.

5. Zimbelman J, Lefkowitz J, Schaeffer C, Hays T, Manco-Johnson M, Mannhalter C, Nuss R. Unusual complications of warfarin therapy: skin necrosis and priapism. J Pediatr 2000;136446–53.

6. Gruppo RA, Leimer P, Francis RB, Marlar RA, Silberstein E. Protein C deficiency resulting from possible double heterozygosity and its response to danazol. Blood 1988;71:370–4.

7. Tait RC, Walker ID, Reitsma PH, Islam SI, McCall F, Poort SR, Conkie JA, Bertina RM. Prevalence of protein C deficiency in the healthy population. Thromb Haemost 1995;73:87–93.

8. Miletich J, Sherman L, Broze G Jr. Absence of thrombosis in subjects with heterozygous protein C deficiency. N Engl J Med 1987;317:991–6.

9. Reitsma PH. Protein C deficiency: summary of the 1995 database update. Nucleic Acids Res 1996;24:157–9.

10. Junge U, Wienke, Schüler A. Acute Budd-Chiari syndrome, portal and splenic vein thrombosis in a patient with ulcerative colitis associated with antiphospholipid antibodies and protein C deficiency. Gastroenterol 2001;39:845–52.

11. Devilat M, Toso M, Morales M. Childhood stroke associated with protein C or S deficiency and primary antiphospholipid syndrome. Pediatr Neurol 1993;9:67–70.

12. Gruppo R, DeGrauw A, Fogelson H, Glauser T, Balasa V, Gartside P. Protein C deficiency related to valproic acid therapy: a possible association with childhood stroke. J Pediatr 2000;137:14–18.

13. Farah RA, Jalkh KS, Farhat HZ, Sayad PE, Kadri AM. Acquired protein C deficiency in a child with acute myelogenous leukemia, splenic, renal and intestinal infarction. Blood Coagul Fibrinolysis 2011;22:140–3.

14. Bernard G, Vincent J-L, Laterre P-F, LaRosa SP, Dhainaut J-F, Lopez-Rodriquez A, Steingrub JS, Garger GE, Helterbrand JD, Ely EW, Fisher CJ Jr, Efficacy and safety of recombinant human activated protein C worldwide evaluation in severe sepsis (PROWESS) study group. New Engl J Med 2001;344:699–709.

15. Nadel S, Goldstein B, Williams MD, DAlton H, Peters M, Macias WL, Abd-Allah SA, Levy H, Angle R, Wang D, Sundin DP, Giroir B. REsearching severe Sepsis and Organ dysfunction in children: a gLobal perspective (RESOLVE) study group. Lancet 2007;369:836–43.

16. Manco-Johnson MJ, Knapp-Clevenger R. Activated protein C concentrate reverses purpura fulminans in severe genetic protein C deficiency. J Pediatr Hematol/Oncol 2004;26:25–7.

17. Mahasandana C, Suvatte V, Marlar RA, Manco-Johnson MJ, Jacobson L, Hathaway WE. Neonatal purpura fulminans associated with homozygous protein S deficiency. Lancet 1990;335:61–2.

18. Martinelli I, Bucciarelli P, Artoni A, Fossali EF, Passamonti SM, Tripodi A, Peyvandi F. Anticoagulant treatment with rivaroxaban in severe protein S deficiency. Pediatrics 2013;132:e1435.

19. Mintz-Hittner HA, Miyashiro MJ, Knight-Nanan DM, O'Malley RE, Marlar RA. Vitreoretinal findings similar to retinopathy of prematurity in infants with compound heterozygous protein S deficiency. Ophthalmology 1999;106:1525–30.

20. Pung-Amritt P, Poort SR, Vos HL, Bertina RM, Mahasandana C, Tanphaichitr VS, Veerakul G, Kankirawatana S, Suvatte V. Compound heterozygosity for one novel and one recurrent mutation in a Thai patient with severe protein S deficiency. Thromb Haemost 1999;81:189–92.

21. Köner Ö, Tekin S, Soybir N, Gülcan F, Karaoğlu K. Cardiac operation in a patient with combined homozygous protein C and protein S deficiency. J Cardiothor Vasc Anesth 2000;14:188–90.

22. Gandrille S, Borgel D, Ireland H, Lane DA, Simmonds R, Reitsma PH, Mannhalter C, Pabinger I, Saito H, Suzuki K, Formstone C, Cooper DN, Espinoza Y, Sala N, Bernardi F, Aiach M. Protein S deficiency: a database of mutations. For the Plasma Coagulation Inhibitors Subcommittee of the Scientific and Standardization Committee of the International Society on Thrombosis and Haemostasis. Thromb Haemost 1997;77:1201–14.

23. Manco-Johnson MJ, Nuss R, Key N, Moertel C, Jacobson L, Meech S, Weinberg A, Lefkowitz J. Lupus anticoagulant and protein S deficiency in children with postvaricella purpura fulminans or thrombosis. J Pediatr 1996;128:319–23.

24. Josephson C, Nuss R, Jacobson L, Hacker MR, Murphy J, Weinberg A, Manco-Johnson MJ. The varicella–autoantibody syndrome. Pediatr Res 2001;50:345–52.

25. Orlando C, Lissens W, Hasaerts D, Jochmans K. Identification of two de novo mutations responsible for type I antithrombin deficiency. Thromb Haemost 2012;107:187–9.

26. Kumar R, Moharir M, Yau I, Williams S. A novel mutation in the Serpin C1 gene presenting as unprovoked cerebral sinus venous thrombosis in a kindred. Pediatr Blood Cancer 2013;60:133–6.

27. Chowdhury V, Lane DA, Mille B, Auberger K, Gandenberger-Bachem S, Pabinger I, Olds RJ, Thein SL. Homozygous antithrombin deficiency: report of two new cases (99 Leu to Phe) associated with arterial and venous thrombosis. Thromb Haemost 1994;72:198–202.

176

28. Olivieri M, Bidlingmaier C, Schetzeck S, Borggräfe I, Geisen C, Kurnik K. Arterial thrombosis in homozygous antithrombin deficiency. Hamostaseologie 2012;**32** Suppl 1:S79–82.

29. Pascaul C, Muñoz C, Huerta AR, Rus GP, Ortega V, Corral J, Diez-Martin JL. A new case of successful outcome of pregnancy in a carrier of homozygous type II (L99F) antithrombin deficiency. Blood Coagul Fibrinolysis 2014;**25**:74–6.

30. Patnaik MM, Moll S. Inherited antithrombin deficiency: a review. Haemophilia 2008;**14**:1229–39.

31. Lane DA, Bayston R, Olds RJ, Fitches AC, Cooper DN, Millar DS, Jochmans K, Perry DJ, Okajima K, Thein SL, Emmerich J. Antithrombin mutation database: 2nd (1997) update. For the Plasma Coagulation Inhibitors Subcommittee of the Scientific and Standardization Committee of the International Society on Thrombosis and Haemostasis. Thromb Haemost 1997;**77**:1979–211.

32. Bucur SZ, Levy JH, Despotis GJ, Spiess BD, Hillyer CD. Uses of antithrombin III concentrate in congenital and acquired deficiency states. Transfusion 1998;**38**:481–98.

33. Sheridan-Pereira M, Porreco RP, Hays T, Burke MS. Neonatal aortic thrombosis associated with the lupus anticoagulant. Obstet Gynecol 1988;**71**:1016–18.

34. Menache D, O'Malley JP, Schorr JB, Wagner B, Williams C, and the Cooperative Study Group: Alving BM, Ballard JO, Goodnight SH, Hathaway WE, Hultin MB, Kitchens CS, Lessner HE, Makary AZ, Manco-Johnson M, McGhee WG, Penner JA, Sanders JE. Evaluation of the safety, recovery, half-life, and clinical efficacy of antithrombin III (human) in patients with hereditary antithrombin III deficiency. Blood 1990;**75**:33–9.

35. Wong TE, Huang Y-S, Weiser J, Brogan TV, Shah SS, Witmer CM. Antithrombin concentrate use in children: a multicenter cohort study. J Pediatr 2013;**163**:1329–34.

36. Bornikova L, Peyvandi F, Allen G, Bernstein J, Manco-Johnson MJ. Fibrinogen replacement therapy for congenital fibrinogen deficiency. J Thromb Haemost 2011;**9**:1687–704.

37. Mosesson MW. Antithrombin I. Inhibition of thrombin regulation in plasma by fibrin formation. Thromb Haemost 2003;**89**:9–12.

38. Ni H, Denis CV, Subbarao S, Degen JL, Sato TN, Hynes RO, et al. Persistence of platelet thrombus formation in arterioles of mice lacking both von Willebrand factor and fibrinogen. J Clin Invest 2000;**106**:385–92.

39. Dupuy E, Soria C, Molho P, Zini JM, Rosenstingl S, Laurian C, Bruneval P, Tobelem G. Embolized ischemic lesions of toes in an afibrinogenemic patient:

possible relevance to in vivo circulating thrombin. Thromb Res 2001;**102**:211–19.

40. Niwa K, Mimuro J, Miyata M, Sugo T, Ohmori T, Madoiwa S, Tei C, Sakata Y. Dysfibrinogenemia Kagoshima with the amino acid substitution γThr-314 to Ile: Analysis of molecular abnormalities and thrombophilic nature of this abnormal molecule. Thromb Res 2008;**121**:773–80.

41. Niwa K, Yaginuma A, Nakanishi M, Wada Y, Sugo T, Asakura S, Watanabe N, Matsuda M. Fibrinogen Mitaka II: a hereditary dysfibrinogen with defective thrombin binding caused by an A alpha Glu-11 to Gly substitution. Blood 1993;**82**:3658–63.

42. Ramanathan R, Gram J, Feddersen S, Nybo M, Larsen A, Sidelmann JJ. Dusart syndrome in a Scandinavian family characterized by arterial and venous thrombosis at young age. Scand J Clin Lab Invest 2013;**73**:585–90.

43. Huang ZF, Higuchi D, Lasky N, Broze GJ, Jr. Tissue factor pathway inhibitor gene disruption produces intrauterine lethality in mice. Blood 1997;**90**:944–51.

44. Kentsis A, Bradwin G, Miller DT, Trenor CC III. Venous thrombosis associated with gene deletion of tissue factor pathway inhibitor. Am J Hematol 2009;**84**:775–6.

45. Mudd SH, Skovby F, Levy HL, Pettigrew KD, Wilcken B, Pyeritz RE, Andria G, Boers GH, Bromberg IL, Cerone R, Fowler B, Gröbe H, Schmidt H, Schweitzer L. The natural history of homocystinuria due to cystathionine beta-synthase deficiency. Am J Hum Genet 1985;**37**:1–31.

46. Undas A, Brozek J, Szczeklik A. Homocysteine and thrombosis: from basic science to clinical evidence. Thromb Haemost 2005;**94**:907–15.

47. Linssen M, Mohamed M, Wevers RA, Lefeber DJ, Morava E. Thrombotic complications in patients with PMM2-CDG. Mol Genet Metab 2013;**109**:107–11.

48. Tsai H-M. Untying the knot of thrombotic thrombocytopenic purpura and atypical hemolytic uremic syndrome. Am J Med 2013;**126**:200–9.

49. Zipfel PF, Wolf G, John U, Kentouche K, Skerka C. Novel developments in thrombotic microangiopathies: is there a common link between hemolytic uremic syndrome and thrombotic thrombocytopenic purpura? Pediatr Nephrol 2011;**26**:1947–56.

50. Lowe EJ, Werner EJ. Thrombotic thrombocytopenic purpura and hemolytic uremic syndrome in children and adolescents. Semin Thromb Hemost 2005;**31**:717–29.

51. Gruppo RA, Rother RP. Eculizumab for congenital atypical hemolytic-uremic syndrome. NEJM 2009;**360**:544–6.

52. Carreras L, Romero R, Requesens C, Oliver AJ, Carrera M, Clavo M, Alsina J. Familial hypocomplementemic hemolytic uremic syndrome with HLA-A3,B7 haplotype. JAMA 1981;**245**:602–4.

53. Skerka C, Chen Q, Fremeaux-Bacchi V, Roumenina LT. Complement factor H proteins (CFHRs). Mol Immunol 2013;**56**:170–80

54. Zheng XL, Sadler JE. Pathogenesis of thrombotic microangiopathies. Ann Rev Pathol Mech Dis. 2008;**3**:249–77.

55. Levy GG, Nichols WC, Lian EC, Foroud T, McClintick JN, McGee BM, Yang AY, Siemieniak DR, Stark KR, Gruppo R, Sarode R, Shurin SB, Chandrasekaran V, Stabler SP, Sabio H, Bouhassira EE, Upshaw JD, Jr, Ginsburg D, Tsai HM. Mutations in a member of the ADAMTS gene family cause thrombotic thrombocytopenia purpura. Nature 2001;**413**:488–94.

56. Franchini M, Zaffanello M, Veneri O. Advances in the pathogenesis, diagnosis and treatment of thrombotic thrombocytopenic purpura and hemolytic uremic syndrome. Thromb Res 2006;**118**:177–84.

57. Shibagaki Y, Matsumoto M, Kokame K, Ohba S, Miyata T, Fujimura Y, Fujita T. Novel compound heterozygote mutations (H234Q/R1206X) of the *ADAMTS* gene in an adult patient with Upshaw-Shulman syndrome showing predominant episodes of repeated acute renal failure. Nephrol Dial Transplant 2006;**21**:1289–92.

58. Barbot J, Costa E, Guerra M, Barreirinho MS, Isvarlal P, Robles R, Gerritesen HE, Lämmle B, Furlan M. Ten years of prophylactic treatment with fresh-frozen plasma in a child with chronic relapsing thrombotic thrombocytopenic purpura as a result of a congenital deficiency of von Willebrand factor-cleaving protease. Br J Haematol 2001;**113**:649–51.

59. Uvaraj P, Rathisharmila R, Ilamaran V. Protein C and protein S deficiency presenting as Budd-Chiari syndrome. Blood Coag Fibrinolysis 2013;**24**:652–4.

60. Köller H, Stoll G, Sitzer M, Burk M, Schöttler B, Freund HJ. Deficiency of both protein C and protein S in a family with ischemic strokes in young adults. Neurology 1994;**44**:1238–40.

61. Laczika K, Lang IM, Quehenberger P, Mannhalter C, Muhm M, Klepetko W, Kyrle PA. Unilateral chronic thromboembolic pulmonary disease associated with combined inherited thrombophilia. Chest 2002;**121**:286–9.

62. Kosch A, Junker R, Wermes C, Nowak-Göttl U. Recurrent pulmonary embolism in a 13-year-old male homozygous for the prothrombin G20210A mutation combined with protein S deficiency and increased lipoprotein (a). Thromb Res 2002;**105**(1):49–53.

63. Inbal A, Kenet G, Zivelin A, Yermiyahu T, Bronstein T, Sheinfeld T, Tamari H, Gitel S, Eshel G, Duchemin J, Aiach M, Seligsohn U. Purpura fulminans induced by disseminated intravascular coagulation following infection in 2 unrelated children with heterozygosity for factor V Leiden and protein S deficiency. Thromb Haemost 1997;**77**(6):1086–9.

64. Salomon O, Steinberg DM, Zivelin A,Gitel S, Dardik R, Rosenberg N, Berliner S, Inbal A, Many A, Lubetsky A, Varon D, Martinowitz U, Seligsohn U. Single and combined prothrombotic factors in patients with idiopathic venous thromboembolism: prevalence and risk assessment. Arterioscler Thromb Vasc Biol 1999;**19**:511–18.

65. Asherson RA. The primary, secondary, catastrophic and seronegative variants of the antiphospholipid syndrome: a personal history long in the making. Semin Thromb Hemost 2008;**34**:227–35.

66. Cervera R, Espinosa G. Update on the Catastrophic antiphospholipid syndrome and the "CAPS Registry". Semin Thromb Hemost 2012;**38**:333–8.

67. Cervara R and CAPS Registry Project Group. Catastrophic antiphospholipid syndrome (CAPS): update from the 'CAPS Registry'. Lupus 2010;**19**:412–18.

68. Erkan D, Asherson RA, Espinosa G, Cervera R, Font J, Piette J-C, Lockshin MD. Long term outcome of catastrophic antiphospholipid syndrome survivors. Ann Rheum Dis 2003;**62**:530–3.

69. Camacho-Lovillo S, Bernabeu-Wittel J, Iglesias-Jimenez E, Falcón-Neyra D, Neth O. Pediatr Dermatol 2013;**30**:e63–64.

70. Olivier C, Blondiaux E, Blanc T, Borg J-Y, Dacher J-N. Catastrophic antiphospholipid syndrome and pulmonary embolism in a 3-year-old child. Pediatr Radiol 2006;**36**:870–73.

71. Ortel TL, Kitchens CS, Erkan D, Brandão LR, Hahn S, James AH, Kulkarni R, Manco-Johnson MJ, Pericak-Vance MJ, Vance J. Clinical causes and treatment of the thrombotic storm. Expert Rev Hematol 2012;**5**:653–9.

72. Manco-Johnson MJ, Wang M, Goldenberg NA. Treatment, survival and thromboembolic outcomes of thrombotic storm in children. J Pediatr 2012;**161**:682–8.e1.

73. Karpman D, Sartz L, Johnson S. Pathophysiology of typical hemolytic uremic syndrome. Semin Thromb Hemost 2010;**36**:575–85.

74. Amirlak I, Amirlak B. Haemolytic uraemic syndrome: an overview. Nephrology 2006;**11**:213–18.

75. Bouw MC, Dors N, van Ommen H, Ramakers-van Woerden NL. Thrombotic thrombocytopenia in childhood. Pediatr Blood Cancer 2009;**53**:537–42.

76. Moake J. Thrombotic thrombocytopenia purpura (TTP) and other thrombotic microangiopathies. Best Prac Res Clin Haematol 2009;**22**:567–76.

77. Hill A, Kelly RJ, Hillmen P. Thrombosis in paroxysmal nocturnal hemoglobinuria. Blood 2013;**121**:4985–96

78. Borowitz MJ, Craig FE, Digiuseppe JA, Illingworth AJ, Rosse W, Sutherland DR, Wittwer CT, Richards SJ; on behalf of the Clinical Cytometry Society. Guidelines for the diagnosis and monitoring of paroxysmal nocturnal hemoglobinuria and related disorders by flow cytometry. Cytom B Clin Cyt 2010;**78B**:211–30.

Thrombolysis

Donald L. Yee, Catherine M. Amlie-Lefond, and Peter H. Lin

I. Introduction

Therapeutic application of the physiologic process of fibrinolysis (thrombolysis) was first attempted in the late 1950s in individuals with various thrombotic lesions, comprising peripheral venous, arterial, central nervous system (CNS) and coronary involvement [1]. Over time and after rigorous clinical study, intravascular thrombolysis has come to occupy a critical role in the management of thrombotic disease in adults, with clear, approved indications for acute myocardial infarction, stroke and massive pulmonary embolism (PE). Its utility has also been investigated recently via controlled clinical trials in adults with occlusive lower extremity deep vein thrombosis (DVT), with promising results [2]; current guidelines also suggest its use in selected patients with this common condition [3].

For many reasons, however, including the lower incidence of thrombotic disease, consequent difficulty in completing high-quality clinical trials and heightened concerns for bleeding risks in young infants and children, the indications, dosing regimens and safety profiles for thrombolysis in pediatric patients are not as well established. Overall, the quality of evidence supporting the clinical management of pediatric patients via thrombolysis remains low given that a large proportion of the existing literature consists of individual case reports and small case series. Most series have reported on clinically heterogeneous groups of patients, with varied sites of vascular involvement using a variety of thrombolytic dosing regimens and modalities. Several comprehensive literature reviews have been published compiling available safety, efficacy and dosing data from several hundred infants and children [4–6]. Other recent review articles [7–9] summarize experience, expert opinion and important clinical management principles, while practice guidelines [10,11] are available to provide formal recommendations based on existing evidence.

This chapter begins with brief introductions to physiologic fibrinolysis and specific pharmacologic agents used for therapeutic thrombolysis. The next section addresses the major clinical considerations that are important in managing patients undergoing thrombolysis, including patient selection principles and important adjunctive care measures such as monitoring requirements and treatment of bleeding complications. These critical clinical management concepts apply regardless of the specific choices of thrombolytic dosing regimen and mode of therapy, which in turn are important topics discussed in the last part of that section. The final section summarizes by site of involvement the current information on some of the more common types of venous, arterial and CNS thrombotic lesions considered for thrombolytic therapy, and is intended to aid the reader in the approach to thrombolysis at specific anatomic sites.

II. Overview of fibrinolysis

A. Description of normal physiology

Anticoagulants target prevention of clot formation or extension, but have no known effect on removing an existing thrombus. Although many thrombi resolve, either with or without anticoagulant therapy, this occurs due to fibrinolysis, which will be described in this section.

During fibrinolysis, the zymogen plasminogen, synthesized mainly in the liver, is converted to its active form, plasmin (Figure 14.1). Plasmin cleaves fibrinogen and insoluble fibrin polymers at specific locations, releasing soluble fibrinogen and fibrin degradation products that vary in molecular weight and size, including moieties containing the D-dimer antigen. Sufficient formation and activity of plasmin leads to sustained fibrin degradation and eventual

Pediatric Thrombotic Disorders, ed. Neil A. Goldenberg and Marilyn J. Manco-Johnson. Published by Cambridge University Press. © Cambridge University Press 2015.

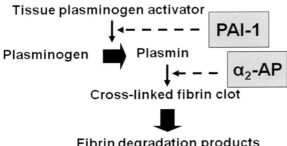

Figure 14.1 Tissue plasminogen activator converts plasminogen to plasmin, which in turn breaks down thrombus. PAI-1 and α₂-AP (grey boxes) inhibit the action of tissue plasminogen activator and plasmin, respectively (dashed lines). Reproduced with permission from J Pediatr Adolesc Gynecol. 2010 Dec;23(6 Suppl):S38–42.

dissolution of thrombus. This process is regulated by several key proteins:

- Plasminogen activators (including the primary physiologic activator known as tissue-type plasminogen activator [tPA]) bind to plasminogen, catalyzing its conversion to plasmin. This catalysis is greatly enhanced (at least 1000-fold) by fibrin, which increases affinity between plasminogen and tPA [12].
- Plasminogen activator inhibitor (PAI-1) is a serpin and acute-phase reactant with a circadian variation; it binds to fibrin-bound tPA and other plasminogen activators such as urokinase-type plasminogen activator (u-PA – see below), leading to their inactivation. PAI-1 is thus the major regulator of tPA.
- Plasminogen contains lysine-binding sites on its kringle-like domains, facilitating its interaction with and incorporation on to lysine-rich fibrin polymers, which occurs during fibrin formation. Activated thrombin activatable fibrinolysis inhibitor (TAFI; synthesized in the liver) removes C-terminal lysine residues from degraded fibrin, leading to decreased interaction with plasminogen, thus impairing plasmin formation [13].
- Circulating plasmin is negatively regulated by the serpin alpha-2 antiplasmin. Interaction between the two molecules depends on the presence of free lysine-binding sites on plasmin and results in the formation of an inactive complex [14].

B. Developmental hemostasis: Impact on physiologic and pharmacologic fibrinolysis

The age-related features of developmental hemostasis apply not just to coagulation and anticoagulant proteins, but also to the proteases and serpins regulating fibrinolysis (Table 14.1). Such age-dependent changes in plasma concentrations of fibrinolytic proteins hold important potential implications for thrombolytic therapies. For example, at birth, plasminogen concentrations are approximately half that of typical adult levels [15]. Premature infants exhibit even lower concentrations. Infants typically attain adult plasminogen levels by about 6 to 12 months of age. Qualitative differences in the plasminogen molecule also exist at birth, including a decreased activation rate by tPA and altered cell surface binding, leading to decreased functional activity of the protein in newborns [16]. Plasma concentrations of tPA, PAI-1 and alpha-2 antiplasmin also vary according to age (Table 14.1) and are described in further detail in Chapters 8 and 9 (Developmental hemostasis I and II). Given these developmental differences in fibrinolytic parameters between infants, children and adults (Table 14.1), and equally compelling differences with respect to other hemostatic parameters, direct extrapolation to infants and children of dosing guidelines derived from studies of thrombolytic agents in adults should be approached very cautiously.

To what degree hypofibrinolytic effects such as decreased plasminogen concentration and activity may be counterbalanced by hyperfibrinolytic effects, such as decreased inhibition by alpha-2 antiplasmin in neonates [17], is poorly understood. Nevertheless, due to the known relative plasminogen deficiency in young infants, routine supplementation with plasminogen via plasma infusion is suggested by current guidelines [11] prior to initiating pharmacologic thrombolysis (section IV.D.1).

III. Pharmacologic agents

A variety of agents have been developed over the years to facilitate the conversion of plasminogen to plasmin, thereby inducing supraphysiologic fibrinolysis, for the purpose of thrombolysis. Early agents (streptokinase, urokinase) were non-specific activators of plasminogen, leading to systemic conversion of plasminogen to plasmin, subsequent consumption of circulating

Table 14.1 Reference values for components of the fibrinolytic system in healthy full-term infants and adults by age

Fibrinolytic component	Day 1	Day 5	Day 30	Day 90	Day 180	Adults
Plasminogen (U/ml)	1.95 (1.25–2.65)	2.17 (1.41–2.93)	1.98 (1.26–2.70)	2.48 (1.74–3.22)	3.01 (2.21–3.81)	3.36 (2.48–4.24)
tPA (ng/ml)	9.6 (5.0–18.9)	5.6 (4.0–10.0)[a]	4.1 (1.0–6.0)[a]	2.1 (1.0–5.0)[a]	2.8 (1.0–6.0)[a]	4.9 (1.4–8.4)
Alpha-2 antiplasmin (U/ml)	0.85 (0.55–1.15)	1.00 (0.70–1.30)[a]	1.00 (0.76–1.24)[a]	1.08 (0.76–1.40)[a]	1.11 (0.83–1.39)[a]	1.02 (0.68–1.36)
PAI-1 (U/ml)	6.4 (2.0–15.1)	2.3 (0.0–8.1)[a]	3.4 (0.0–8.8)[a]	7.2 (1.0–15.3)	8.1 (6.0–13.0)	3.6 (0.0–11.0)

Values presented as means and ranges encompassing 95% of the population.
[a] Values that are indistinguishable from those of the adult. Adapted from [71], with permission.

Table 14.2 Approved recombinant thrombolytic agents

Agent	Year of approval	Half-life	Label indication(s)	Distinctive features	Fibrin specificity
Alteplase	1996	Initial: < 5 minutes	Acute myocardial infarction, acute ischemic stroke, pulmonary embolism	Recombinant human tPA; most commonly used thrombolytic in pediatrics	Yes; (DD)E is another substrate
Reteplase	1996	13–16 minutes	Acute myocardial infarction	Non-glycosylated, truncated mutant form of human tPA; but not more effective	Reduced fibrin affinity
Tenecteplase	2000	Initial: 20–24 minutes Terminal: 90–130 minutes	Acute myocardial infarction, pulmonary embolism and other arteriovenous occlusions	Most fibrin-specific agent, accounting for decreased fibrinogenolysis and lower bleeding risk; more resistant to inhibition by PAI-1	Increased compared to alteplase
Desmoteplase*	Not approved	3 hours	N/A	Derivative from vampire bat saliva; being studied in acute ischemic stroke with potentially less neurotoxicity and effect on blood–brain barrier	Increased compared to alteplase

* Not FDA approved.

fibrinogen and increased risk for clinical bleeding. A recombinant form of tPA (rt-PA) was eventually developed (alteplase) which, like native tPA, featured relative fibrin specificity and targeted plasminogen activation to the fibrin clot, leading to more limited systemic plasmin generation. More recent recombinant agents (Table 14.2) have attempted to further increase fibrin specificity in order to minimize bleeding risk, but through design and genetic engineering have also acquired other desirable properties, such as extended plasma half-life, decreased susceptibility to inactivation by native inhibitors (PAI-1) and a longer therapeutic window for acute stroke (section V.C.1). There is no published pediatric experience with the newer agents, but key features of currently known recombinant agents are outlined in Table 14.2 for current and future reference. The pediatric literature describing clinical experience with thrombolytic

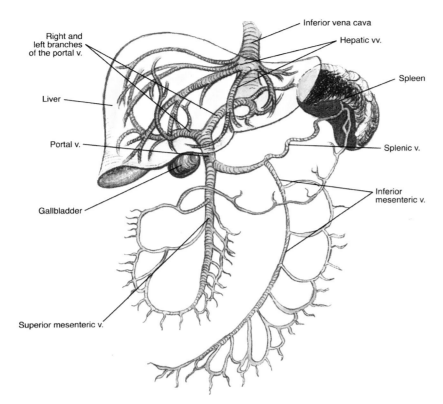

Figure 4.1 Mesenteric and portal vein system.

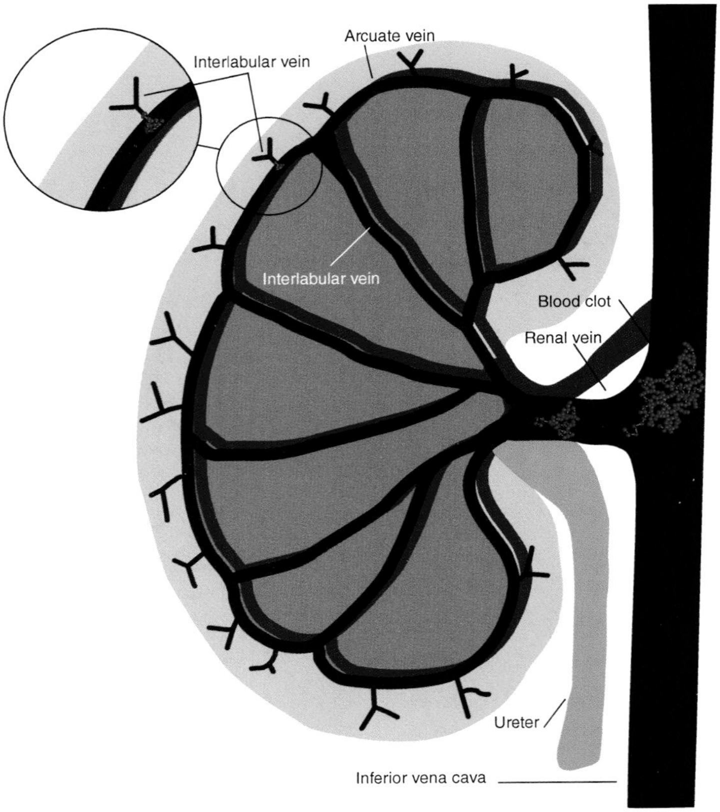

Inferior vena cava

Hepatic vv.

Right and left branches of the portal v.

Spleen

Liver

Portal v.

Splenic v.

Gallbladder

Inferior mesenteric v.

Superior mesenteric v.

Figure 5.1 Most cases of RVT originate in the interlobular and arcuate veins and less commonly in the IVC, extending into the renal vein.

Arcuate vein

Interlabular vein

Interlabular vein

Blood clot

Renal vein

Ureter

Inferior vena cava

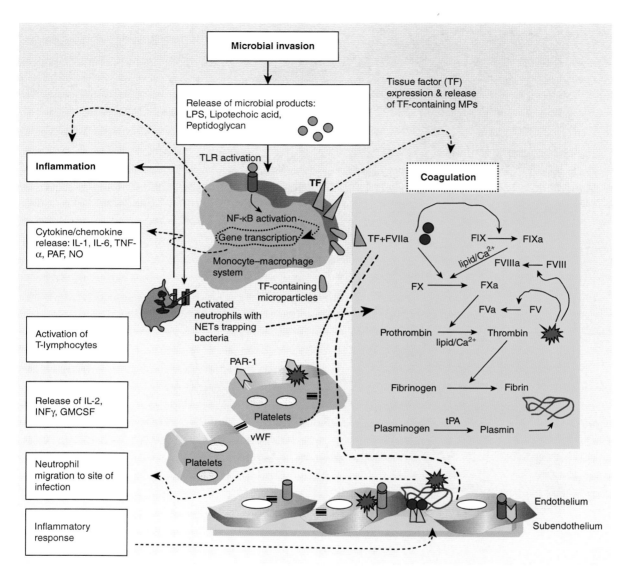

Figure 7.1 Cross-talk between inflammation and coagulation: Upon microbial invasion, release of microbial antigens activate monocytes/ macrophages via toll-like receptors. Activated monocytes/macrophages release cytokines/chemokines and tissue factor containing microparticles. Tissue factor serves as an interface between inflammation and coagulation; it activates factor VII, which in turn activates the coagulation cascade leading to thrombin generation. Inflammatory cytokines cause neutrophil migration at the site of inflammation. These cytokines mount an inflammatory response, which in turn increases tissue factor expression and activation of coagulation. Thrombin generation causes platelet activation through PAR-1 receptors and further amplifies the coagulation cascade. Endothelium secretes von Willebrand factor and causes platelet adhesion and aggregation. The activated platelets and damaged endothelium provide a phospholipid surface for the deposition of coagulation cascade. Additionally activated neutrophils develop neutrophil extracellular traps, which help with trapping bacteria and causing neutrophil apoptosis.

Abbreviations and symbols: IL: Interleukin; INFy: Interferon gamma; PAF: Platelet activating factor; NO: Nitric oxide; NET: Neutrophil extracellular trap; vWF: von Willebrand factor; PAR-1: protease activated receptor-1; PAI-1: plasminogen activator inhibitor-1.

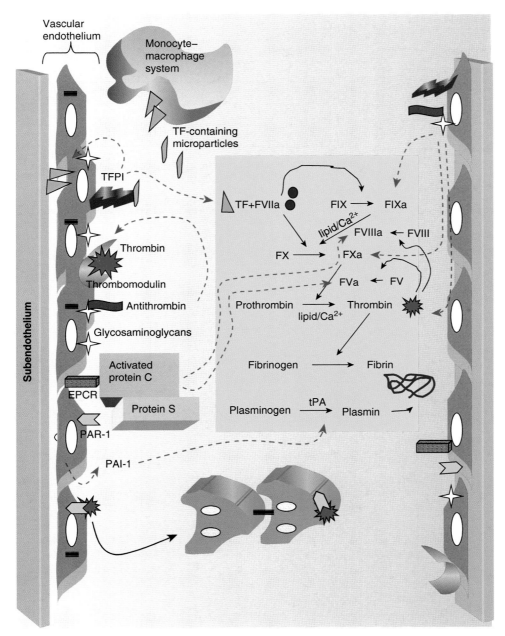

Figure 7.2 Schematic representation of the role of endothelium in hemostasis. Vascular endothelium serves as anticoagulant and procoagulant functions. On the anticoagulant side, it expresses TFPI (**T**issue **F**actor **P**athway **I**nhibitor), thrombomodulin, EPCR (**E**ndothelial **P**rotein **C R**eceptors), glycosaminoglycans, and PAI-1(plasminogen activator inhibitor-1). On the procoagulant side, endothelial cells synthesize vWF (von Willebrand factor), TF (tissue factor), thrombin receptor or **P**roease **A**ctivated **R**eceptor-1 (PAR-1). Red lines represent anticoagulant/ inhibition loops while black lines represent procoagulant/activation loops.

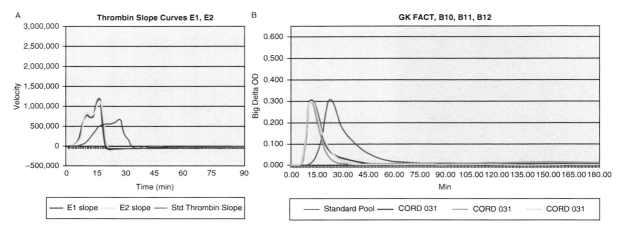

Figure 9.2 Thrombin generation and plasma coagulability in the newborn infant and adult. **A:** First derivative (velocity) of thrombin generation in the newborn infant (yellow/blue) and adult standard pooled plasma (red). **B:** Plasma clot formation and lysis (CloFAL) in the newborn infant (blue/green/yellow) and adult standard pooled plasma (red).

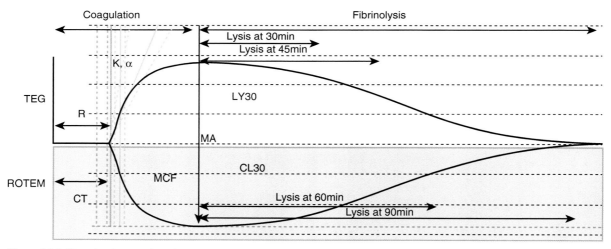

Figure 11.2 Thromboelastograph tracing.

agents is limited to streptokinase, urokinase and rt-PA (alteplase). These three agents are thus briefly reviewed below.

Streptokinase

Streptokinase is derived from certain species of hemolytic streptococcal bacteria and was the first thrombolytic agent used in children. Unlike other plasminogen activators, it has no direct lytic activity against plasminogen itself, but forms a stoichiometric complex with plasminogen; the complex has plasmin-like activity. As one of the primary agents in the early years of thrombolysis in pediatric patients, its use, along with limited safety and efficacy data, have been summarized in previous reviews [4–6]. However, it is no longer used commonly in pediatrics due to its immunogenicity and allergenicity. Streptokinase can induce neutralizing antibodies after recent streptococcal infection or exposure to the drug and is associated with a significant incidence of allergic reactions, which can be severe.

Urokinase (u-PA)

Native urokinase is produced in the kidney and endothelial cells, and most recently was manufactured via cell culture of human neonatal kidney cells. Its fibrinolytic activity depends on urokinase-type plasminogen activator receptor on cell surfaces, and thus urokinase has no fibrin specificity. Although it, like streptokinase, has a substantial history of use in pediatrics (4–6,18), it fell out of favor in the last decade due initially to concerns raised by the Food and Drug Administration (FDA) about infectious risk related to the drug's manufacturing processes. It currently is not being marketed.

Alteplase (rt-PA)

Tissue-type plasminogen activator (tPA) is a natural glycoprotein produced in endothelial cells that selectively binds to fibrin-bound plasminogen, catalyzing its conversion to plasmin. The recombinant form of this molecule (alteplase; rt-PA) became FDA approved in 1996. Its use in pediatrics dates back to at least 1990 [19]. Alteplase currently holds FDA-approved indications for acute myocardial infarction, stroke and massive pulmonary embolism in adults. It is cleared hepatically and has a half-life of less than 5 minutes. Despite its relative fibrin specificity, a clear advantage of rt-PA in terms of lower bleeding risk has not

been consistently observed in clinical studies of children. The fibrin specificity of rt-PA is not absolute, as some bleeding complications probably occur secondary to a lytic state induced by the drug's action on plasminogen attached to certain circulating fibrin degradation products, resulting in free circulating plasmin. However, in vitro studies show that rt-PA appears to be more effective than streptokinase or urokinase at lysing thrombi suspended in plasma containing lower concentrations of plasminogen, as occurs in neonates [20]. Trials directly comparing rt-PA with streptokinase or urokinase are not available, and comprehensive literature reviews have not clearly identified superior efficacy or safety of rt-PA [5,6]. Nevertheless, it has become the most widely used thrombolytic agent in pediatrics. Given this historical shift and rt-PA's recommended use in published guidelines (6,10,11), the remainder of this chapter will focus on rt-PA as the thrombolytic agent of choice.

IV. General clinical considerations

A. Indications for thrombolysis in pediatric patients

1. Intravascular thrombosis

Intravascular thrombosis in its various forms is the primary indication for thrombolytic therapy. Successful thrombolysis results in reduction of pathologic clot burden. Benefits of intravascular thrombolysis thus include increased rates and earlier restoration of vessel patency, which may lead to decreased risk for post-thrombotic syndrome (in the setting of venous thrombosis) [2,3], improved organ or extremity viability and reduced symptoms from acute thrombosis. Most reports describing outcomes have utilized restoration of flow or thrombus resolution as a primary efficacy endpoint. These have featured widely varied success rates which could reasonably be expected to depend on patient population, dosing regimen, modality of administration and thrombus location, among many other clinical variables. In the most comprehensive literature review to date involving 413 patients who had undergone pharmacologic thrombolysis, Albisetti described an overall 64% rate of complete thrombus resolution, with 21% having no response and 15% having partial resolution [6]. This group of patients comprised newborns, infants and children, and involved arterial and venous (non-CNS) events treated with either systemic or catheter-directed thrombolysis.

According to current guidelines and expert opinion [8,11], specific types of intravascular thrombosis for which thrombolysis can or should be considered include:

- Life-, organ- or limb-threatening conditions due to thrombosis, including arterial or venous thrombosis causing tissue ischemia – examples may include severe superior vena cava syndrome and phlegmasia cerulea dolans
- Massive pulmonary embolism with significant right ventricular dysfunction or hypotension
- Extensive or progressive arterial or venous thrombosis not responding to acute anticoagulation therapy or with high-risk features – for example, completely occlusive, lower extremity DVT with elevated factor VIII and D-dimer [21]
- Bilateral renal vein thrombosis with evident renal impairment
- Acute arterial ischemic stroke in the setting of a specific research protocol (section V.C.1)
- Severe (e.g., with complications related to increased intracranial pressure) cerebral sinovenous thrombosis without improvement on anticoagulation
- Large (> 2 cm) mobile atrial thrombi
- Congenital heart disease with clinically (e.g., hemodynamically) significant shunt obstruction
- Acute obstructive thrombosis of iliofemoral veins or inferior vena cava
- Anatomic compressive conditions such as May–Thurner or Paget–Schroetter syndromes
- Kawasaki disease with giant aneurysm and acute coronary artery thrombosis

See section V for additional details.

2. Restoring catheter patency

Thrombolytic agents have been used for many years to treat occluded central venous catheters; rt-PA is described in published pediatric guidelines and is generally regarded as safe and efficacious for this indication [10,11]. Usual practice is to instill 0.5 to 2 mg of rt-PA in an affected lumen for time periods of up to 4 hours or more [22], but an interval between 30 minutes and 1–2 hours appears most typical. Clearance rates of 85–97% with only rare bleeding complications have been reported in children [6]. Regular prophylactic instillation of thrombolytic

agents into central venous catheters may reduce rates of infection, thrombosis or both [23,24].

B. Contraindications: Bleeding risk

Bleeding is the primary complication of pharmacologic thrombolysis. Reported bleeding frequencies have varied widely between studies, which is likely due to heterogeneous patient populations, treatment regimens and case definitions of bleeding. The most comprehensive review comprising 413 newborns and children analyzed bleeding rates according to mode of drug administration (systemic versus catheter-directed) and by agent (streptokinase, urokinase, rt-PA). For systemic therapy (320 patients), frequency of minor bleeding (including mucosal bleeding and bleeding at puncture sites) was reported as 22% and of major bleeding (into CNS or organ, or requiring transfusion) was 15% for all agents in aggregate; the figures were 9% and 7%, respectively, for catheter-directed therapy [6]. The fatal bleed rate was reported as 1.25%.

The largest single-center study to date described a major bleeding complication rate of 40% and a minor rate of 30% among 80 consecutive patients treated mostly with systemic rt-PA, at an average dose of 0.5 mg/kg/hour and a median duration of 6 hours [25]. Most cases involved arterial thrombi (Table 14.3). In contrast, the largest single-center study using an alternative low-dose rt-PA regimen (section IV.E.1), described major bleeding in 9% and minor bleeding in 22% of 23 patients, all with venous thrombi [26]. Another recent single-center study utilizing the higher dose of rt-PA described major bleeding in 12% and minor bleeding in 42% of 26 patients with either arterial or venous thrombosis [27]. Minor bleeding thus appears quite commonly and typically involves oozing from wound or puncture sites. Although studies have been limited by small numbers of patients, major bleeding rates may have declined in recent years due to more judicious patient selection and increased experience with thrombolytic agents and interventions. Catheter-directed thrombolysis offers the potential for lower bleeding risk (section IV.E.2) and should be considered in centers with appropriate experience.

Most contraindications to pharmacologic thrombolysis pertain to bleeding risk. Specific considerations have been suggested by various authors [8,28] and are summarized below:

- Known allergy to the agent
- Active bleeding

Table 14.3 Summary of individual series of thrombolytic treatment using rt-PA in children (minimum ten patients)

Age range	Number	Site	Dosing regimen	Lysis	Bleeding	Year of publication
1 day–17 years	12	Mixed	0.1–0.5 mg/kg/h for 2h–3days	7 C 4 P	7 total	1991 [50]
2 days–47 months	17	Arterial	0.5 mg/kg/h first hour then 0.25 mg/h until clot lysis or bleeding	16 C	3 major 6 minor	1993 [72]
1–14 days	16	Mixed	0.1 mg/kg/h for 10 minutes then 0.3 mg/kg/h for 3 hours. Up to 4 repeat infusions every 12–24 hours	7 C 7 P	"Satisfactory" 1 ICH	1998 [49]
3–21 days	14	Arterial	0.7 mg/kg first hour then 0.1–0.3 mg/kg/h for 1–5 days	11 C 2 P	2 minor	2001 [73]
2 days–17.8 years	80	Mixed	Mean 0.5 mg/kg/h for median of 6 hours; local or systemic or both	52 C 16 P	54 total 31 transfused	2001 [25]
1 day–3 years	21	Arterial[a]	0.1 mg/kg bolus then 0.5 mg/kg/h for 2 hours, repeat once if needed	15 C 6 P	6 total 2 transfused	2003 [74]
1 day–17 years	35	Mixed	0.1–0.5 mg/kg/h for 1–24 hours (14 patients) or 0.03–0.06 mg/kg/h for 4–48 hours (21 patients) local or systemic	29 C 6 P	1 major 8 minor	2003 [37]
1 day–15 years	26	Mixed	0.5 mg/kg/h for 6 hours, repeated 12–24 hours later if needed	13 C 5 P	3 major 11 minor	2007 [27]
0.5–21 years	23	Venous	0.03–0.06 mg/kg/h for 12–48 hours increased to 0.12 mg/kg/h if needed	4 C 9 P	2 major 5 minor	2010 [26]

C = complete; P = partial; [a]persistent loss of pedal pulse after cardiac catheterization. Adapted from [9] with permission.

- Major surgery within 7 to 14 days
- CNS ischemia, or bleeding, or neurosurgical procedures within 30 days; birth asphyxia within 7 to 14 days
- Invasive procedure within 3 days
- Seizures within 48 hours
- Recent, severe trauma
- Inability to maintain fibrinogen concentration > 100 mg/dl or platelet count > 50,000 to 100,000/μl
- Prematurity (corrected age < 32 weeks)
- Uncontrolled hypertension
- Other risk factors for bleeding (e.g., presence of arteriovenous malformation, sepsis, solid tumor)

Many of the above should be considered as relative contraindications since a particular scenario may dictate use of thrombolysis even with significant bleeding risk. Under certain circumstances, the need for thrombolytic therapy may necessitate treatment despite contraindications.

Premature infants appear to be at particularly high risk for severe bleeding complications, but the proportion of risk that can be ascribed to thrombolytic therapy is uncertain given the high baseline rate of intracranial hemorrhage (ICH) in this age group. A literature review comprising 929 pediatric patients treated with thrombolysis suggested that risk of ICH may be related to age, since premature infants had the highest frequency (14%) compared to term neonates (1.2%) and children beyond the neonatal period (0.4%) [29]. The study acknowledged, however, the difficulty in interpreting the data given the high rate of ICH in premature babies not receiving thrombolysis.

C. Suitability: Age of thrombus

There exists a general perception that attempts at thrombolysis become less effective with increasing thrombus age. A retrospective study of 85 adults with DVT treated with thrombolysis showed progressively lower clot resolution rates as duration of symptoms prior to treatment initiation increased [30]. Some experts thus suggest an age of 2 weeks or less for an acute thrombus as a general criterion for appropriate initiation of thrombolytic therapy [7,8], although others have employed a cut-off of 4 weeks in children [31]. For older, more chronic clots with a delayed presentation, the risks versus benefits of attempted thrombolysis should be carefully considered.

D. Adjunctive and supportive care measures

From a clinical management perspective, several steps can be taken to minimize complication risks and maximize the likelihood of successful treatment in a patient undergoing thrombolytic therapy. These precautions and considerations are categorized according to their primary relevance to either: (1) general care of the patient undergoing thrombolysis, (2) monitoring of laboratory or imaging parameters or (3) treatment of bleeding complications.

1. General care considerations

- Adequate informed consent for treatment should be obtained.
- Patients should be managed in an intensive care unit or alternative setting in which the staff has adequate experience with thrombolytic therapy.
- Clear communication among all staff regarding the patient's clinical status and potential bleeding risk should be ensured, such as via a sign at the head of the bed and/or an alert in the electronic medical record indicating the patient is receiving thrombolytic therapy.
- According to the clinical status of the patient, activity and care restrictions should be directed at minimizing bleeding risk. Examples to consider include strict bedrest and minimizing patient manipulation, such as through limitations on bathing, physiotherapy, intramuscular injections, arterial punctures, rectal temperatures and urinary catheters.
- Patients should be monitored closely for bleeding signs and symptoms, including frequent, periodic neurologic assessments.
- In the appropriate clinical setting (e.g., limb ischemia, renal impairment), careful and frequent clinical monitoring of tissue and organ perfusion is mandatory.

- The need to rule out pre-existing CNS bleeding via imaging study should be considered prior to initiating thrombolytic therapy.
- Thrombocytopenia or coagulopathy should be corrected via blood product replacement or other means as appropriate. Adequate anticipatory communication and coordination should occur with the blood bank to ensure timely and reliable supply of blood products as needed.
- Thrombolytic agents do not inhibit clot formation. Evidence suggests that plasmin formation can lead to thrombin generation, possibly through activation of the contact pathway [32]. In addition to increased thrombin generation, there is evidence that clot-bound thrombin is less susceptible to inactivation by antithrombin; thus free thrombin with procoagulant activity is released during the process of fibrinolysis [33]. For these reasons, and since anticoagulation is evidence-based for prevention of thromboembolism, concomitant anticoagulation with unfractionated heparin (UFH) at a low or prophylactic dose (e.g., 10 units/kg/h) has been a commonly employed adjunctive practice during thrombolysis; this appears safe and is described in current guidelines [11] and expert recommendations [7,18,28]. Therapeutic anticoagulation is typically initiated or resumed after completion of thrombolytic therapy.
- Given the dependence of pharmacologic thrombolysis on an adequate supply of plasminogen (section II.B), empiric administration of plasma (or assessment of plasma plasminogen concentration) prior to initiating therapy, especially in young infants, should be strongly considered. Since plasminogen is further consumed by thrombolytic therapy ("plasminogen steal") [34], repletion should also be considered with prolonged or repeated courses of thrombolysis, or if radiographic or biochemical evidence of effective thrombolysis is lacking (section IV.D.2).
- If evidence of effective thrombolysis is lacking, thrombolytic dose escalation, a repeat treatment course or alternative salvage therapies may merit consideration (sections IV.D.2 and IV.E.2). However, since the impact of increasing thrombolytic drug exposure and its timing on bleeding risk may be uncertain, decisions about dose changes and how soon after a treatment course to pursue a repeat attempt must be carefully considered.

- In adults, periprocedural IVC filter placement is strongly discouraged in most patients undergoing drug-only thrombolysis, either systemically or via catheter (see section IV.E.3). In certain selected cases, preprocedure placement and post-procedure removal of a retrievable IVC filter may be reasonable depending on the thrombus site and extent, patient factors and the specific clot-removal methods to be used [3].

2. Monitoring requirements

Laboratory measures: Laboratory parameters such as D-dimer, fibrin degradation products (FDP) and fibrinogen activity correlate poorly with the degree of in vivo thrombolytic effect [35]; there exists no target therapeutic range for any of these parameters. However, each does reflect the presence of lytic activity (via increases in the former two and decline in fibrinogen) such that their monitoring is recommended [8].

- Given the need for frequent laboratory monitoring, placement of an intravenous catheter dedicated to blood sampling should be considered.
- Prior to initiating thrombolytic therapy, a baseline assessment of complete blood count (CBC) and coagulation parameters, including prothrombin time, activated partial thromboplastin time, fibrinogen activity, and D-dimer or FDP, should be obtained, along with a sample for matching for possible blood products.
- After thrombolytic therapy has been initiated, monitoring of CBC and coagulation parameters at regular intervals should occur to assess for occult bleeding and thrombocytopenia, and for biochemical confirmation of a thrombolytic effect. In the presence of a thrombolytic effect, fibrinogen activity typically declines by 25–50% and D-dimer and FDP increase. If these changes in surrogate markers do not occur and thrombolysis is deemed ineffective, options to consider include dose escalation, plasminogen repletion and alternative therapies (sections IV.D.1 and IV.E.2)
- Low fibrinogen concentration (< 100 mg/dl) or platelet count (< 50,000 to 100,000/μl) suggests the need for repletion with blood products.

Imaging studies: In addition to imaging to rule out pre-existing CNS bleed prior to initiating thrombolytic therapy, follow-up CNS imaging should also be considered during therapy, especially in the critically ill patient whose neurologic status is difficult to assess

clinically. Repeat imaging of the thrombus site should occur at regular intervals after starting therapy to assess therapy effectiveness and guide treatment decisions. The optimal monitoring regimen may be highly individualized and best formulated in close multidisciplinary consultation with experts in radiology or other interventional services, and may include angiographic imaging dictated by required interventions.

3. Treatment of bleeding complications

As discussed above (section IV.B), bleeding occurs commonly during thrombolytic therapy, especially from wound and puncture sites. Minor superficial bleeding can be treated with local pressure and supportive care. For more significant bleeding, holding or discontinuing infusion of the thrombolytic agent (rt-PA half-life < 5 minutes) and any concurrent heparin being administered can be considered, along with use of pressure dressings and topical adjunctive agents such as fibrin sealants, other thrombin preparations and antifibrinolytic agents. Systemic use of antifibrinolytics and repletion with cryoprecipitate and/or plasma can be considered for severe bleeding.

E. Modes of therapy

Thrombolytic agents can be administered either systemically (through a peripheral vein) or locally (via a catheter located in close proximity to the targeted thrombus). In the setting of catheter-associated thrombosis, therapy may be administered through a previously placed intravascular catheter left *in situ* after thrombosis has been diagnosed, or, as is more often the case, through a catheter placed specifically to deliver thrombolytic therapy to the targeted site. Moreover, interventional catheters may hold additional features designed to augment thrombolytic effectiveness, such as multiple side holes to deliver drug more uniformly throughout a thrombus and certain mechanical capabilities to aid in clot breakdown or removal (section IV.E.3). Surgical thrombectomy offers another general therapeutic approach to rapid resolution of pathologic thrombi, but because of perceived risks for long-term vascular damage, is generally reserved for very specific, and often extreme, clinical scenarios [11].

There currently exists no conclusive evidence to favor one mode of thrombolytic drug delivery (systemic versus catheter-directed) over the other in children, but technical feasibility (e.g., dependence on patient size) and availability of appropriate institutional expertise, tools and equipment necessarily bear on which modality is selected [11]. Systemic and catheter-based approaches are summarized below followed by a brief discussion of surgical thrombectomy.

1. Systemic thrombolytic infusion

Historically, systemic drug delivery has been the route of administration most commonly described for pediatric patients; 320 cases involving systemic thrombolysis were reported in the most comprehensive pediatric literature review, compared with 93 cases of catheter-directed thrombolytic infusion (CDT) [6]. In this review, the overall response rate for systemic thrombolysis was reported as 79% (64% complete, 15% partial response) and minor, major and fatal bleeding rates were reported as 22%, 15% and 1.25%, respectively. No pediatric studies have directly compared systemic thrombolysis to CDT; comparative studies in adults are also relatively lacking. However, because of technical limitations imposed by patient size and because CDT requires a specific set of interventionalist skills and equipment, systemic thrombolysis may be the only modality available in certain settings, especially for infants and small children.

Dosing regimens: A wide variety of dosing regimens have been employed for systemic (non-CNS) administration of rt-PA in infants and children (Table 14.3), but no controlled trials are available to clearly support one regimen over another [6,9]. Ranges for reported systemic infusion dose, duration and loading dose of rt-PA vary from 0.01 to 3.75 mg/kg/h (median 0.435), 1 hour to 8 days (median 7.5 hours) and 0 to 0.8 mg (median 0.2), respectively [6].

Current guidelines do not recommend a particular dose or duration for systemic thrombolysis [11], but two distinct dosing regimens have emerged as primary approaches from literature reports. The first calls for rt-PA infusion at 0.1 to 0.6 mg/kg/h for 6 hours (without a loading dose) and has been described as the most commonly used systemic dose regimen in pediatric patients [36]. Several case series have utilized similar dosing strategies. The largest single-center pediatric case series of rt-PA use involved 80 consecutive children, most of whom received systemic thrombolysis according to this regimen for arterial thrombosis; the average dose was 0.5 mg/kg/h and median infusion duration was 6 hours. Complete resolution was reported in 65% and partial resolution in 20%; bleeding complications occurred in 71% of patients who received systemic rt-PA, about half of which were classified as major [25]. Factors associated with major bleeding complications included longer duration of thrombolytic therapy, lower body weight and greater decline in fibrinogen level after therapy [25]. Other case series of systemic rt-PA use in infants or children are considerably smaller (Table 14.3).

Distinct from the "standard" dosing strategy described above is a "low-dose" regimen initiating rt-PA at 0.03 to 0.06 mg/kg/h infused over 12 to 48 hours or more [26,37], intended to reduce drug exposure and hence bleeding risk. Dose escalation strategies were not uniform between studies, but response rates were reported as 59% and 71%. Major bleeding complications occurred in three of the 40 cases initiated on a low-dose regimen in the two largest published case series, which appears favorable compared to standard dosing. Importantly, given the prolonged infusion duration of the low-dose regimen, no relationship was identified between rt-PA infusion duration and bleeding events [26,37], in contrast to the study by Gupta *et al.* [25]. An initial maximum dose rate of 2 mg/h has been suggested for this dosing regimen [7,38].

Another important difference relevant to the studies describing the low-dose regimen is that they involved a higher percentage of patients affected by venous, as opposed to arterial, thrombosis. Of note, a small cohort study utilizing the standard dose rt-PA regimen reported an 81% clot resolution rate among children with arterial thrombosis, but 0% resolution among children with venous thrombosis [27]. These observations, coupled with the typical infusion durations planned for the standard versus low-dose rt-PA regimens may suggest that standard dosing is more appropriate for clinical scenarios such as limb-compromising arterial thrombosis, in which re-establishing adequate perfusion expeditiously is particularly critical.

2. Catheter-directed thrombolytic infusion

Catheter-directed thrombolytic infusion (CDT) has been reported less frequently as a means of thrombolytic drug administration in pediatric patients compared to systemic thrombolysis [6], but its use and acceptance appear to be increasing based on recent literature [31,38]. Although no studies have rigorously compared systemic to CDT for thrombolysis in pediatrics, CDT holds the theoretical advantage of direct delivery of the thrombolytic agent to the thrombus, thus enhancing drug concentration at the thrombus surface and minimizing systemic exposure, perhaps leading to decreased bleeding risk. Use of CDT also permits alternative mechanical treatment modalities that may enhance treatment effectiveness (section IV.E.3). There exists as yet no conclusive evidence that mode of delivery confers advantages with respect to safety or efficacy. However, aggregate, small, uncontrolled studies suggest that catheter-directed regimens may be associated with less bleeding and comparable or better efficacy. In a systematic review, Albisetti reported complete thrombus resolution in 76% and partial resolution in 15% of pediatric patients who received CDT with rt-PA; this was accompanied by a major bleed rate of 6.5%, a minor bleed rate of 15% and no fatal bleeds, which compares favorably to the efficacy and safety parameters reported for systemic thrombolysis [6] (section IV.E.1). These data must be interpreted cautiously however, in light of the small, uncontrolled and heterogeneous nature of the reviewed studies.

Dosing regimens: Historical dosing of rt-PA in CDT has been described as a weight-based infusion, ranging from 0.015 to 0.2 mg/kg/h (median 0.08) [6], but typical rt-PA dosing in CDT is often fairly empiric, with infusion rate increasing by 0.25 to 0.5 mg/h increments from 0.5 up to 1–2 mg/h based on the general size of the patient and depending on interventionalist preference. Duration of CDT rt-PA infusions have been reported to range from 2 hours up to 10 days with a median of 24 hours [6]; rt-PA infusion at 1–2 mg/h for 24 to 48 hours is a published pediatric dosing regimen for CDT [7,38]. As an adjunct to mechanical thrombectomy (section IV.E.3), somewhat lower infusion rates have been described (0.5 to 1 mg/h for subsequent CDT for 12 to 24 hours) [31]. Of note, recent studies in adults have utilized an infusion rate of 0.01 mg/kg/h for CDT [2].

3. Other catheter-based interventions

Recent technological advances have significantly broadened the therapeutic armamentarium for percutaneous removal of intravascular thrombus. While the vast majority of available clinical reports focus on the adult population, these endovascular treatment modalities are potentially applicable to pediatric patients, subject to limitations imposed by body and vessel size. Having institutional access to appropriate interventionalist experience, adequate tools and equipment, and a collaborative, multidisciplinary team of interventionalists, intensivists, hematologists, nurses and technologists are other crucial factors impacting feasibility and the likelihood of successful outcomes. Available endovascular treatment modalities include ultrasound-accelerated CDT, mechanical thrombectomy, and pharmacomechanical CDT, each of which is described briefly. It should be emphasized that published pediatric experience with each of these modalities is limited.

Ultrasound-accelerated CDT: The application of ultrasound to disrupt intravascular thrombus was first reported by Rosenschein and colleagues in the 1990s when it was noted that ultrasonic energy was effective in disrupting the fibrin matrix within thrombi [39]. A differential in tissue absorption rate of ultrasonic energy was observed, attributed to differences in tissue elasticity, conferring increased sensitivity of thrombus to ultrasonic energy compared to the surrounding vessel wall. Various mechanisms have been proposed to explain how ultrasonic energy can facilitate thrombolysis, including acoustic cavitation, mechanical defragmentation, microstreaming effects and thermal warming [40].

The EkoSonic Endovascular System® (EKOS Corp, Bothell, WA) is an ultrasound-accelerated thrombolytic system that combines high-frequency, low-power ultrasound with simultaneous CDT to accelerate intravascular clot dissolution (Figure 14.2). Ultrasound-enhanced thrombolytic therapy achieves its effect first by disrupting the fibrin mesh to increase the thrombus surface area of the fibers in contact with the thrombolytic agent. Acoustic microstreaming induced by ultrasonic waves then facilitates diffusion of the thrombolytic agent away from the catheter deep into the macerated clot. A potential advantage of the EkoSonic system is that ultrasonic energy emanating from the transducers appears to penetrate venous valves, allowing dissolution of thrombus located behind these valves. Thrombus located in this hard-to-reach region is typically inaccessible to other mechanical thrombectomy systems. Because the entire segment of the venous thrombus can be exposed to the ultrasound energy, it potentially reduces infusion time and required dosing of thrombolytic agents. Clinical experience using ultrasound-accelerated CDT to remove either arterial or venous thrombus has been well documented, with favorable results compared to standard CDT [41], but experience in pediatric patients is limited.

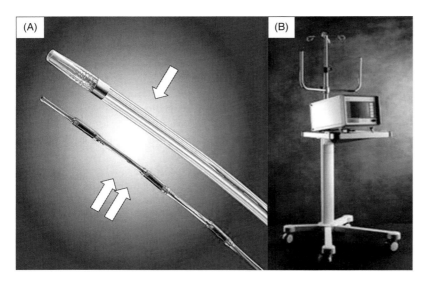

Figure 14.2 (A) The EkoSonic® system consists of a multilumen catheter for thrombolytic delivery (single arrow) with one central lumen and three separate infusion ports. Each drug lumen incorporates a series of laser-cut, microinfusion pores that focus drug delivery for coordinated interface with the ultrasound waves. Each catheter has a matched ultrasound core wire (double arrows) that incorporates a series of miniature ultrasound transducers spaced at approximately 1 cm intervals to deliver ultrasonic energy evenly along the entire infusion pathway. (B) The system is driven by a control unit that automatically adjusts the power for each of the ultrasound transducers based on ambient conditions in the vessel. Reproduced with permission from Perspect Vasc Surg Endovasc Ther. 2010 Sep;22(3):152–63.

Percutaneous mechanical and pharmacomechanical thrombectomy: A variety of mechanical thrombectomy devices for use either in isolation or in concert with simultaneous pharmacologic thrombolysis have been developed. Combining percutaneous mechanical thrombectomy (PMT) with pharmacologic thrombolysis, also known as pharmacomechanical CDT (PCDT), holds appeal because it can potentially reduce overall exposure to thrombolytic agents (via decreased dose and duration) [42] as well as reduce procedure time, length of stay and treatment costs as compared with conventional systemic or CDT [43]. Major bleeding events and acute symptomatic PE appear to be relatively uncommon with PMT/PCDT, although these outcomes have not been widely assessed [31]. A limited number of studies in adults suggest PCDT can effect thrombus removal in a single procedure session, but no prospective studies have rigorously validated this possibility, and increased mechanical manipulation associated with such interventions may carry additional risk [3]. A comprehensive discussion of all devices relevant to PMT/PCDT is beyond the scope of this chapter, but two of the most commonly used will be described briefly.

The AngioJet® (Medrad Inc, Warrendale, PA) rheolytic mechanical thrombectomy system applies Bernoulli's principle, directing high-velocity saline jets retrograde within the catheter, from the tip of the device toward outflow channels in a coaxial fashion, generating a vacuum force at the tip which draws macerated thrombus into an effluent lumen of the catheter for evacuation (Figure 14.3). The thrombectomy catheter can be delivered through a small-bore introducer sheath, which reduces access site trauma and avoids operative vessel exposure required with surgical thromboembolectomy. Clinical studies in adults demonstrate this system's effectiveness in thrombus removal, restoration of vessel patency and relieving symptoms of vessel thrombosis. Secondary benefits of pharmacomechanical utilization of this device have included decreased length of stay and lower costs compared with CDT [43].

The Trellis® (Covidien, Mansfield, MA) system is designed specifically for pharmacomechanical use, employing localized thrombolytic infusion followed by mechanical disruption and aspiration of the thrombus. Initially, thrombolytic agent is infused in between proximal and distal occlusion balloons, which isolate the intervening thrombus from the adjacent vasculature. A dispersion wire is inserted within the catheter between the two occlusion balloons and is then activated and rotated rapidly by an electrically powered drive unit, thereby creating a mechanical dispersion of the thrombolytic agent (Figure 14.4). The advantage of this thrombectomy and infusion system is that it directs administration of the thrombolytic agent to the isolated segment of vessel containing thrombus, thus minimizing systemic dispersion and potentially

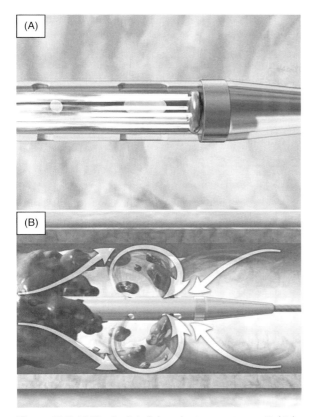

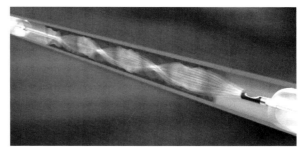

Figure 14.4 To activate the thrombectomy function using the Trellis® system, a dispersion wire is inserted within the catheter between the two occlusion balloons. The dispersion wire is rotated rapidly by the electrically powered drive unit at 500 to 3,000 rpm. This rapid rotation mechanically disperses the thrombolytic agent and facilitates thrombus resolution. Reproduced with permission from Perspect Vasc Surg Endovasc Ther. 2010 Sep;22(3):152–63.

Figure 14.3 (A) The AngioJet® thrombectomy system emits high-velocity saline jets that are directed retrograde within the catheter from the tip of the device to outflow channels in a coaxial fashion. (B) This generates a vacuum force which draws the thrombus into the catheter, achieving the rheolytic thrombectomy effect. Reproduced with permission from Perspect Vasc Surg Endovasc Ther. 2010 Sep;22 (3):152–63.

bleeding risk. Clinical studies in adults suggest that use of this device is associated with favorable rates of vessel patency, both acutely and on follow-up, reduced exposure to thrombolytic agents and a high rate of successful thrombectomy after a single session [44].

4. Surgical thrombectomy

Surgical thrombectomy requires an open incision whereby arterial or venous thrombus is surgically removed using a balloon catheter, and is often associated with significant blood loss and operative morbidity. In the longer term, it is generally regarded to be associated with high risk for thrombus recurrence, long-term vascular injury and other complications. Currently, surgical thrombectomy should be considered as a last resort for urgent restoration of circulatory flow, such as when there

exists imminent threat to limb or life due to thrombus formation and pharmacologic thrombolysis is contraindicated [11].

V. Specific approaches based on thrombus location

Much of the existing literature on pediatric thrombolysis consists of case reports or small case series featuring considerable variation in patient age, thrombus site, mode of thrombolytic delivery, dose and duration. Taken together, such reports must be viewed with caution, given the likelihood of a positive reporting bias and that a large percentage of patients being considered for thrombolysis are critically ill, with imminent threat to limb, organ or life.

A. Venous thromboembolism (VTE)

1. Venous thrombosis

Current guidelines suggest that thrombolysis in this clinical setting be reserved for life- or limb-threatening VTE [11]. However, post-thrombotic syndrome (PTS) is a recognized complication of limb DVT in children and adolescents, affecting nearly 25% of patients and conferring significant morbidity in the form of functional limitations and cosmetic impact [45]. Some pediatric patients appear to be at even higher risk for PTS based on the extent of vascular occlusion and acute elevations in plasma biomarkers at clinical presentation [21,38]. Moreover, either thrombus extension or symptom progression in the face of anticoagulation therapy that otherwise appears adequate would seem to present clinical scenarios for which alternative therapeutic options, such as additional efforts to rapidly restore venous patency, must be considered.

The utility of thrombolysis in improving outcomes in selected patients with DVT, especially those with extensive iliofemoral involvement, appears supported by limited trial data in adults. As summarized in a recent scientific statement from the AHA, numerous adult studies link the presence of residual thrombus at the time of follow-up with increased risk for DVT recurrence and PTS [3]. These findings suggest that early restoration of venous patency in the setting of lower extremity DVT ought to lead to lower risk of PTS. Indeed, a Cochrane review of 12 randomized trials comparing additional thrombolysis (systemic or CDT) to anticoagulation alone for acute DVT reported improved venous patency and decreased PTS in patients who received thrombolytic therapy, although the latter was based on only two randomized studies reporting this outcome. Patients undergoing thrombolysis also had more bleeding complications [46]. Current ACCP recommendations suggest anticoagulation alone for acute proximal DVT of the leg over both systemic and CDT [47]. However, the associated strength of recommendation is weak and characteristics to identify individuals who are most likely to benefit from thrombolysis are presented, including iliofemoral DVT, good functional status, low risk of bleeding and symptom duration of less than 14 days [47]. Furthermore, alternate published guidelines from the AHA are nuanced to a slightly different stance on this point, suggesting that CDT/PCDT is reasonable as first-line treatment for selected young patients with iliofemoral DVT who are at low risk of bleeding [3].

A recent randomized, multicenter trial of over 200 adults with acute iliofemoral DVT comparing initial CDT using rt-PA added to standard therapy with standard therapy alone, showed that patients who received CDT had a higher frequency of venous patency at 6 months and a lower frequency of PTS at 2 years. Patients in the experimental arm received rt-PA at 0.01 mg/kg/h. The associated major bleed rate was 3%, compared to 0% for the control arm [2]. Importantly, recent retrospective studies in adults using similar rt-PA dosing regimens report major bleeding rates in the range of 2–4%, suggesting that major bleeding risk associated with CDT has decreased compared with earlier studies using alternate agents and regimens [3].

As described above, PCDT may hold additional advantages compared with CDT by decreasing thrombolytic drug exposure and consequent bleeding risk, procedure time, length of stay and costs of care [43]. An ongoing study with underlying hypothesis and aims similar to the study by Enden et al. described above is the Acute Venous Thrombosis: Thrombus Removal with Adjunctive Catheter-directed Thrombolysis (ATTRACT) trial, a prospective, multicenter, randomized trial of adult patients with acute, symptomatic proximal DVT (ClinicalTrials.gov Identifier NCT00790335). The ATTRACT trial will assess the impact of pharmacomechanical intervention by comparing PCDT using rt-PA followed by standard care, to standard care alone. The primary endpoint is occurrence of PTS at 2 years of follow-up.

A retrospective study showed that children and adolescents with acute, occlusive DVT and high-risk features who underwent thrombolysis according to an institutional protocol had significantly reduced odds of PTS after 18 to 24 months compared with those who received standard therapy via anticoagulation alone (22% versus 77% frequency, respectively). Major bleeding occurred in one patient, judged unlikely to be related to thrombolytic therapy [38]. The institutional protocol typically consisted of low-dose systemic rt-PA (section IV.E.1) with salvage PMT or PCDT for persistent occlusion. A follow-up prospective study of 16 older children and adolescents with occlusive, high-risk DVT, PMT or PCDT in conjunction with approximately 24 hours of adjunctive CDT using rt-PA resulted in a relatively low frequency of functionally significant PTS at 1 to 2 years (13%) and no major periprocedural bleeding events. One patient however, had symptomatic periprocedural pulmonary embolism. Early and late DVT recurrence rate were not insignificant in this high-risk cohort (40% and 27%, respectively), but the early events were generally responsive to repeat lysis [31]. Early clot resolution and restoration of venous patency via thrombolysis may thus be important therapeutic goals in selected patients. Risk-targeted lytic strategies are the focus of a planned clinical trial in pediatrics, currently being refined via a planning grant from NIH NHLBI [48].

Other descriptions of systemic thrombolysis for venous thrombosis in pediatrics report success rates varying between 0 and 100% [18,25–27,37,49–51]. Of note, two of the more recent studies describe general success using a low-dose regimen of systemic rt-PA [26,37]. These results contrast markedly with those reported by Newall *et al.*, who uniformly utilized the higher, standard rt-PA dosing regimen [27], suggesting that lower doses and longer infusion times may be more effective for venous clots. However, differences in patient selection, thrombus age and validity of outcome assessments may also contribute to the discrepant results, as no randomized trial has compared the two dosing regimens. Anatomic compressive syndromes such as May–Thurner and Paget–Schroetter merit brief mention due to the emergence of thrombolysis, and especially CDT/PCDT, as a key component of optimal initial therapy for affected patients, based on the premise that such approaches improve long-term outcomes compared with initial anticoagulation alone.

2. Pulmonary embolism

Massive PE is a labeled indication for rt-PA, but the optimal role for thrombolysis in PE during childhood remains undefined. Current ACCP recommendations make no specific mention of thrombolysis in the setting of PE other than implied as part of the general suggestion to restrict thrombolysis to cases of VTE that threaten life, limb or organ [11]. Literature descriptions in pediatrics are restricted to either case reports or small subgroups of patients analyzed as part of a larger case series [9]. Two reports from the same institution reported a total of 14 patients with PE treated with thrombolysis [25,52]. These patients typically had substantial cardiorespiratory compromise and poor outcomes. In the largest case series of pediatric patients with PE, eight patients were treated with rt-PA at a median dose and duration of 0.5 mg/kg/h and 6 hours, respectively. One patient had a complete response and three showed no response. Major bleeding occurred in 50%. Four patients received repeat courses of thrombolysis but none had improvement with subsequent doses. Based on these findings, the authors recommended no more than a single course attempt of thrombolytic therapy for childhood PE [52].

Current adult guidelines suggest systemic thrombolysis for massive PE as defined by the presence of sustained hypotension. There is clinical equipoise for submassive PE, characterized by right ventricular dysfunction or myocardial necrosis in normotensive patients, with guidance to consider thrombolysis specifically for patients with "clinical evidence of adverse prognosis" [3]. Results from two ongoing trials of submassive PE in adults should help address this question [3]. The dose for PE in adults on the drug label for rt-PA is 100 mg IV given over 2 hours.

Catheter-based interventions for PE have been reported in adults and children, but are not currently recommended as a first-line therapy [3,9,53]. The senior author of this chapter and colleagues have previously reported treatment efficacy with ultrasound-accelerated thrombolytic therapy in adult patients with massive PE, who demonstrated reduced infusion times and bleeding complications compared with CDT alone [41]. Based on this experience, we have also utilized this modality with relative success and safety in carefully selected pediatric patients with acute massive PE at higher risk for bleeding.

Until further evidence becomes available, systemic thrombolysis appears reasonable for children with PE with hypotension, significant right ventricular dysfunction or worsening cardiorespiratory status attributable to PE unresponsive to anticoagulation. Systemic drug delivery is the current standard of care in adults and is the modality most commonly described in the pediatric literature. However, CDT/PCDT may be considered subject to institutional capabilities, especially in patients at higher risk for bleeding.

B. Arterial thrombosis

Non-CNS arterial thrombi have been described as the most common reported indication for thrombolytic therapy, accounting for just over half of reported cases; about 80% were catheter-related [6]. Thrombosis of the aorta, femoral and/or iliac arteries is most often related to recent catheter use, either umbilical or due to cardiac catheterization. Other arterial sites of involvement include brachial and radial arteries after catheterization, Blalock–Taussig shunts in children with congenital heart disease and coronary arteries in patients with Kawasaki disease.

Current guidelines recommend thrombolysis for femoral artery thrombosis that threatens limb or organ, if response to anticoagulation has been inadequate and there exist no contraindications [11]. For this and other indications involving peripheral arteries, systemic administration of rt-PA at standard dosing (section IV.E.1) appears to be the most commonly described regimen [25,27], although other successful approaches have been reported (Table 14.3). A specific algorithm has been published for brachial artery thrombosis in infants, which incorporates standard systemic dosing for rt-PA, but also describes intra-arterial infusion for selected cases [54]. Specific guidelines are also available for pharmacologic thrombolysis of acute coronary artery thrombosis in children with Kawasaki disease and giant aneurysms [11].

C. Central nervous system (CNS) thrombosis

1. Arterial ischemic stroke

Thrombolysis is used acutely in arterial ischemic stroke (AIS) to dissolve intracerebral arterial thrombi and restore blood flow to brain parenchyma, thereby salvaging tissue that is not yet infarcted. Intravenous (IV) rt-PA at a dose of 0.9 mg/kg (maximum total dose 90 mg), with 10% given as a bolus over the first minute and the remainder given over the next hour, is FDA-approved for use in adults within 3 hours of stroke onset; this regimen was shown to improve outcome at 3 months, but was associated with symptomatic ICH in 6.4% of treated adults [55]. The benefits appeared to be reduced and offset by bleeding complications if given beyond 3 hours [56]; however, subsequent studies suggested thrombolysis beyond this window may be beneficial in selected patients [56,57]. This was further investigated in the European Cooperative Acute Stroke Study (ECASS) III, in which IV rt-PA at a dose of 0.9 mg/kg initiated 3 to 4.5 hours after stroke onset also improved clinical outcomes and was associated with a rate of symptomatic ICH of 2.4% in a group of patients selected for lower bleeding risk [58]. Based on these findings, an advisory panel in 2009 recommended extending the time window for IV rt-PA to 4.5 hours in selected patients [59]. It should be noted however, that this extension is not currently FDA-approved.

With respect to pediatric patients, approximately one-fifth of children presenting for evaluation of suspected acute stroke have a "stroke mimicker," such as migraine, seizure, tumor, infection or a psychogenic diagnosis [60]. Evaluation for these conditions often contributes to delayed stroke recognition and a lost opportunity to initiate thrombolysis within the currently recommended time window for adult stroke. Current consensus-based guidelines recommend against rt-PA treatment of acute childhood AIS due to the lack of safety and efficacy studies: "Until there are additional published safety and efficacy data, rt-PA generally is not recommended for children with AIS outside a clinical trial," [61] a recommendation echoed by other experts [11].

Despite the lack of pediatric safety and efficacy data, thrombolysis with rt-PA has been used in clinical practice in children with stroke. For example, nine children receiving IV rt-PA for AIS were reported to the International Pediatric Stroke Study (IPSS) from 2003–2007 [62]. Among these nine children, IV rt-PA treatment was initiated within the 3 hours of stroke onset recommended in adults in only three. Moreover, total rt-PA dose ranged widely between 0.02 and 0.9 mg/kg, and less than half of the cases received rt-PA as a 10% bolus followed by the remaining dose (90%) over 1 hour. Outcomes were poor, and included one death due to middle cerebral artery dissection and stroke; the remaining eight children had neurological deficits; two asymptomatic ICH were noted [62]. In addition, there exist 11 published English-language case reports of children who received IV rt-PA for acute stroke treatment (Table 14.4). In contrast to the patients reported to the IPSS, treatment was started within 3 hours in nine of 11 patients, at 4 hours in one patient, and "promptly" in one patient. All but one received the FDA-recommended rt-PA dose regimen for adults. Five had a normal outcome and four had only mild deficit. Overall, when compared qualitatively with the IPSS cohort, the case reports were characterized by shorter times until rt-PA initiation and better outcomes.

Other acute, urgent therapies used in adults with AIS include intra-arterial thrombolytic administration and endovascular clot-retrieval devices. Despite reports of the successful use of intra-arterial thrombolytics in childhood stroke [63,64], data are insufficient for making recommendations. Good outcome despite extended time to treatment has been reported in intra-arterial thrombolysis of basilar artery occlusion [65], which otherwise frequently results in death or severe morbidity. Review of the literature and the IPSS database yields seven individual published case reports of pediatric AIS treated with intra-arterial rt-PA, in addition to six cases reported to the IPSS [62].

Information from the Nationwide Inpatient Sample database revealed that between 2000 and 2003, 46 of 2904 (1.6%) children diagnosed with ischemic stroke received thrombolysis. Of these, 24 received thrombolysis intravenously and 19 intra-arterially [66]. These data are limited by its dependence on ICD-9 codes, which often lack accuracy and sensitivity for childhood stroke, and information about the specific indication for thrombolysis.

Reports of endovascular device use for pediatric AIS have been rare, with varied outcomes, and usually followed other attempts at thrombolysis. Consistent with

Table 14.4 IV rt-PA in acute childhood stroke

Report	Age in years/sex	Given according to drug label for adults?	Hours since awake and at neurological baseline at time of initiation	Neurologic outcome
Cannon et al., 2001 [75]	12 F	Yes	2.5	Normal
Carlson et al., 2001 [76]	13 F	Yes	< 3	Minimal deficit
Cremer et al., 2008 [77]	15 F	Yes	2.5	Minimal deficit
Heil et al., 2008 [78]	16 F	Yes	4	Normal
Jain and Morton, 2008 [79]	15 F	Yes	< 3	Minimal deficit
Losurdo et al., 2006 [80]	4 M	No	"Promptly started"	Neurologic deficit
Muñiz, 2012 [81]	15 M	Yes	1.72	Normal
Noser et al., 2001 [82]	16 F	Yes	2.8	Neurologic deficit
Sampaio et al., 2011 [83]	14 M	Yes	2	Minimal deficit
Shuayto et al., 2006 [84]	16 M	Yes	2.7	Normal
Thirumalai & Shubin, 2000 [85]	16 F	Yes	1.75	Normal

current consensus guidelines, mechanical thrombectomy via endovascular intervention is not recommended for pediatric stroke outside of specific research protocols [11]. Furthermore, until its safety has been established in childhood stroke via rigorous clinical trials, systemic rt-PA cannot be routinely recommended.

2. Cerebral venous sinus thrombosis

A multicenter cohort study of 70 pediatric patients with cerebral sinovenous thrombosis (CSVT) identified only three who had been treated with thrombolysis [67]. A recent literature review of catheter-directed thrombolysis for CSVT in adults found that intracranial hemorrhages occurred in 7.6%, over half of whom died [68]. Endovascular treatment of CSVT in children has been reported as well, including use of continuous and repeated rt-PA infusion and mechanical disruption [69,70]. However, precise indications and optimal therapeutic dose and duration of treatment are unknown. Recent guidelines suggest "thrombolysis, thrombectomy, or surgical decompression only in children with severe CSVT in whom there is no improvement" with initial anticoagulant therapy [11].

VI. Conclusion

Of the approximately one dozen current ACCP recommendations pertaining to thrombolysis in pediatric patients, all are based on low-quality evidence and nearly all offer only a weak level of recommendation [11]. In the absence of more compelling evidence supporting additional indications, thrombolysis in infants, children and adolescents, with only a few exceptions, is largely regarded as a salvage-level therapy for patients with limb-, organ- or life-threatening manifestations of thrombotic disease. Through ongoing or planned trials, generation of more robust data regarding thrombolytic therapy will help to better define optimal use, especially given the perceived substantial risk-to-benefit ratio in many cases. In the meantime, careful, individualized, risk–benefit assessment and detailed discussion of these potential risks and benefits with patients and families are paramount for clinical decision-making regarding thrombolysis in pediatrics.

References

1. Ouriel K. A history of thrombolytic therapy. *J Endovasc Ther* 2004 Dec;**11**(Suppl 2):II128–II133.

2. Enden T, Haig Y, Klow NE, Slagsvold CE, Sandvik L, Ghanima W, et al. Long-term outcome after additional catheter-directed thrombolysis versus standard treatment for acute iliofemoral deep vein thrombosis (the CaVenT study): a randomised controlled trial. *Lancet* 2012 Jan 7;**379**(9810):31–8.

3. Jaff MR, McMurtry MS, Archer SL, Cushman M, Goldenberg N, Goldhaber SZ, et al. Management of massive and submassive pulmonary embolism, iliofemoral deep vein thrombosis, and chronic thromboembolic pulmonary hypertension: a scientific statement from the American Heart Association. *Circulation* 2011 Apr 26;**123**(16):1788–830.

4. Leaker M, Massicotte MP, Brooker LA, Andrew M. Thrombolytic therapy in pediatric patients: a comprehensive review of the literature. *Thromb Haemost* 1996 Aug;**76**(2):132–4.

5. Nowak-Gottl U, Auberger K, Halimeh S, Junker R, Klinge J, Kreuz WD, et al. Thrombolysis in newborns and infants. *Thromb Haemost* 1999 Sep;**82**(Suppl 1):112–16.

6. Albisetti M. Thrombolytic therapy in children. *Thromb Res* 2006;**118**(1):95–105.

7. Manco-Johnson MJ. How I treat venous thrombosis in children. *Blood* 2006 Jan 1;**107**(1):21–9.

8. Raffini L. Thrombolysis for intravascular thrombosis in neonates and children. *Curr Opin Pediatr* 2009 Feb;**21**(1):9–14.

9. Williams MD. Thrombolysis in children. *Br J Haematol* 2010 Jan;**148**(1):26–36.

10. Manco-Johnson MJ, Grabowski EF, Hellgreen M, Kemahli AS, Massicotte MP, Muntean W, et al. Recommendations for tPA thrombolysis in children. On behalf of the Scientific Subcommittee on Perinatal and Pediatric Thrombosis of the Scientific and Standardization Committee of the International Society of Thrombosis and Haemostasis. *Thromb Haemost* 2002 Jul;**88**(1):157–8.

11. Monagle P, Chan AK, Goldenberg NA, Ichord RN, Journeycake JM, Nowak-Gottl U, et al. Antithrombotic therapy in neonates and children: Antithrombotic Therapy and Prevention of Thrombosis, 9th edn: American College of Chest Physicians Evidence-Based Clinical Practice Guidelines. *Chest* 2012 Feb;**141**(2 Suppl):e737S–801S.

12. Hoylaerts M, Rijken DC, Lijnen HR, Collen D. Kinetics of the activation of plasminogen by human tissue plasminogen activator. Role of fibrin. *J Biol Chem* 1982 Mar 25;**257**(6):2912–19.

13. Bouma BN, Marx PF, Mosnier LO, Meijers JC. Thrombin-activatable fibrinolysis inhibitor (TAFI, plasma procarboxypeptidase B, procarboxypeptidase R, procarboxypeptidase U). *Thromb Res* 2001 Mar 1;**101**(5):329–54.

14. Albisetti M. The fibrinolytic system in children. *Semin Thromb Hemost* 2003 Aug;**29**(4):339–48.

15. Andrew M, Paes B, Milner R, Johnston M, Mitchell L, Tollefsen DM, et al. Development of the human coagulation system in the full-term infant. *Blood* 1987 Jul;**70**(1):165–72.

16. Edelberg JM, Enghild JJ, Pizzo SV, Gonzalez-Gronow M. Neonatal plasminogen displays altered cell surface binding and activation kinetics. Correlation with increased glycosylation of the protein. *J Clin Invest* 1990 Jul;**86**(1):107–12.

17. Ries M, Easton RL, Longstaff C, Zenker M, Morris HR, Dell A, et al. Differences between neonates and adults in carbohydrate sequences and reaction kinetics of plasmin and alpha(2)-antiplasmin. *Thromb Res* 2002 Feb 1;**105**(3):247–56.

18. Manco-Johnson MJ, Nuss R, Hays T, Krupski W, Drose J, Manco-Johnson ML. Combined thrombolytic and anticoagulant therapy for venous thrombosis in children. *J Pediatr* 2000 Apr;**136**(4):446–53.

19. Kennedy LA, Drummond WH, Knight ME, Millsaps MM, Williams JL. Successful treatment of neonatal aortic thrombosis with tissue plasminogen activator. *J Pediatr* 1990 May;**116**(5):798–801.

20. Andrew M, Brooker L, Leaker M, Paes B, Weitz J. Fibrin clot lysis by thrombolytic agents is impaired in newborns due to a low plasminogen concentration. *Thromb Haemost* 1992 Sep 7;**68**(3):325–30.

21. Goldenberg NA, Knapp-Clevenger R, Manco-Johnson MJ. Elevated plasma factor VIII and D-dimer levels as predictors of poor outcomes of thrombosis in children. *N Engl J Med* 2004 Sep 9;**351**(11):1081–8.

22. Choi M, Massicotte MP, Marzinotto V, Chan AK, Holmes JL, Andrew M. The use of alteplase to restore patency of central venous lines in pediatric patients: a cohort study. *J Pediatr* 2001 Jul;**139**(1):152–6.

23. Ragni MV, Journeycake JM, Brambilla DJ. Tissue plasminogen activator to prevent central venous access device infections: a systematic review of central venous access catheter thrombosis, infection and thromboprophylaxis. *Haemophilia* 2008 Jan;**14**(1):30–8.

24. Dillon PW, Jones GR, Bagnall-Reeb HA, Buckley JD, Wiener ES, Haase GM. Prophylactic urokinase in the management of long-term venous access devices in children: a Children's Oncology Group study. *J Clin Oncol* 2004 Jul 1;**22**(13):2718–23.

25. Gupta AA, Leaker M, Andrew M, Massicotte P, Liu L, Benson LN, et al. Safety and outcomes of thrombolysis with tissue plasminogen activator for treatment of intravascular thrombosis in children. *J Pediatr* 2001 Nov;**139**(5):682–8.

26. Leary SE, Harrod VL, de Alarcon PA, Reiss UM. Low-dose systemic thrombolytic therapy for deep vein thrombosis in pediatric patients. *J Pediatr Hematol/Oncol* 2010 Mar;**32**(2):97–102.

27. Newall F, Browne M, Savoia H, Campbell J, Barnes C, Monagle P. Assessing the outcome of systemic tissue plasminogen activator for the management of venous and arterial thrombosis in pediatrics. *J Pediatr Hematol/Oncol* 2007 Apr;**29**(4):269–73.

28. Manco-Johnson MJ, Grabowski EF, Hellgreen M, Kemahli AS, Massicotte MP, Muntean W, et al. Recommendations for tPA thrombolysis in children. On behalf of the Scientific Subcommittee on Perinatal and Pediatric Thrombosis of the Scientific and Standardization Committee of the International Society of Thrombosis and Haemostasis. *Thromb Haemost* 2002 Jul;**88**(1):157–8.

29. Zenz W, Arlt F, Sodia S, Berghold A. Intracerebral hemorrhage during fibrinolytic therapy in children: a review of the literature of the last thirty years. *Semin Thromb Hemost* 1997;**23**(3):321–32.

30. Theiss W, Wirtzfeld A, Fink U, Maubach P. The success rate of fibrinolytic therapy in fresh and old thrombosis of the iliac and femoral veins. *Angiology* 1983 Jan;**34**(1):61–9.

31. Goldenberg NA, Branchford B, Wang M, Ray C, Jr., Durham JD, Manco-Johnson MJ. Percutaneous mechanical and pharmacomechanical thrombolysis for occlusive deep vein thrombosis of the proximal limb in adolescent subjects: findings from an institution-based prospective inception cohort study of pediatric venous thromboembolism. *J Vasc Interv Radiol* 2011 Feb;**22**(2):121–32.

32. Hoffmeister HM, Szabo S, Helber U, Seipel L. The thrombolytic paradox. *Thromb Res* 2001 Sep 30;**103**(Suppl 1):S51–55.

33. Gast A, Tschopp TB, Schid G, Hilpert K, Ackermann J. Inhibition of clot-bound and free (fluid-phase thrombin) by a novel synthetic thrombin inhibitor (Ro 46–6240), recombinant hirudin and heparin in human plasma. *Blood Coag Fibrinolysis* 1994;**5**:879–87.

34. Torr SR, Nachowiak DA, Fujii S, Sobel BE. "Plasminogen steal" and clot lysis. *J Am Coll Cardiol* 1992 Apr;**19**(5):1085–90.

35. Bovill EG, Becker R, Tracy RP. Monitoring thrombolytic therapy. *Prog Cardiovasc Dis* 1992 Jan;**34**(4):279–94.

36. Monagle P, Chalmers E, Chan A, deVeber G, Kirkham F, Massicotte P, et al. Antithrombotic therapy in neonates and children: American College of Chest Physicians Evidence-Based Clinical Practice Guidelines (8th Edn). *Chest* 2008 Jun;**133**(6 Suppl):887S–968S.

37. Wang M, Hays T, Balasa V, Bagatell R, Gruppo R, Grabowski EF, et al. Low-dose tissue plasminogen activator thrombolysis in children. *J Pediatr Hematol/Oncol* 2003 May;**25**(5):379–86.

38. Goldenberg NA, Durham JD, Knapp-Clevenger R, Manco-Johnson MJ. A thrombolytic regimen for high-risk deep venous thrombosis may substantially reduce the risk of post-thrombotic syndrome in children. *Blood* 2007 Jul 1;**110**(1):45–53.

39. Rosenschein U, Rozenszajn LA, Kraus L, Marboe CC, Watkins JF, Rose EA, et al. Ultrasonic angioplasty in totally occluded peripheral arteries. Initial clinical, histological, and angiographic results. *Circulation* 1991 Jun;**83**(6):1976–86.

40. Atar S, Rosenschein U. Perspectives on the role of ultrasonic devices in thrombolysis. *J Thromb Thrombolysis* 2004 Apr;**17**(2):107–14.

41. Lin PH, Annambhotla S, Bechara CF, Athamneh H, Weakley SM, Kobayashi K, et al. Comparison of percutaneous ultrasound-accelerated thrombolysis versus catheter-directed thrombolysis in patients with acute massive pulmonary embolism. *Vascular* 2009 Nov;**17**(Suppl 3):S137–147.

42. Vedantham S, Vesely TM, Parti N, Darcy M, Hovsepian DM, Picus D. Lower extremity venous thrombolysis with adjunctive mechanical thrombectomy. *J Vasc Interv Radiol* 2002 Oct;**13**(10):1001–8.

43. Lin PH, Zhou W, Dardik A, Mussa F, Kougias P, Hedayati N, et al. Catheter-direct thrombolysis versus pharmacomechanical thrombectomy for treatment of symptomatic lower extremity deep venous thrombosis. *Am J Surg* 2006 Dec;**192**(6):782–8.

44. O'Sullivan GJ, Lohan DG, Gough N, Cronin CG, Kee ST. Pharmacomechanical thrombectomy of acute deep vein thrombosis with the Trellis-8 isolated thrombolysis catheter. *J Vasc Interv Radiol* 2007 Jun;**18**(6):715–24.

45. Goldenberg NA, Donadini MP, Kahn SR, Crowther M, Kenet G, Nowak-Gottl U, et al. Post-thrombotic syndrome in children: a systematic review of frequency of occurrence, validity of outcome measures, and prognostic factors. *Haematologica* 2010 Nov;**95**(11):1952–9.

46. Watson LI, Armon MP. Thrombolysis for acute deep vein thrombosis. *Cochrane Database Syst Rev* 2004;(**4**):CD002783.

197

47. Kearon C, Akl EA, Comerota AJ, Prandoni P, Bounameaux H, Goldhaber SZ, et al. Antithrombotic therapy for VTE disease: Antithrombotic Therapy and Prevention of Thrombosis, 9th edn: American College of Chest Physicians Evidence-Based Clinical Practice Guidelines. *Chest* 2012 Feb;**141**(2 Suppl): e419S–e494S.

48. Manco-Johnson MJ, Goldenberg NA. 2–10–2013. (Personal Communication.)

49. Farnoux C, Camard O, Pinquier D, Hurtaud-Roux MF, Sebag G, Schlegel N, et al. Recombinant tissue-type plasminogen activator therapy of thrombosis in 16 neonates. *J Pediatr* 1998 Jul;**133**(1):137–40.

50. Levy M, Benson LN, Burrows PE, Bentur Y, Strong DK, Smith J, et al. Tissue plasminogen activator for the treatment of thromboembolism in infants and children. *J Pediatr* 1991 Mar;**118**(3):467–72.

51. Smets K, Vanhaesebrouck P, Voet D, Schelstraete P, Govaert P. Use of tissue type plasminogen activator in neonates: case reports and review of the literature. *Am J Perinatol* 1996 May;**13**(4):217–22.

52. Biss TT, Brandao LR, Kahr WH, Chan AK, Williams S. Clinical features and outcome of pulmonary embolism in children. *Br J Haematol* 2008 Sep;**142**(5):808–18.

53. Kuo WT, Gould MK, Louie JD, Rosenberg JK, Sze DY, Hofmann LV. Catheter-directed therapy for the treatment of massive pulmonary embolism: systematic review and meta-analysis of modern techniques. *J Vasc Interv Radiol* 2009 Nov;**20**(11):1431–40.

54. Coombs CJ, Richardson PW, Dowling GJ, Johnstone BR, Monagle P. Brachial artery thrombosis in infants: an algorithm for limb salvage. *Plast Reconstr Surg* 2006 Apr 15;**117**(5):1481–8.

55. Tissue plasminogen activator for acute ischemic stroke. The National Institute of Neurological Disorders and Stroke rt-PA Stroke Study Group. *N Engl J Med* 1995 Dec 14;**333**(24):1581–7.

56. Marler JR, Tilley BC, Lu M, Brott TG, Lyden PC, Grotta JC, et al. Early stroke treatment associated with better outcome: the NINDS rt-PA stroke study. *Neurology* 2000 Dec 12;**55**(11):1649–55.

57. Uyttenboogaart M, Vroomen PC, Stewart RE, De KJ, Luijckx GJ. Safety of routine IV thrombolysis between 3 and 4.5 h after ischemic stroke. *J Neurol Sci* 2007 Mar 15;**254** (1–2):28–32.

58. Hacke W, Kaste M, Bluhmki E, Brozman M, Davalos A, Guidetti D, et al. Thrombolysis with alteplase 3 to 4.5 hours after acute ischemic stroke. *N Engl J Med* 2008 Sep 25;**359**(13):1317–29.

59. Del Zoppo GJ, Saver JL, Jauch EC, Adams HP, Jr. Expansion of the time window for treatment of acute ischemic stroke with intravenous tissue plasminogen activator: a science advisory from the American Heart Association/American Stroke Association. *Stroke* 2009 Aug;**40**(8):2945–8.

60. Shellhaas RA, Smith SE, O'Tool E, Licht DJ, Ichord RN. Mimics of childhood stroke: characteristics of a prospective cohort. *Pediatrics* 2006 Aug;**118**(2):704–9.

61. Roach ES, Golomb MR, Adams R, Biller J, Daniels S, deVeber G, et al. Management of stroke in infants and children: a scientific statement from a Special Writing Group of the American Heart Association Stroke Council and the Council on Cardiovascular Disease in the Young. *Stroke* 2008 Sep;**39**(9):2644–91.

62. Amlie-Lefond C, deVeber G, Chan AK, Benedict S, Bernard T, Carpenter J, et al. Use of alteplase in childhood arterial ischaemic stroke: a multicentre, observational, cohort study. *Lancet Neurol* 2009 Jun;**8** (6):530–6.

63. Byrnes JW, Williams B, Prodhan P, Erdem E, James C, Williamson R, et al. Successful intra-arterial thrombolytic therapy for a right middle cerebral artery stroke in a 2-year-old supported by a ventricular assist device. *Transpl Int* 2012 Mar;**25**(3):e31–e33.

64. Tan M, Armstrong D, Birken C, Bitnun A, Caldarone CA, Cox P, et al. Bacterial endocarditis in a child presenting with acute arterial ischemic stroke: should thrombolytic therapy be absolutely contraindicated? *Dev Med Child Neurol* 2009 Feb;**51**(2):151–4.

65. Kirton A, Wong JH, Mah J, Ross BC, Kennedy J, Bell K, et al. Successful endovascular therapy for acute basilar thrombosis in an adolescent. *Pediatrics* 2003 Sep;**112**(3 Pt 1): e248–e251.

66. Janjua N, Nasar A, Lynch JK, Qureshi AI. Thrombolysis for ischemic stroke in children: data from the nationwide inpatient sample. *Stroke* 2007 Jun;**38**(6):1850–4.

67. Wasay M, Dai AI, Ansari M, Shaikh Z, Roach ES. Cerebral venous sinus thrombosis in children: a multicenter cohort from the United States. *J Child Neurol* 2008 Jan;**23**(1):26–31.

68. Dentali F, Squizzato A, Gianni M, De Lodovici ML, Venco A, Paciaroni M, et al. Safety of thrombolysis in cerebral venous thrombosis. A systematic review of the literature. *Thromb Haemost* 2010 Nov;**104** (5):1055–62.

69. Mallick AA, Sharples PM, Calvert SE, Jones RW, Leary M, Lux AL, et al. Cerebral venous sinus thrombosis: a case series including thrombolysis. *Arch Dis Child* 2009 Oct;**94**(10):790–4.

70. Waugh J, Plumb P, Rollins N, Dowling MM. Prolonged direct catheter thrombolysis of cerebral venous sinus thrombosis in children: a case series. *J Child Neurol* 2012 Mar;**27**(3):337–45.

71. Andrew M, Paes B, Johnston M. Development of the hemostatic system in the neonate and young infant. *Am J Pediatr Hematol/Oncol* 1990;**12**(1):95–104.

72. Zenz W, Muntean W, Beitzke A, Zobel G, Riccabona M, Gamillscheg A. Tissue plasminogen activator (alteplase) treatment for femoral artery thrombosis after cardiac catheterisation in infants and children. *Br Heart J* 1993 Oct;**70**(4):382–5.

73. Hartmann J, Hussein A, Trowitzsch E, Becker J, Hennecke KH. Treatment of neonatal thrombus formation with recombinant tissue plasminogen activator: six years experience and review of the literature. *Arch Dis Child Fetal Neonatal Ed* 2001 Jul;**85**(1):F18–F22.

74. Balaguru D, Dilawar M, Ruff P, Radtke WA. Early and late results of thrombolytic therapy using tissue-type plasminogen activator to restore arterial pulse after cardiac catheterization in infants and small children. *Am J Cardiol* 2003 Apr 1;**91**(7):908–10.

75. Cannon BC, Kertesz NJ, Friedman RA, Fenrich AL. Use of tissue plasminogen activator in a stroke after radiofrequency ablation of a left-sided accessory pathway. *J Cardiovasc Electrophysiol* 2001 Jun;**12**(6):723–5.

76. Carlson MD, Leber S, Deveikis J, Silverstein FS. Successful use of rt-PA in pediatric stroke. *Neurology* 2001 Jul 10;**57**(1):157–8.

77. Cremer S, Berliner Y, Warren D, Jones AE. Successful treatment of pediatric stroke with recombinant tissue plasminogen activator (rt-PA): a case report and review of the literature. *CJEM* 2008 Nov;**10**(6):575–88.

78. Heil JW, Malinowski L, Rinderknecht A, Broderick JP, Franz D. Use of intravenous tissue plasminogen activator in a 16-year-old patient with basilar occlusion. *J Child Neurol* 2008 Sep;**23**(9):1049–53.

79. Jain SV, Morton LD. Ischemic stroke and excellent recovery after administration of intravenous tissue plasminogen activator. *Pediatr Neurol* 2008 Feb;**38**(2):126–9.

80. Losurdo G, Giacchino R, Castagnola E, Gattorno M, Costabel S, Rossi A, et al. Cerebrovascular disease and varicella in children. *Brain Dev* 2006 Jul;**28**(6):366–70.

81. Muniz AE. Thrombolytic therapy for acute stroke in a teenager. *Pediatr Emerg Care* 2012 Feb;**28**(2):170–3.

82. Noser EA, Felberg RA, Alexandrov AV. Thrombolytic therapy in an adolescent ischemic stroke. *J Child Neurol* 2001 Apr;**16**(4):286–8.

83. Sampaio I, Abecasis F, Quintas S, Moreno T, Camilo C, Vieira M, et al. Successful intravenous thrombolysis in a 14-year-old boy with ischemic stroke. *Pediatr Emerg Care* 2011 Jun;**27**(6):541–3.

84. Shuayto MI, Lopez JI, Greiner F. Administration of intravenous tissue plasminogen activator in a pediatric patient with acute ischemic stroke. *J Child Neurol* 2006 Jul;**21**(7):604–6.

85. Thirumalai SS, Shubin RA. Successful treatment for stroke in a child using recombinant tissue plasminogen activator. *J Child Neurol* 2000 Aug;**15**(8):558.

New anticoagulants in children: A review of recent studies and a look to the future

Guy Young and Neil A. Goldenberg

Introduction

The incidence of venous thromboembolism (VTE) in children is steadily rising [1,2]. While some of this increase may be due to increased recognition, it is likely that this represents a true increase in incidence. Much of the increase is due to the advancements in the management of critically ill children and particularly the widespread use of central venous catheters, which are the leading cause for the development of VTE. Treatment of VTE in children involves the use of anticoagulation and occasionally, thrombolytic agents. Treatment guidelines for the management of VTE in children have been published; however, these are largely based on low levels of evidence in the published literature, and relevant to this chapter, do not discuss the use of newer anticoagulants [3]. This chapter will provide a brief overview of the current (standard) anticoagulants in use in children (details can be found in other chapters), in particular discussing their limitations as they relate to the properties of the newer agents. This will be followed by a discussion of the data available regarding the use of new anticoagulants. Table 15.1 provides a historical context of anticoagulant clinical use and studies in children.

Standard anticoagulants

The so-called standard or conventional anticoagulants currently in widespread use in children include unfractionated heparin, low molecular weight heparins (LMWH), of which there are several available around the world, and vitamin K antagonists (VKA), of which warfarin is the most commonly available. Despite a long history of use in pediatrics (Table 15.1) and an accumulated clinical experience among practitioners, very few large (e.g., multicenter) prospective studies have been performed and none are

sufficiently powered randomized studies to definitively compare safety and efficacy between/among agents. Nevertheless, it is recognized that treatment of such patients is required to help resolve the VTE as well as to prevent complications such as pulmonary embolism and post-thrombotic syndrome. A brief discussion of the properties of these agents is described below.

Unfractionated heparin

Unfractionated heparin is a polysaccharide compound derived from porcine intestine and functions as an anticoagulant by potentiating the inhibitory effects of antithrombin on thrombin and factor Xa. Unfractionated heparin is most often used for the treatment and prevention of thrombosis in critically ill children, and is also used to maintain the patency of extracorporeal circuits and venous and arterial catheters [4]. The major advantages of unfractionated heparin include the many years of clinical experience in using it, the short half-life (i.e., rapid extinction of anticoagulant effect), and easy reversibility, both of which are useful in the critical care and surgical setting where the risk for bleeding is higher than in clinically stable or otherwise healthy children. Conversely, unfractionated heparin has several significant limitations. First, laboratory monitoring of heparin in children is challenging due to the frequency of monitoring deemed necessary (every 24–48h in the absence of bleeding or change in clinical status). Due to this frequency, monitoring is often performed via blood sampling from a heparinized intravenous catheter, wherein inaccuracies may occur even with substantial discard volumes (in itself a concern, given pediatric blood sampling volume constraints) prior to collection of the specimen for testing. Second, there is a high degree of inter- and even intrapatient variability in

Pediatric Thrombotic Disorders, ed. Neil A. Goldenberg and Marilyn J. Manco-Johnson. Published by Cambridge University Press. © Cambridge University Press 2015.

Table 15.1 Historical context of new anticoagulants in children

Anticoagulant	Discovery	First clinical use in adults	First published use in children	First prospective study in children
Heparin	1916	1934	1954	1994[48]
Warfarin	1929	1954	1976	1994[17]
LMWH	1970s	1980s	1993	1996[8]
Direct thrombin inhibitors intravenous	1884	1997	1999	2007[30]
Fondaparinux	1985	2001	2004	2010[37]
New oral agents	2005	2010	None	Ongoing (began in 2010)

Reproduced from: Young G. New anticoagulants in children: A review of recent studies and a look to the future. Thromb Res. 2011; 27(2): 70–4, with permission from Elsevier Ltd.

dosing leading to poor maintenance of therapeutic levels, which can lead to the potential for worsening thrombosis or bleeding [5]. Furthermore, unfractionated heparin can cause heparin-induced thrombocytopenia, which can lead to devastating consequences. The occurrence of heparin-induced thrombocytopenia in children has been systematically reviewed and reported at approximately 0.3% in children who undergo cardiopulmonary bypass [6]. Lastly, as unfractionated heparin is a biologic compound processed from porcine intestine, it is subject to potential contamination, which could lead to severe complications as was seen several years ago [7]. Despite these limitations, unfractionated heparin is widely used in children, and is still considered the first-line therapy (although without formal indication in children) for the prevention of thrombosis in patients undergoing cardiac catheterization, cardiopulmonary bypass surgery, and for anticoagulation of extracorporeal circuits. It has been supplanted by low molecular weight hpearin as the first-line therapy for VTE in non-critically ill children.

Low molecular weight heparin

Several different low molecular weight heparin preparations are in clinical use throughout the world, and a number of pediatric pharmacokinetic and dose-finding studies have been published [8–19]. The low molecular weight heparins are derived from unfractionated heparin, and comprised of shorter lengths of the polysaccharide chains. This feature changes several of this agent's properties. First, low molecular weight heparins have a more profound effect on factor Xa than on thrombin with ratios ranging from an anti-Xa to thrombin effect of 1.5 to > 10 [8,9]. In addition, the low molecular weight heparins have stable pharmacokinetics and a more predictable pharmacodynamic dose response than unfractionated heparin. Furthermore, these agents have a longer half-life, making them particularly useful in the outpatient setting. As a result, there has been a substantial increase in the use of low molecular weight heparins in children over the past decade and these agents have replaced unfractionated heparin as the agent of choice in the acute treatment of VTE in non-critically ill children, and have replaced warfarin as the agent of choice for subacute/long-term VTE management in the USA [1]. Although the longer half-life when compared to unfractionated heparin allows for outpatient use, treatment of VTE requires twice daily dosing as demonstrated by a detailed pharmacokinetic study of enoxaparin [14]. Furthermore, LMWH is also a biologic product and can also lead to HIT though at lower rates than unfractionated heparin. More relevant perhaps is the effect of low molecular weight heparin on bone metabolism, and while there are no studies in children addressing this issue, it is well known that long-term use over months as is common in pediatrics could lead to osteopenia [20]. Lastly, while unfractionated heparin has an excellent antidote in protamine, this agent is only partially effective at reversing the anticoagulant effect of low molecular weight heparin. The most studied LMWH in children is enoxaparin [14], although published studies have used reviparin [17], dalteparin [18] and tinzaparin [19]. Active multicenter clinical trials on low molecular weight heparins in children, as registered in clinicaltrials.gov, include

FRAG-201/DaVINCI (NCT00952380, dalteparin) and Dalteparin Sub-study of the Kids-DOTT trial (NCT00687882).

Vitamin K antagonists

Compared to heparin and low molecular weight heparin, the major advantage of the vitamin K antagonists is that they are administered orally. Most of the published data in children with oral agents utilize warfarin [21,22] although there are some data with acenocoumarol [23] and phenprocoumon [24,25]. The major advantage of warfarin is the oral route of administration and long half-life allowing for once daily dosing; however, warfarin has several significant disadvantages. Most important is its narrow therapeutic index leading to a high risk for serious bleeding. In adults, the risk for serious bleeding approximates to 2% per year [27]. In addition, warfarin has numerous drug interactions and is affected by vitamin K intake, further complicating the ability to maintain a therapeutic anticoagulant effect. This problem is exacerbated in children due to the often changing diet in young children and the need for intermittent antibiotic therapy in many children who have developed VTE in association with other illnesses – both of which can significantly affect the INR. Very little outcomes data have been published with specific pediatric warfarin dosing and monitoring nomograms, and recent work indicates that age is a major determinant of weight-based initial therapeutic dose (with minimal contribution from VKORC1 and CYP2C9 genotypes) [27,28]. In addition, the use of warfarin in infants is difficult due to their inability to swallow whole tablets and to

challenges in compounding warfarin tablets into a liquid formulation. Crushing the tablets (a common practice in pediatrics) may lead to inconsistent dosing leading to additional variations in the INR and is not in general recommended. Furthermore, a well-designed study demonstrated that the target INR is not met on a sufficiently consistent basis in children and in particular in infants [21]. Due to the narrow therapeutic index, there is a premium on compliance which is often problematic in children during the teenage years. Finally, routine and frequent monitoring of the INR can be difficult especially in infants due to poor venous access and poor acceptability of frequent venipuncture in young children. For all these reasons, there is a clear need for more reliable and pragmatic anticoagulants for children.

New anticoagulants

A rather small body of published work addresses dosing and outcomes of anticoagulants that lie outside of the standard (i.e., conventional) anticoagulants discussed above [29,30]. For the sake of simplicity, we will refer to these non-conventional agents as "new" or "novel" anticoagulants, although we recognize that some of them (e.g., the intravenous direct thrombin inhibitors) have been in use for decades in adults. These agents can be classified in a variety of ways, including according to their mechanism of action, route of administration, half-life (which in part impacts route and frequency of administration), and others. As demonstrated in Table 15.2, a pragmatic approach is to group agents by route of administration, allowing comparison of other characteristics

Table 15.2 Clinically relevant features of several anticoagulants available for VTE treatment in children

Anticoagulant	Route of administration	Administration interval*	Half-life	Antithrombin dependence	Antidote
Heparin	IV	Bolus followed by continuous infusion*	30 minutes	Yes	Protamine
Enoxaparin	Subcutaneous	Q12 hours*	6 hours	Yes	Protamine (partial)
Bivalirudin	IV continuous infusion	Bolus followed by continuous infusion	25 minutes	No	None
Argatroban	IV continuous infusion	Continuous infusion	40 minutes	No	None
Fondaparinux	Subcutaneous	Once-daily*	17 hours	Yes	None

* Once-daily use has also been reported.

between the standard and new anticoagulants administered via the same route (i.e., intravenous, subcutaneous, oral). As such, unfractionated heparin (which is given by continuous intravenous infusion) may be compared to the direct thrombin inhibitors lepirudin, bivalirudin, and argatroban, which are likewise each administered by continuous infusion. Similarly, fondaparinux can be compared to LMWH, both administered subcutaneously. Lastly, the new oral direct thrombin and direct factor Xa inhibitors may be compared with warfarin.

Parenteral agents: Lepirudin, bivalirudin, argatroban

Use of three intravenous direct thrombin inhibitors has been published in children: lepirudin, bivalirudin, and argatroban. For a detailed description of their properties from the pediatric perspective, the reader is pointed to previous publications [29,30]. There are a number of case reports and case series describing the use of these agents in children [31–35]. Recently, clinical trials have been completed and published on the use of bivalirudin and argatroban in children.

The first trial of a DTI in children described the use of bivalirudin in a single arm, open-label, dose-finding, safety, and efficacy study of VTE treatment in children less than 6 months of age [36]. This age group was preferentially selected since infants have physiologically low levels of antithrombin and therefore were felt to have the best opportunity to benefit from an alternative to intravenous unfractionated heparin, whose efficacy (as noted above) is antithrombin-dependent. The study led to several important findings. First, the dosing regimen for children of this age was established (see Table 15.3). Second, the bivalirudin regimen was suggested to be safe, as there were no clinically serious bleeding events or other treatment-related adverse events. Third, the study demonstrated

the potential for rapid clot resolution as six of 16 patients had either complete (3) or significant partial (3) resolution of their thrombi at 48–72 hours. This finding may relate to the fact that DTIs inhibit both circulating and clot-bound thrombin, offering a theoretical advantage over heparin that could translate into earlier clot resolution. Of note, a retrospective study of bivalirudin for VTE treatment in children of all ages demonstrated rapid clot resolution in nearly all patients [37]. Most recently, a second clinical trial of VTE treatment in children between 6 months and 18 years of age demonstrated similar findings with 9 of 18 patients demonstrating partial or complete clot resolution by 48–72 hours [38]. In addition, a trial of bivalirudin for the prevention of thrombosis in children undergoing percutaneous coronary interventions (PCI) was recently completed [39]. This was a single-arm, safety, efficacy and dose-finding study in children from birth to 16 years of age divided into four age cohorts and enrolled 110 patients using dosing similar to that for the adult licensed indication of bivalirudin. The results demonstrated a high degree of safety with only two of 110 patients experiencing protocol-defined major bleeding events, both of which remitted without reversal agents or other hemostatic interventions.

A single clinical trial has addressed the use of argatroban in children [40]. This study evaluated the safety, efficacy, and pharmacokinetics of argatroban in 18 children, most of whom had confirmed or suspected heparin-induced thrombocytopenia. The study established dosing guidelines for children that are now included in the prescribing information in the USA (a first among anticoagulants) [41]. Regarding safety, two of the 18 patients had major bleeding events, both of which were fatal intracranial hemorrhages in critically ill children undergoing extracorporeal membrane oxygenation. The independent Data and Safety Monitoring Board reviewed both events and determined that the study should

Table 15.3 Suggested dosing and monitoring for new anticoagulants

Anticoagulation	Dose	Interval	Monitoring test	Target range
Bivalirudin	0.125mg/kg 0.125mg/kg/h	Bolus Continuous infusion	PTT	1.5–2.5 baseline PTT
Argatroban	0.75mcg/kg/min	Continuous infusion	PTT	1.5–2.5 baseline PTT
Fondaparinux†	0.1mg/kg	Once daily	Anti-Xa level**	0.5–1 mg/l

† Fondaparinux dosing has not been evaluated in children < 1 year of age. ** Fondaparinux-based anti-Xa assay with results expressed as mg/l.

continue without any amendments. Argatroban was effective at preventing thrombosis, as only two of the 18 developed clots while on argatroban, a rate which is generally similar to that in adult patients similarly treated with argatroban for heparin-induced thrombocytopenia [42]. A detailed pharmacokinetic analysis was undertaken in a separate publication [43] and from which the dosing recommendations arose.

Fondaparinux is a synthetic pentasaccharide (the core structure of heparins) that correspondingly shares the antithrombin potentiation mechanism of action and the subcutaneous administration route of the LMWH molecules. Its main differences from heparins are as follows. First, as a synthetic compound not derived from porcine intestine, it is less subject to concerns of contamination as has happened with heparin and LMWH in the past. Second, fondaparinux selectively inhibits factor Xa, with no direct inhibition of thrombin. Several case reports have described its pediatric use in the past several years [44–47]; however, only one prospective study has been published in children [48]. This was a single-arm, open label, dose-finding, and safety trial that enrolled 24 VTE patients between 1–18 years of age in three age cohorts. The study did not enroll patients less than a year of age due to an investigational new drug (IND) restriction imposed by the FDA. This study demonstrated excellent safety with only one serious bleeding event, an intracranial hemorrhage, which was noted after the study drug was begun on a surveillance MRI for a child with a neurological disorder, but which had occurred prior to study drug initiation based on the MRI report. The pharmacologic analysis demonstrated that nearly all patients were therapeutic after the first dose and that once-daily dosing led to therapeutic anticoagulation for 24 hours in all the patients. Dosing recommendations are provided in Table 15.3. While the study was not designed to assess efficacy, a follow-up study evaluating the long-term safety, efficacy, and dosing is underway, and preliminary data from this analysis were recently presented in abstract form [49]. The follow-up study demonstrated stable dosing (only seven dose adjustments required in greater than 5,000 patient-days of treatment), no further bleeding episodes, and excellent efficacy, with 94% of patients achieving a complete or partial resolution of thrombosis at a median follow-up time of 63 days. Twice-daily fondaparinux dosing has also been reported in small case series [50].

Oral direct factor IIa (thrombin) and factor Xa inhibitors

Several novel oral direct thrombin (e.g., dabigatran) and factor Xa (e.g., apixaban and rivaroxaban) inhibitors are currently in clinical development for a variety of antithrombotic indications in adults [51]. Dabigatran, apixaban, and rivaroxaban are all FDA- and/or EMA-approved for VTE prevention following elective knee or hip replacement surgery in adults, as well as for the prevention of stroke in adult patients with non-valvular atrial fibrillation. As a result of new regulations in Europe and stricter adherence to existing regulations in the USA, the manufacturers of these agents are required to have a drug development program for pediatrics. A Canadian open-label safety and tolerability trial of dabigatran given for 3 days at the end of standard anticoagulant therapy in adolescents was recently completed (NCT00844415; results not yet published), and a similar study of children aged 1–12 years is underway internationally outside the USA (NCT01083732). In addition, an international single-dose study is planned to evaluate the pharmacokinetics, pharmacodynamics, safety, and tolerability of apixaban in children (neonate to 18 years of age) at risk for a venous or arterial thrombotic disorder, including patients with central venous catheters (NCT01707394). Lastly, a single-dose, pharmacokinetic/pharmacodynamic study of rivaroxaban is underway in pediatric subjects (6 months to 18 years of age) at the end of their VTE treatment (NCT01145859), and a second study is planned for rivaroxaban given for the last 30 days of a 3-month intended course for VTE treatment in children aged 6–18 years (NCT01684423). Given that no pediatric trial findings have been published, a detailed discussion of these agents is beyond the scope of this review, and the reader is referred to an excellent review [51].

Conclusions

The standard anticoagulants used in children, unfractionated heparin, low molecular weight heparin, and vitamin K antagonists all have significant limitations. Preliminary pediatric evidence suggests that argatroban is useful for heparin-induced thrombocytopenia in children (or bivalirudin in the setting of cardiopulmonary bypass), that bivalirudin may be a suitable alternative to unfractionated heparin in children with

VTE, and that fondaparinux is a viable option in lieu of low molecular weight heparin. Devoted pediatric trials have led to pediatric dosing recommendations for each of these agents. Furthermore, although dose-finding trials are not yet complete, pediatric development programs are underway for the oral direct thrombin and factor Xa inhibitors, as potential future alternatives to warfarin.

In conclusion, a new era has recently emerged with respect to pediatric anticoagulation. After nearly 15 years since the widespread use of low molecular weight heparins in children began, trials of several new anticoagulants have been conducted or are underway. With the ever more stringent US and European regulations requiring pediatric studies for such drugs, a period of fruitful research in this field can be anticipated for many years to come, leading to improved management of pediatric thrombosis.

References

1. Raffini L, Huang Y, Witmer C, Feudtner C. Dramatic increase in venous thromboembolism in children's hospitals in the United States from 2001–2007. Pediatrics 2009;**124**:1001–8.

2. Setty BA, O'Brien SH, Kerlin BA. Pediatric venous thromboembolism in the United States: a tertiary care complication of chronic diseases. Pediatr Blood Cancer 2012;**59**:258–64.

3. Monagle P, Chan AK, Goldenberg NA, Ichord RN, Journeycake JM, Nowak-Gottl U, Vesley SK. Antithrombotic therapy in neonates and children: Antithrombotic therapy and prevention of thrombosis, 9th edn: American College of Chest Physicians Evidence-Based Clinical Practice Guidelines. Chest 2012;**141**(Suppl 2):e737S–801S.

4. Newall F, Johnston L, Ignjatovic V, Monagle P. Unfractionated heparin therapy in infants and children. Pediatrics 2009;**123**:e510–18.

5. Sutor AH, Massicotte P, Leaker M, Andrew M. Heparin therapy in pediatric patients. Semin Thromb Hemost 1997;**23**:303–19.

6. Avila ML, Shah V, Brandão LR. Systematic review on heparin-induced thrombocytopenia in children: a call to action. J Thromb Haemost 2013;**11**:660–9.

7. Kishimoto TK, Viswanathan K, Ganguly T, et al. Contaminated heparin associated with adverse clinical events and activation of the contact system. N Eng J Med 2008;**358**:2457–67.

8. Hirsh J, Levine MN. Low molecular weight heparin. Blood 1992;**79**:1–17.

9. Samama MM, Gerotziafas GT. Comparative pharmacokinetics of LMWHs. Semin Thromb Hemost 2000;**26**(Suppl 1):S31–8.

10. Massicotte P, Julian JA, Marzinotto V, et. al. Dose-finding and pharmacokinetic profiles of prophylactic doses of a low molecular weight heparin (reviparin-sodium) in pediatric patients. Thromb Res 2003;**109**:93–9.

11. Massicotte P, Adams M, Marzinotto V, Brooker LA, Andrew M. Low-molecular-weight heparin in pediatric patients with thrombotic disease: a dose-finding study. J Pediatr 1996;**128**:313–18.

12. Punzalan RC, Hillery CA, Montgomery RR, Scott CA, Gill JC. Low-molecular-weight heparin in thrombotic disease in children and adolescents. J Pediatr Hematol/Oncol 2000;**22**:137–42.

13. Albisetti M, Andrew M. Low molecular weight heparin in children. Eur J Pediatr 2002;**161**:71–7.

14. O'Brien SH, Lee H, Ritchey AK. Once-daily enoxaparin in pediatric thromboembolism: a dose finding and pharmacodynamics/pharmacokinetics study. J Thromb Haemost 2007;**5**:1985–7.

15. Trame MN, Mitchell L, Krumpel A, et al. Population pharmacokinetics of enoxaparin in infants, children, and adolescents during secondary thromboembolic prophylaxis: a cohort study. J Thromb Haemost 2010;**8**:195–8.

16. Massicotte MP. Low-molecular-weight heparin therapy in children. J Pediatr Hematol/Oncol 2000;**22**:98–9.

17. Massicotte P, Julian JA, Marzinotto V, et al. Dose-finding and pharmacokinetic profiles of prophylactic doses of a low molecular weight heparin (reviparin-sodium) in pediatric patients. Thromb Res 2003;**109**:93–9.

18. Nohe N, Flemmer A, Rumler R, Praun M, Auberger K. The low molecular weight heparin dalteparin for prophylaxis and therapy of thrombosis in childhood: a report on 48 cases. Eur J Pediatr 1999;**158**(Suppl 3):S134–9.

19. Kuhle S, Massicotte P, Dinyari M, et al. Dose-finding and pharmacokinetics of therapeutic doses of tinzaparin in pediatric patients with thromboembolic events. Thromb Haemost 2005;**94**:1164–71.

20. Rajgopal R, Bear MK, Shaugnessy SG. The effects of heparin and low molecular weight heparin on bone. Thromb Res 2008;**122**:293–8.

21. Andrew M, Marzinotto V, Brooker LA, et. al. Oral anticoagulation therapy in pediatric patients: a prospective study. Thromb Haemost 1994;**71**:265–9.

22. Streif W, Andrew M, Marzinotto V, et al. Analysis of warfarin therapy in pediatric patients: A prospective cohort study of 319 patients. Blood 1999;**94**:3007–14.

23. Woods A, Vargas J, Berri G, Kreutzer G, Meschengieser S, Lazzari MA. Antithrombotic therapy in children and adolescents. Thromb Res 1986;**42**:289–301.

24. Gunther T, Mazzitelli D, Schreiber C, et. al. Mitral-valve replacement in children under 6 years of age. Eur J Cardiothorac Surg 2000;**17**:426–30.

25. Wermes C, Bergmann F, Reller B, Sykora KW. Severe protein C deficiency and aseptic osteonecrosis of the hip joint: a case report. Eur J Pediatr 1999;**158**(Suppl 3): S159–61.

26. Hirsh J. Oral anticoagulant drugs. N Engl J Med 1991;**324**:1865–75.

27. Nowak-Gottl U, Dietrich K, Schaffranek D, et al. In pediatric patients, age has more impact on dosing of vitamin K antagonists than VKORC1 or CYP2C9 genotypes. Blood 2010;**116**:6101–5.

28. Goldenberg NA, Crowther MA. The "age" of understanding VKA dose. Blood 2010;**116**:5789–90.

29. Young G. New anticoagulants in children: A review of recent studies and a look to the future. Thromb Res 2010;**127**:70–4.

30. Chan VHT, Monagle P, Massicotte P, Chan AKC. Novel paediatric anticoagulants: a review of the current literature. Blood Coag Fibrin 2010;**21**:144–51.

31. Deitcher SR, Topoulos AP, Bartholomew JR, Kichuk-Chrisant MR. Lepirudin anticoagulation for heparin-induced thrombocytopenia. J Pediatr 2002;**140**:264–6.

32. Cetta F, Graham LC, Wrona LL, Arruda MJ, Walenga JM. Argatroban use during pediatric interventional cardiac catheterization. Catheter Cardiovasc Interv 2004;**61**:147–9.

33. Kawada T, Kitagawa H, Hoson M, Okada Y, Shiomura J. Clinical application of argatroban as an alternative anticoagulant for extracorporeal circulation. Hematol Oncol Clin North Am 2000;**14**:445–57.

34. Severin T, Zieger B, Sutor AH. Anticoagulation with recombinant hirudin and danaparoid sodium in pediatric patients. Semin Thromb Hemost 2002;**28**:447–54.

35. Deitcher SR, Topoulos AP, Bartholomew JR, Kichuk-Chrisant MR. Lepirudin anticoagulation for heparin-induced thrombocytopenia. J Pediatr 2002;**140**:264–6.

36. Young G, Tarantino MD, Wohrley J, Weber LC, Belvedere M, Nugent DJ. Pilot dose-finding and safety study of bivalirudin in infants < 6 months of age with thrombosis. J Thromb Haemost 2007;**5**:1654–9.

37. Rayapudi S, Torres A, Deshpande GG, et al. Bivalirudin for anticoagulation in children. Pediatr Blood Cancer 2008;**51**:798–801.

38. O'Brien SH, Yee D, Lira J, Goldenberg NA, Young G. Prospective open-label clinical trial of bivalirudin in children with venous thrombosis. Blood (abstract) 2012;**120**:1165.

39. Forbes TJ, Hijazi Z, Young G, Ringewald JM, Aquino PM, Vincent RN, et al. Pediatric catheterization laboratory anticoagulation with bivalirudin. Catheter and Cardiovasc Interv 2011;**77**:671–9.

40. Young G, Boshkov LK, Sullivan JE, et al. Argatroban therapy in pediatric patients requiring nonheparin anticoagulation: An open-label, safety, efficacy, and pharmacokinetic study. Pediatr Blood Cancer 2011;**56**:1103–9.

41. Argatroban prescribing information. Available at www.argatroban.com (accessed May 27, 2010).

42. Lewis BE, Wallis DE, Leya F, et al. Argatroban anticoagulation in patients with heparin-induced thrombocytopenia. Arch Intern Med 2003;**163**:1849–56.

43. Madabushi R, Cox DS, Hossain M, et al. Pharmacokinetic and pharmacodynamic basis for effective argatroban dosing in pediatrics. J Clin Pharm 2011;**51**:19–28.

44. Young G, Nugent DJ. Use of argatroban and fondaparinux in a child with heparin-induced thrombocytopenia. Pediatr Blood Cancer (abstract) 2004;**42**:S542.

45. Boshkov LK, Kirby A, Shen I, et al. Recognition and management of heparin-induced thrombocytopenia in pediatric cardiopulmonary bypass patients. Ann Thorac Surg 2006;**81**:S2355–9.

46. Grabowski EF, Bussell JB. Pediatric experience with fondaparinux in deep vein thrombosis. Blood (abstract) 2006;**108**:916.

47. Sharatkumar AA, Crandall C, Lin JJ, et al. Treatment of thrombosis with fondaparinux (Arixtra) in a patient with end-stage renal disease receiving hemodialysis therapy. J Pediatr Hematol/Oncol 2007;**29**:581–4.

48. Young G, Yee DL, O'Brien S, Khanna R, Nugent DJ. FondaKIDS: A prospective dose-finding, pharmacokinetic, and safety study of fondaparinux in children between 1–18 years of age. Pediatr Blood Cancer 2011;**57**:1049–54.

49. Ko RH, Michieli C, Bernardini L, Young G. FondaKIDS II: Long-term follow up data of children receiving fondaparinux for treatment of venous thrombotic events. Blood (abstract) 2012;**120**:3415.

50. Manco-Johnson MJ, Wang M, Goldenberg NA, Soep J, Gibson E, Knoll CM, Mourani PM. Treatment, survival, and thromboembolic outcomes of thrombotic storm in children. J Pediatr 2012;**161**:682–8.

51. Garcia D, Libby E, Crowther MA. The new oral anticoagulants. Blood 2010;**115**:15–20.

Chapter 16

Prevention of VTE in children

Brian R. Branchford and Leslie Raffini

Introduction

In-hospital venous thromboembolism (VTE) represents a significant, yet preventable, public health burden, which was recognized in 2008 by the USA Surgeon General's Call-to-Action [1]. Prophylactic anticoagulation for VTE prevention has been proven to be safe and effective, and has become standard care in hospitalized adults [2,3]. As providers become increasingly aware of the growing problem of VTE in hospitalized children, attention is starting to focus on prevention in this population.

The available data regarding utility and safety of primary prophylaxis is sparse, likely due to the relative infrequency of VTE in children compared to their adult counterparts. Since high-quality evidence in this area is lacking, clinical care is often formulated by expert consensus and extrapolation from adult studies. Two important considerations are clinician awareness of in-hospital VTE, and risk-stratified approaches to prevent unnecessary exposure of low-risk patients to potentially serious side effects. While this is an area expected to evolve greatly, this chapter provides a contemporary review of pertinent background information, risk factors for in-hospital VTE development, and existing recommendations for pharmacologic and non-pharmacologic VTE prophylaxis in children.

Although the incidence of in-hospital VTE is considerably lower in children than adults, it is an increasing problem particularly in pediatric tertiary care hospitals, with potential for severe consequences [4]. Possible explanations for the rising incidence include advances in tertiary care, prolonged survival of medically complex patients, increased utilization of central venous access devices (CVADs), improved imaging sensitivity, and increased awareness. Of children with VTE, 16% to 20% have objectively

confirmed pulmonary embolism (PE) [5], and retrospective data from the Hospital for Sick Children indicates a VTE-specific mortality rate of 9% among pediatric PE cases [6]. The risks of long-term pulmonary insufficiency and chronic thromboembolic pulmonary hypertension following PE in children remain undefined. Additionally, a systematic review has demonstrated that at least 20% of children with extremity VTE develop post-thrombotic syndrome (PTS), a syndrome of chronic venous insufficiency that may be associated with limitation in physical activities [7].

Recommendations for prevention of hospital-acquired VTE in adult patients are well established [8–10] and have been informed by evidence from randomized controlled clinical trials. In pediatrics, such recommendations and data are largely lacking, historically attributable to the rarity of VTE in this population. A non-selective approach would undoubtedly expose an excess of young patients to bleeding risks in order to prevent relatively few deaths and long-term sequelae from VTE. While registries and cohort studies have identified numerous risk factors as highly prevalent among pediatric VTE cases, few well-designed cases–control studies have identified independent risk factors that would allow for a selective approach to VTE prevention in hospitalized children. The development of such evidence, and its substantiation via subsequent multicenter studies, would provide the basis for future risk-stratified RCTs of pediatric VTE prevention.

Risk factors

One of the basic tenets of in-hospital VTE prevention in children is awareness of the risk factors, since early recognition and intervention may help prevent morbidity and mortality. It is important to distinguish

Pediatric Thrombotic Disorders, ed. Neil A. Goldenberg and Marilyn J. Manco-Johnson. Published by Cambridge University Press. © Cambridge University Press 2015.

Table 16.1 Risk factors for pediatric VTE

Prior VTE [48]
Intensive care unit stay [48,55]
Mechanical ventilation [55]
Systemic infection [48,55,64–66]
Hospitalization >/= 5 days [48,55,64,66,67]
Central venous catheterization [48,64–66,68,69]
Parenteral nutrition [68]
Deep sedation [68]
Neuromuscular blockade [68]
Inotropic support [68]
Recombinant FVIIa administration [68]
Immobilization > 72 hours [64]
Estrogen-containing contraceptive [64]
Malignancy [48,65–67,69]
Neurologic disability [65]
Cardiac disease [65]
Nephrotic syndrome [65,69]
Autoimmune disease [65]

between associated factors (underlying conditions found in conjunction with VTE in some patients) and risk factors (underlying conditions found significantly more frequently in children with VTE than in a comparable control population). For example, asthma is a condition with high frequency among children and, therefore, may often be found as an associated factor. A VTE in an otherwise healthy child with asthma, however, would still be considered unprovoked since there is not a known statistically significant increase in VTE found in children with asthma. The concept of VTE provocation is important, as discussed below, as it has bearing on length of therapy. Unprovoked, or spontaneous, VTE are considered to be those without an identifiable proximate clinical trigger. In contrast to adults in whom VTE is unprovoked in up to 40%, the vast majority of children with VTE (90%) have identifiable risk factors [11], and most have several risk factors. Table 16.1 lists the most common risk factors, some of which are discussed in more depth below.

The presence of a central venous access device (CVAD) is the single most common risk factor for VTE in pediatric patients, and they are found in up to 90% of neonates with VTE and 60% of older children

with VTE [12]. This risk is likely related to vessel wall trauma and endothelial cell damage at the insertion site and/or obstruction of venous flow [13–15]. Prospective pediatric studies have suggested that the incidence of VTE is independent of CVAD type (peripheral, tunneled, subcutaneous, etc.), right or left side, or duration of placement [16], but the proportion of VTE cases in any pediatric cohort does appear to vary by anatomic location (e.g., femoral: 32%, subclavian: 27%, brachial: 12%, jugular: 8%) [16]. The reported incidence of CVAD-related VTE varies greatly depending on the population studied and the imaging modality used to detect thrombosis [17–21]. A prospective, multicenter cohort study of children with acute lymphoblastic leukemia utilizing screening venography and ultrasound found CVAD-related VTE in 29 of 85 (34%) patients within the first month after CVAD placement [22]. Although most of these (86%) were asymptomatic, these "subclinical" VTEs may dislodge and cause fatal pulmonary embolism [23,24]. In addition, VTEs can severely limit life-saving/sustaining venous access for patients who have chronic medical conditions requiring multiple CVADs over time. There is also increasing evidence that CVAD-related VTE predisposes patients to bacteremia and sepsis [25–27]. Thus, subclinical VTE are clearly clinically relevant.

The safety and efficacy of pharmacologic thromboprophylaxis to prevent CVAD-related VTE has not been clearly established. The PROphylaxis of ThromboEmbolism in Kids Trial (PROTEKT) was an open-label randomized controlled trial of low molecular weight heparin (LMWH) for the prevention of CVAD thrombosis that closed prematurely due to poor accrual and was underpowered, but did not find a benefit to the use of prophylactic LMWH. In this study, 14.1% (11/78) of the patients who received LMWH developed VTE compared to 12.5% (10/80) of control patients [28]. Similarly, a randomized placebo-controlled single-center study of infants after cardiac surgery determined that although low-dose heparin infusion (10 units/kg/h) was safe, there was no difference between the incidence of CVAD-related VTE between the heparin and placebo groups, 15% vs. 16%, respectively [29].

The use of vitamin K antagonists (VKAs) such as warfarin for CVAD-related thromboprophylaxis has had mixed results. A small prospective cohort study [30] in eight pediatric patients with short-gut syndrome or small intestinal anomalies receiving long-term parenteral nutrition suggested improved catheter survival using vitamin K antagonists (target INR 1.3–1.8 for no previous thrombosis or 2.0–3.0 for previous thrombosis), compared to historical data from the same patient population. However, a randomized study in children with cancer showed no benefit from low-dose warfarin (INR 1.3–1.9) compared to a control group for VTE prevention [31]. Additionally, a principally adult study of 1,590 patients over age 16 from 68 UK clinical centers demonstrated that warfarin did not reduce CVAD-associated VTE in patients with cancer, and a trend toward increased major bleeding events was observed in the warfarin-treated group [32].

Trauma is a well-established risk factor for VTE in adults, with a highly variable 5–63% incidence of VTE following traumatic injury [33]; however, the risk appears to be much lower in children, at least in the absence of CVAD. A recent retrospective study of data from 135,032 pediatric, adolescent, and young adult trauma patients in the National Trauma Data Bank demonstrated that the risk of VTE in patients without a CVAD was < 1% even in adolescents/young adults [34]. In this study, the presence of a CVAD was significantly associated with VTE (OR = 2.24; p < 0.0001). The authors concluded that thromboprophylaxis should be considered only in critically injured adolescents and young adults with a continuing need for central venous access. A Canadian study of severely injured children showed that children with VTE were more likely to have higher injury severity scores. The greatest risk of VTE was in children with CVADs (OR: 64), but other independent risk factors included thoracic (OR: 6.9) and spinal injuries (OR: 37.4) [35].

Children with congenital cardiac abnormalities are a population at unique risk for VTE. This is due to altered circulation dynamics, artificial circulation components (cardiac valves, prosthetic vessel graft material, etc.), and/or frequent procedural needs. Primary VTE prophylaxis is most frequently considered for children with severe cardiac disease (congestive heart failure, endovascular stenting, mechanical valve replacement, surgical correction of single ventricle physiology lesions, or ventricular assist device placement) [36]. A recent multicenter, randomized trial demonstrated that aspirin is as effective as heparin or warfarin anticoagulation as primary thromboembolic prophylaxis following the Fontan cardiac surgical procedure in children [37].

Another specific group of children at risk are those with acute lymphoblastic leukemia (ALL) requiring treatment with L-asparaginase (Asp), whose prothrombotic effects are likely secondary to acquired antithrombin (AT) deficiency [38,39] or dysfibrinogenemia [40]. The Prophylactic Antithrombin Replacement in Kids with ALL treated with L-Asparaginase (PARKAA) study was an open-label, randomized controlled pilot trial to evaluate AT concentrates as primary prophylaxis in children with ALL treated with Asp [41]. Patients randomized to AT had an incidence of thrombosis of 28% (95% CI: 10–46%), compared to 37% (95% CI: 24–49%) in the non-AT treated arm, suggesting a trend toward therapeutic efficacy. However, no definitive RCT has yet been performed in follow-up to this pilot trial.

Inherited thrombophilia increases the risk of first VTE in children [42]. A large meta-analysis of published studies reported pooled odds ratios that range from 2.6 for the factor II G20210A mutation to 9.5 in children with more than one defect [43]. Importantly, in addition to an inherited thrombophilia, the majority of these patients in these studies had additional risk factors for thrombosis [43].

Age also influences the risk of pediatric VTE. The VTE incidence in children is bimodal, with a peak in neonates and again during adolescence [12]. A survey of pediatric intensive care units revealed that providers were more likely to prescribe thromboprophylaxis to adolescents compared with children or infants, but less often than for adults, underscoring the need for rigorous randomized trials to determine the need for thromboprophylaxis in critically ill adolescents and children [44].

Obesity is another factor of increasing importance, responsible for doubling VTE risk compared to adults of normal body mass index [45]. The percentage of the population with a body mass index of 30 or greater has doubled worldwide since 1980, to an estimated 10% of men and 14% of women, according to a recent report from *The Lancet*. This report also identified nearly one-third of Americans as obese, with the expectation to include half of the US population by 2030 if current trends continue [46].

One other important VTE risk factor is infection [47,48]. A recent pediatric study from investigators at Baylor University showed that the predominant community-acquired, methicillin-resistant *Staphylococcus aureus* clone may have unique propensity to cause VTE in association with osteomyelitis [49]. Other studies have demonstrated an association between *Chlamydia pneumonia* and VTE [50,51], which was investigated due to the relationship between chronic *Chlamydia pneumonia* infection and development of atherosclerosis [52]; VTE has also been associated with viral infections such as CMV [53] and HIV [54].

Risk stratification

Although numerous studies have identified risk factors for pediatric VTE (Table 16.1), how best to use this information to stratify patients for thromboprophylaxis has not been determined. A retrospective case–control study employing diagnostic validation from Children's Hospital Colorado [55] was performed in 2010/2011 for this purpose. In this study, patients with three or more putative risk factors had a six-fold increase in odds of in-hospital VTE. A risk factor model that included mechanical ventilation, systemic infection, and length of hospitalization greater than or equal to 5 days had a sensitivity of 45% and specificity of 95% for in-hospital VTE. This translated to a change from pretest VTE probability of 0.35% to a post-test probability of 3.1% in a hospital-wide setting, and a pretest probability of 0.45% to a post-test probability of 0.95% in the PICU setting. Prospective validation of this model is, however, required. A substantive issue following validation will be whether the number-needed-to-treat with anticoagulation in order to prevent one VTE is perceived to favorably offset the bleeding risk (number-needed-to-harm) associated with the intervention. Ultimately, this can best be assessed through a well-designed clinical trial.

A UK guideline for perioperative thromboprophylaxis in children focuses particularly on those with multiple risk factors for VTE [56]. According to the guideline, low-risk patients (based on a system that assigns points for risk factors such as age, underlying disease, medications, and the nature of the surgery) should undergo early mobilization and receive adequate hydration; moderate-risk patients undergoing major general surgery should receive elastic stockings and compression devices; and high-risk patients undergoing major general or orthopedic surgery should also receive LMWH.

A single-center patient safety and quality improvement study demonstrated increased use of VTE prophylaxis in high-risk adolescent patients by using risk-based guidelines that were extrapolated from adult studies [57]. This quality improvement study provides a useful algorithm for inpatient VTE risk assessment and prophylaxis initiation for patients aged 14 years and older. These findings, if substantiated, could provide the basis for greater risk stratification for pediatric in-hospital VTE.

In addition to awareness of the risk factors for VTE, clinicians must also have an effective means of assessing these risk factors. This has proven to be a challenge in adult settings and is one explanation as to why implementation of recommended thromboprophylaxis may be suboptimal, even when there is strong evidence [58]. An observational study of a pediatric point-based VTE risk assessment tool demonstrated only fair to moderate inter-rater reliability, with suboptimal adherence to the protocol [59]. Concern exists that these findings may suggest potential under-utilization of VTE prevention strategies, and inter-rater reliability of risk assessment tools should be emphasized during future efforts to generate prospective evidence on pediatric VTE prevention.

Prophylaxis

Options for preventing VTE include both pharmacologic and non-pharmacologic measures. General non-pharmacologic approaches include maintenance of adequate hydration, early post-operative mobilization, and early removal of CVADs. Physical methods such as graduated compression stockings (GCS) or intermittent pneumatic compression (IPC) devices help to increase venous outflow and reduce stasis within the leg veins [60]. These devices should be considered in older children and adolescents at increased risk of VTE, usually those over 40 kg [61], and should be size-selected based upon manufacturers' recommendations. In post-pubertal girls undergoing surgery, consideration should be given to withholding the combined contraceptive pill for 4 weeks prior to planned surgery, particularly if there is a strong family history of thrombosis or a known thrombophilic risk factor [61]. These physical methods are particularly helpful in patients with high risk of bleeding, or as a complement to pharmacologic prophylaxis in patients at particularly high VTE risk.

Children, especially adolescents, with multiple risk factors merit consideration for pharmacologic thromboprophylaxis [57,61]. Many of the recommendations for pediatric VTE prevention are adapted from existing adult evidence-based guidelines. Pharmacologic VTE prophylaxis without significant bleeding risk or renal dysfunction is typically achieved using LMWH. In cases of high bleeding risk, or those in which bleeding could be catastrophic, (hemodynamic instability, recent or imminent surgery) unfractionated heparin may be preferred over other agents since the effect is short acting and can be easily reversed. Dosing of LMWH for VTE prophylaxis in children has not been independently validated. The recommended prophylactic dose of enoxaparin, the most widely used LMWH in children, is 0.5 mg/kg subcutaneous twice daily (0.75 mg/kg for infants < 2mo) [36]. For patients weighing more than 60 kg, one could adapt adult dosing strategies: enoxaparin 30 mg subcutaneous twice daily (accepted dose for adult orthopedic surgery patients) or 40 mg once daily (accepted dose for adult medical patients) [36]. Extrapolating from adult studies, anticoagulant prophylaxis can be initiated within 12–24 hours following a high-risk surgery [36]. Anti-Xa levels are not routinely monitored

in pediatric patients receiving prophylactic anticoagulation, except in cases of renal insufficiency, bleeding complications, or weight change in excess of 10 percent of total body weight. Contraindications to prophylactic anticoagulation generally include acute stroke or bleeding, intracranial hemorrhage within the previous 7 days, coagulopathy (except disseminated intravascular coagulopathy at some centers), incomplete spinal cord injury with suspected or proven paraspinal hematoma, allergy to pork products (heparins) or other components of the anticoagulant medication being prescribed, or (for heparins) a history of heparin-induced thrombocytopenia [36].

In the strictly pediatric setting, the importance of clinical guidelines in the absence of high-quality evidence cannot be underestimated. The limited data on the use of thromboprophylaxis in children necessitate the consideration of risk/benefit ratios on an individual patient basis. The quality of evidence in the ACCP antithrombotic therapy guidelines is rated according to the ACCP Guideline Grading Recommendations [62]. Grade 1 recommendations

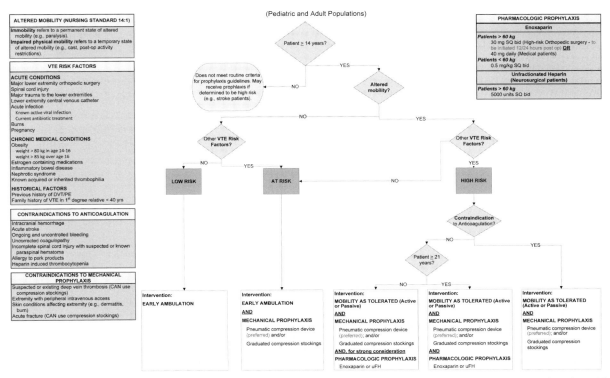

Figure 16.1 Algorithm for inpatient VTE risk assessment and prophylaxis – Children's Hospital Philadelphia [57]. DVT, deep vein thrombosis; PE, pulmonary embolism; SQ, subcutaneous; BID, twice daily; uFH, unfractionated heparin.

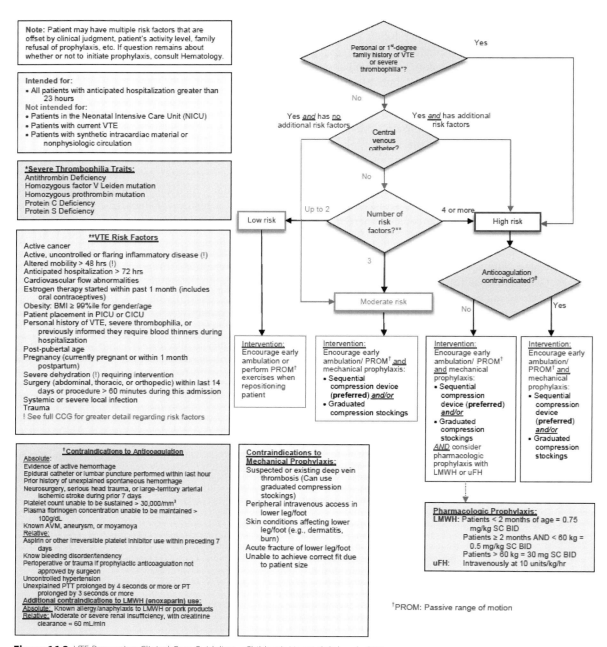

Figure 16.2 VTE Prevention Clinical Care Guideline – Children's Hospital Colorado [55].

are strong recommendations in which the benefits clearly outweigh the associated risk. Typically, 1A evidence comes from randomized control trials (RCTs) without limitations, while 1B evidence comes from RCTs with limitations, and 1C evidence typically comes from observational studies or case series. Grade 2 recommendations are weaker recommendations where the benefits are closely balanced with associated risks. Generally, 2A evidence comes from RCTs without important limitations, 2B

Table 16.2 Adult medical and surgical thromboembolism prophylaxis guidelines

Patient type	Subtype	Recommendation and evidence grade*
Medical [8]	Acutely ill hospitalized medical patients at increased VTE risk	Anticoagulant thromboprophylaxis with LMWH, low-dose unfractionated heparin (LDUH) bid/tid, or fondaparinux (grade 1B) for only the duration of immobilization or hospital stay (2B)
		Mechanical prophylaxis alone, such as graduated compression stockings (GCS) or intermittent pneumatic compression devices (IPCD) (2C), for patients who are bleeding or at high risk for major bleeding
		No mechanical or pharmacologic prophylaxis for patients at low risk of thrombosis
	Critically ill medical patients	LMWH or LDUH thromboprophylaxis (2C)
		Mechanical prophylaxis alone for patients who are bleeding or at high risk for major bleeding, until bleeding risk decreases (2C)
	Outpatients with cancer or chronic immobility without additional VTE risk factors	No routine prophylaxis with LMWH or LDUH (grade 2B) or vitamin K antagonists (1B)
Non-orthopedic surgical [9]	All risk groups	No inferior vena cava filters (2C) or compression ultrasonography surveillance (2C)
	Very low VTE risk (< 0.5%)	No specific pharmacologic (1B) or mechanical (2C) prophylaxis except early ambulation
	Low VTE risk (1.5%)	Mechanical prophylaxis with IPCD (2C)
	Moderate VTE risk (~ 3%) not at high risk for major bleeding complications	LMWH (2B), LDUH (2B), or mechanical prophylaxis with IPCD (2C)
	High VTE risk (~ 6%) not at high risk for major bleeding complications	LMWH (1B) or LDUH (1B) and mechanical prophylaxis with GCS or IPCD (2C)
	High VTE risk undergoing abdominal or pelvic cancer surgery	Extended duration, post-operative, pharmacologic prophylaxis (4 weeks) with LMWH (1B)
	Moderate to high VTE risk with high risk for major bleeding complications or those in whom the consequences of bleeding are believed to be particularly severe	Mechanical prophylaxis with IPCD until bleeding risk diminishes and pharmacologic prophylaxis may be initiated (2C)
Orthopedic surgical [10]	Major orthopedic surgery	LMWH (preferred, 2C/2B); fondaparinux; dabigatran, apixaban, rivaroxaban (total hip arthroplasty or total knee arthroplasty but not hip fracture surgery); LDUH; adjusted-dose VKA; aspirin (all 1B) extended up to 35 days (2B); or an IPCD (1C) for a minimum of 10 to 14 days
	Patients at increased bleeding risk	IPCD or no prophylaxis (2C)
	Patients who decline injections	Apixaban or dabigatran (1B)
	Contraindications to both pharmacologic and mechanical thromboprophylaxis	No inferior vena cava filter placement (2C) or Doppler (or duplex) ultrasonography screening before hospital discharge (1B)
	Isolated lower extremity injuries requiring immobilization	No thromboprophylaxis required (2B)
	Patients undergoing knee arthroscopy without a history of VTE	No thromboprophylaxis required (2B)

* The ACCP Grading System for Guideline Recommendation: Relationship of Strength of the Supporting Evidence to the Balance of Benefits to Risks and Burdens [62].

Table 16.3 Balance of benefits to risks and burdens

		Benefits outweigh risks/burdens	Risks/burdens outweigh benefits	Evenly balanced	Uncertain
Strength of evidence	High	1A	1A	2A	
	Moderate	1B	1B	2B	
	Low or very low	1C	1C	2C	2C

evidence comes from RCTs with important limitations, and 2C evidence comes from observational studies or case series where there is uncertainty in the estimates of benefits and risk. Grade 1 recommendations can be applied uniformly to most patients whereas grade 2 recommendations require a more individualized application.

Currently, the ACCP guidelines recommend that, for acutely ill hospitalized pediatric patients, treatment should vary according to the risk of thrombosis [8]. Based on available evidence however, there are a small number of clinical guidelines that can provide a rational basis for VTE prevention in children. For children receiving long-term home TPN, these guidelines suggest thromboprophylaxis with VKAs (grade 2C) [36]. For pediatric patients with cardiomyopathy, the guidelines suggest VKAs no later than their activation on a cardiac transplant waiting list (grade 2C). For children after Fontan surgery, they recommend either [1] aspirin or [2] therapeutic UFH followed by VKAs (as opposed to no antithrombotic therapy) (grade 1C). For children with biologic or mechanical prosthetic heart valves, they recommend that clinicians follow the relevant recommendations from the adult population. For children with short- or medium-term CVADs, they recommend against the use of routine systemic thromboprophylaxis (grade 1B) [36].

To address the lack of robust evidence-based recommendations for VTE prevention in children, some pediatric institutions have implemented their own algorithms for risk assessment and risk-stratified intervention as part of institutional quality and safety improvement initiatives. Children's Hospital of Philadelphia, for example, has developed a tool for inpatient VTE assessment and prophylaxis (Figure 16.1) [57]. Children's Hospital Colorado has also implemented a similar tool into the computerized

physician order entry section of the electronic medical record, based upon, and adapted from, a recent institutional case–control study of VTE risk factors (Figure 16.2) [55].

Another important concept is that of careful periprocedural management of anticoagulant dosing to prevent bleeding side effects as well as thrombus progression or recurrence. When adults with high VTE risk who are receiving warfarin require invasive procedures, LMWH bridging is recommended, based mainly upon observational evidence. A recent institution-based prospective inception cohort study of 17 children (23 bridging events) at Children's Hospital Colorado reported a median preprocedure duration of LMWH administration of 6 days (range, 4–10 days) and a median duration without anticoagulation periprocedurally of 1.5 days (range, 1–2 days), with low risks of major bleeding (4.3%), recurrent VTE (0%), and arterial thromboembolism (0%) at 30 days post-procedure. [63]

Conclusions

In-hospital VTE is a rare but serious problem in children, often with significant sequelae. Awareness of the problem, and appropriately risk-stratified use of available guidelines regarding general preventative measures and physical and/or pharmacologic prophylaxis, may decrease VTE incidence in certain populations. It is imperative, however, that guideline-based care is continually monitored for compliance, as well as safety and efficacy. Further evaluation by multicenter controlled trials will be required to determine the appropriate prophylactic steps in the pediatric population. In the meantime, consensus-based guidelines and some institution-specific algorithms (risk assessment and risk-stratified intervention) for pediatric VTE prophylaxis can help to inform and standardize clinical decision-making in the face of this growing clinical concern.

References

1. United States Surgeon General's Call-to-Action for Deep Vein Thrombosis 2008 [cited 2012]. Available from: http://www.surgeongeneral.gov/topics/deepvein/calltoaction/call-to-action-ondvt-2008.pdf

2. Sjalander A, Bergqvist D, Eriksson H, Carlberg B, Svensson P. Efficacy and safety of anticoagulant prophylaxis to prevent venous thromboembolism in acutely ill medical inpatients: a meta-analysis. J Int Med. 2008;263(1):52–60.

3. Dentali F, Gianni M, Lim W, Crowther M. Meta-analysis: Anticoagulant prophylaxis to prevent symptomatic venous thromboembolism in hospitalized medical patients. Annals Int Med. 2007;146(4):278–88.

4. Raffini L, Witmer C, Feudtner C. Dramatic increase in venous thromboembolism in children's hospitals in the United States from 2001 to 2007. Pediatrics. 2009;124:1001–8.

5. Journeycake JM, Manco-Johnson MJ. Thrombosis during infancy: what we know and what we do not know. Hematol Oncol Clin North Am. 2004;18:1315–38.

6. Biss TT, Kahr WH, Chan AK, Williams S. Clinical features and outcome of pulmonary embolism in children. Br J Haem. 2008;142:808–18.

7. Goldenberg NA, Kahn SR, Crowther M, Nowak-Göttl U, Manco-Johnson MJ. Post thrombotic syndrome in children: a systematic review of frequency of occurrence, validity of outcome measures, and prognostic factors. Haematologica. 2010;95(11):1952–9.

8. Kahn S, Dunn A, Cushman M, Dentali F, Akl E, Cook D, Balekian A, et al. Prevention of VTE in nonsurgical patients: antithrombotic therapy and prevention of thrombosis, 9th edn: American College of Chest Physicians Evidence-Based Clinical Practice Guidelines. Chest. 2012;141(Suppl 2):e195S–226S.

9. Gould M, Wren S, Karanicolas P, Arcelus J, Heit J, Samama C. Prevention of VTE in Nonorthopedic Surgical Patients: Antithrombotic Therapy and Prevention of Thrombosis, 9th edn: American College of Chest Physicians Evidence-Based Clinical Practice Guidelines. Chest. 2012;141 (Suppl 2):e227S–775.

10. Falck-Ytter Y, Johanson N, Curley C, Dahl O, Schulman S, Ortel T, Pauker S, Colwell C. Prevention of VTE in orthopedic surgery patients: Antithrombotic Therapy and Prevention of Thrombosis, 9th edn: American College of Chest Physicians Evidence-Based Clinical Practice Guidelines Chest. 2012;141 (Suppl 2):e278–325.

11. Goldenberg NA. Venous thromboembolism in children. Hematol Oncol Clin North Am. 2010;24 (1):151–66.

12. Paul Monagle, Michael Mahoney, Kaiser Ali, Dorothy Barnard, Mark Bernstein, Linda Brisson, Michele David, Sunil Desai, Marie-Francis Scully, Jacqueline Halton, Sara Israels, Lawrence Jardine, Michael Leaker, Patricia McCusker, Marianna Silva, John Wu, Ron Anderson, Maureen Andrew, M Patricia Massicotte. Outcome of pediatric thromboembolic disease: a report from the Canadian Childhood Thrombophilia Registry. Pediatric Research. 2000;47(6):763–6.

13. Revel-Vilk S, Bauman M, Massicotte P. Prothrombotic conditions in an unselected cohort of children with venous thromboembolic disease. J Thromb Haemost. 2003;1:915–21.

14. Andrew M, Pencharz P, Zlotkin S, Burrows P, Ingram J, Adams M, Filler R. A cross-sectional study of catheter-related thrombosis in children receiving total parenteral nutrition at home. J Pediatr. 1995;126:358–63.

15. Koksoy C, Erden I, Akkaya A. The risk factors in central venous catheter-related thrombosis. Aust NZ J Surg. 1995;65:796–8.

16. Male C, Massicotte P, Gent M, Mitchell L. Significant association with location of central venous line placement and risk of venous thrombosis in children. Thromb Haemost. 2005;94:516–21.

17. Stanley A. Primary prevention of venous thromboembolism in medical and surgical oncology patients. Brit J Cancer. 2010;13(102 Suppl 1):S10–16.

18. Elice F. Hematologic malignancies and thrombosis. Thromb Research. 2012;129(3):360–6.

19. Takemoto CM. Venous thromboembolism in cystic fibrosis. Pediatr Pulmonology. 2012;47(2):105–12.

20. Higgerson RA, Christie LM, Brown AM, McArthur JA, Totapally BR, Hanson SJ. National Association of Children's Hospitals and Related Institutions Pediatric Intensive Care Unit FOCUS group. Incidence and risk factors associated with venous thrombotic events in pediatric intensive care unit patients. Pediatr Crit Care Med. 2011;12(6):628–34.

21. Male C, Ginsberg JS, Hanna K, Andrew M, Halton J, et al. Comparison of venography and ultrasound for the diagnosis of asymptomatic deep vein thrombosis in the upper body in children: results of the PARKAA study. Thromb Haemost. 2002;87:593–8.

22. Male C, Andrew M, Hanna K, Julian J, Mitchell L; PARKAA Investigators. Central venous line-related thrombosis in children: association with central venous line location and insertion technique. Blood. 2003;101 (11):4273–8.

23. Dollery CM, Bauraind O, Bull C, Milla PJ. Thrombosis and embolism in long-term central venous access for parenteral nutrition. Lancet. 1994;344(8929):1043–5.

24. Derish MT, Frankel LR. Venous catheter thrombus formation and pulmonary embolism in children. Pediatr Pulmonology. 1995;20(6):349–54.

25. Randolph A, Gonzales C, Andrew M. Benefit of heparin in peripheral venous and arterial catheters: systematic review and meta-analysis of randomised controlled trials. BMJ. 1998;316:969–75.

26. Dillon PW, Bagnall-Reeb HA, Buckley JD, Wiener ES, Haase GM. Prophylactic urokinase in the management of long-term venous access devices in children: a Children's Oncology Group study. J Clin Oncol. 2004;22(13):2718–23.

27. Raad I, Khalil S, Costerton J, Lam C, Bodey G. The relationship between the thrombotic and infectious complications of central venous catheters. JAMA. 1884;271(13):1014–16.

28. Massicotte P, Gent M, Shields K, Marzinotto V, Szechtman B, Chan A, Andrew M. An open-label randomized controlled trial of low molecular weight heparin for the prevention of central venous line-related thrombotic complications in children: the PROTEKT trial. Thromb Res. 2003;109(2–3):101–8.

29. Schroeder AR, Silverman NH, Rubesova E, Merkel E, Roth SJ. A continuous heparin infusion does not prevent catheter-related thrombosis in infants after cardiac surgery. Pediatr Crit Care Med. 2010;11(4):489–95.

30. Newall FH, Savoia HF, Campbell J, Monagle P. Warfarin therapy in children requiring long-term total parenteral nutrtion (TPN). Pediatrics. 2003;112(5):e386.

31. Ruud E, De Lange C, Hogstad EM, Wesenberg F. Low-dose warfarin for the prevention of central line-associated thrombosis in children with malignancies: a randomized, controlled study. Acta Paediatr. 2006;95:1053–9.

32. Young A, Begum G, Kerr D, Hughes A, Rea D, Shepherd S, Stanley A, et al. Warfarin thromboprophylaxis in cancer patients with central venous catheters (WARP): an open-label randomised trial. The Lancet. 2009;373(9663):567–74.

33. Toker S, Morgan SJ. Deep vein thrombosis prophylaxis in trauma patients. Thrombosis. 2011;9(1):7–9.

34. O'Brien SH. In the absence of a central venous catheter, risk of venous thromboembolism is low in critically injured children, adolescents, and young adults: Evidence from the National Trauma Data Bank. Pediatr Crit Care Med. 2011;12(3):251–6.

35. Cyr C, Pettersen G, David M, Brossard J. Venous thromboembolism after severe injury in children. Acta Haematol. 2006;115(3–4):198–200.

36. Monagle P, Goldenberg N, Ichord R, Journeycake J, Nowak-Gottl U, Vesely S. Antithrombotic therapy in neonates and children: Antithrombotic Therapy and Prevention of Thrombosis, 9th edn. American College of Chest Physicians Evidence-Based Clinical Practice Guidelines. Chest. 2012;141: e737S–801S.

37. Monagle P, Cochrane A, Roberts R, Manlhiot C, Weintraub R, Szechtman B, et al. A multicenter, randomized trial comparing heparin/warfarin and acetylsalicylic acid as primary thromboprophylaxis for 2 years after the Fontan procedure in children. J Am Coll Cardiol. 2011;58(6):645–51.

38. Grace RF, Neuberg D, Sallan SE, Connors JM, Neufeld EJ, Deangelo DJ, Silverman LB. The frequency and management of asparaginase-related thrombosis in paediatric and adult patients with acute lymphoblastic leukaemia treated on Dana-Farber Cancer Institute consortium protocols. Brit J Haematol. 2011;152(4):452–9.

39. Raetz EA. Tolerability and efficacy of L-asparaginase therapy in pediatric patients with acute lymphoblastic leukemia. J Pediatr Hematol/Oncol. 2010;32(7):554–63.

40. Hirota-Kawadobora M, Ishikawa S, Fujihara N, Wakabayashi S, Kamijo Y, Yamauchi K, et al. Analysis of hypofibrinogenemias found on routine coagulation screening tests and identification of heterozygous dysfibrinogenemia or fibrinogen deficiency. Rinsho byori: The Japanese Journal of Clinical Pathology. 2007;55(11):989–95.

41. Mitchell L Andrew M, Hanna K, Abshire T, Halton J, Wu J, Anderson R, Cherrick I, Desai S, Mahoney D, McCusker P, Chait P, Abdolell M, deVeber G, Mikulis D. Trend to efficacy and safety using antithrombin concentrate in prevention of thrombosis in children receiving L-asparaginase for acute lymphoblastic leukemia. Results of the PAARKA study. Thromb Haemost. 2003;90(2):235–44.

42. Nowak-Gottl U, Manner D, Kenet G. Thrombophilia testing in neonates and infants with thrombosis. Semin Fetal Neonatal Med. 2011;16(6):345–8.

43. Young G, Bonduel M, Brandao L, Chan A, Friedrichs F, Goldenberg NA, Grabowski E, Heller C, Journeycake J, Kenet G, Krumpel A, Kurnik K, Lubetsky A, Male C, Manco-Johnson M, Matthew P, Monagle P, van Ommen H, Simoni P, Svirirn P, Tormene D, Nowak Gottl U. Impact of inherited thrombophilia on venous thromboembolism in children: a systematic review and meta-analysis of observational studies. Circulation. 2008;118(13):1373–82.

44. Faustino E, Thiagarajan R, Cook D, Northrup V, Randolph A. Survey of parmacologic thromboprophylaxis in critically ill children. Critical Care Medicine. 2011;**39**(7):1773–8.

45. MA A-F. Obesity and venous thrombosis: a review. SeminThromb Hemost. 2011;**37**(8):903–7.

46. Wang YC MK, Marsh T, Gortmaker S, Brown M. Health and economic burden of the projected obesity trends in the USA and the UK. The Lancet. 2011;**378** (9793):815–27.

47. Gerotziafas GT. Risk factors for venous thromboembolism in children. International Angiology: A Journal of the International Union of Angiology. 2004;**23**(3):195–205.

48. Sandoval JA, Sheehan MP, Stonerock CE, Shafique S, Rescorla FJ, Dalsing MC. Incidence, risk factors, and treatment patterns for deep venous thrombosis in hospitalized children: an increasing population at risk. J Vasc Surg: Official publication, the Society for Vascular Surgery [and] International Society for Cardiovascular Surgery, North American Chapter. 2008;**47** (4):837–43.

49. Gonazalez B, Mahoney D, Hulten K, Edwards R, Lamberth L, Hammerman W, Mason E, Kaplan S. Venous thrombosis associated with staphylococcal osteomyelitis in children. Pediatrics. 2006;**117** (5):1673–9.

50. Koster T, Lieuw-A-Len DD, Kroes ACM, Emmerich JD, Van Dissel JT. Chlamydia pneumoniae IgG seropositivity and risk of deep-vein thrombosis. Lancet. 2000;**355**:1694–5.

51. Emmerich J. Infection and venous thrombosis. Pathophysiol Haemost Thromb. 2002;**32**:346–8.

52. Lozinguez O, Belec L, Nicaud V, Alhenc-Gelas M, Fiessinger JN, Aiach M, Emmerich J. Demonstration of an association between *Chlamydia pneumoniae* infection and venous thromboembolic disease. Thromb Haemost. 2000;**83**:887–91.

53. Fridlender Z, Leitersdorf E. Association between cytomegalovirus infection and venous thromboembolism. Am J Med Sci. 2007;**334** (2):111–14.

54. Matta F, Stein P. Human immunodeficiency virus infection and risk of venous thormboembolism. Am J Med Sci. 2008;**336**(5):402–6.

55. Branchford B, Bajaj L, Manco-Johnson M, Wang M, Goldenberg NA. Risk factors for in-hospital venous thromboembolism in children: a case-control study employing diagnostic validation. Haematologica. 2011. 2012 Apr;**97**(4):509–15.

56. Jackson PC, Morgan JM. Perioperative thromboprophylaxis in children: development of a guideline for management. Pediatr Anesthes. 2008;**18**:478–87.

57. Raffini L, Beliveau J, Davis D. Thromboprophylaxis in a pediatric hospital: A patient safety and quality improvement initiative. Pediatrics. 2011;**127**:e1326–32.

58. Amin A, Dobesh P, Shorr A, Hussein M, Mozaffari E, Benner JS. Are hospitals delivering appropriate VTE prevention? The venous thromboembolism study to assess the rate of thromboprophylaxis (VTE start). J Thromb Thrombolysis. 2010;**29**:326–39.

59. Beck M, Todoric K, Lehman E, Sciamanna C. Reliability of a point-based VTE risk assessment tool in the hands of medical residents. J Hosp Med. 2011;**6** (4):195–201.

60. Amarigiri S. Elastic compression stockings for prevention of deep vein thrombosis. Cochr Database Syst Rev. 2010;7.

61. Chalmers E, Ganesen V, Liesner R, Maroo S, Nokes T, Saunders D, et al. Guideline on the investigation, management and prevention of venous thrombosis in children. Brit J Haematol. 2011;**154**(2):196–207.

62. Guyatt G, Gutterman D, Baumann M, Addrizzo-Harris D, Hylek E, Phillips B, Raskob G, Zelman Lewis S, et al. Grading strength of recommendations and quality of evidence in clinical guidelines: Report from an American College of Chest Physicians Task Force. Chest. 2006;**129** (1):174–81.

63. Moruf A, Spyropoulos AC, Schardt TQ, Gibson E, Manco-Johnson MJ, Wang M, et al. Peri-procedural bridging with low molecular weight heparin in patients receiving warfarin for venous thromboembolism: a pediatric experience. Thromb Res. 2012;**130**(4):612–15.

64. Sharathkumar AA, Mahajerin A, Heidt L, Doerfer K, Heiny M, Vik T, et al. Risk-prediction tool for identifying hospitalized children with a predisposition for development of venous thromboembolism: Peds-Clot Clinical Decision Rule. J Thromb Haemost. 2012;**10** (7):1326–34.

65. Wright JM, Watts RG. Venous thromboembolism in pediatric patients: epidemiologic data from a pediatric tertiary care center in Alabama. J Pediatr Hematol Oncol. 2011;**33**(4):261–4.

66. Oschman A, Kuhn RJ. Venous thromboembolism in the pediatric population. Orthopedics. 2010;**33** (3):180–4.

217

67. Anderson FA, Jr., Spencer FA. Risk factors for venous thromboembolism. Circulation. 2003;**107**(23 Suppl 1):19–16.

68. Hanson SJ, Punzalan RC, Greenup RA, Liu H, Sato TT, Havens PL. Incidence and risk factors for venous thromboembolism in critically ill children after trauma. J Trauma. 2010;**68**(1):52–6.

69. Spentzouris G, Scriven RJ, Lee TK, Labropoulos N. Pediatric venous thromboembolism in relation to adults. Journal of Vascular Surgery: Official Publication, the Society for Vascular Surgery [and] International Society for Cardiovascular Surgery, North American Chapter. 2012;**55** (6):1785–93.

Arterial ischemic stroke in children

Timothy J. Bernard and Ulrike Nowak-Göttl

Introduction

Childhood arterial ischemic stroke (AIS) has received increasing attention as a cause of morbidity and mortality in the pediatric population. Several population based studies in the USA have demonstrated an incidence of childhood AIS at 0.63–1.2 cases per 100,000 children per year [1,2]. Of the estimated 83,000,000 children in the USA [3], nearly 1,000 will suffer an AIS this year. Extrapolating from the 2012 world population of 2,314,000,000 children [4], approximately 28,000 children will experience an AIS this year worldwide. Despite these increasingly recognized large numbers of childhood AIS cases, the pathogenesis, risk factors and outcomes of childhood AIS have only recently been explored. International networks, such as the International Pediatric Stroke Study (IPSS), have initiated large multicenter series demonstrating the natural history of this disease. Treatment trials, however, are still lacking. As a result, specific prevention and treatment strategies for childhood AIS remain largely unclear in all subtypes except sickle-cell related AIS. The purpose of this chapter is to review the current understanding of childhood AIS by stroke subtype, with a focus upon epidemiology, risk factors, pathophysiology, treatments and outcomes. Particular emphasis will be made on the hematologic risk factors for this disease, with special sections for sickle cell disease thrombotic risk factors.

Epidemiology

Most population-based estimates of childhood-onset AIS are over 20 years old, with the initial estimate coming from a 10-year cohort of children in Rochester Minnesota [1], and the second from the Cincinnati metropolitan area [2]. With the increased availability of magnetic resonance imaging (MRI) with diffusion-weighted imaging in pediatric hospitals,

these previous estimates of incidence (0.63–1.2/ 100,000 children per year [1,2] may actually underestimate the disease. Childhood AIS clearly occurs in males more often than females, with one series of 1,187 children finding that 59% of their cohort was male [5]. Interestingly, known trauma accounts for some of this disparity, as 75% of patients with traumatic dissection are male. Males are over-represented in cases without trauma as well; making it unclear if the gender disparity is the result of known trauma and unrecognized trauma, or if an alternative mechanism is invoked. For unknown reasons, Black children are also at greater risk for childhood AIS. Fullerton et al. described a population-based cohort of 2,278 children with AIS, in whom Black children were at higher risk of stroke than whites (relative risk [RR] 2.59, 95% CI 2.17 to 3.09, p < 0.0001) [6]. Interestingly, the same study found a lower risk for Hispanics and a similar risk for Asians, as compared to Whites [6]. This finding of similar stroke risk between Asian and Caucasian races is despite the association between Japanese heritage and moyamoya syndrome, a high-risk condition for stroke.

The IPSS has published the largest prospective series of childhood AIS. Although this series is not population based, and may be associated with referral bias to tertiary care setting, this series provides a representative sample of the childhood AIS population in this setting. Among 676 children with AIS, the majority of strokes were unilateral (78%) and associated with a single infarct (58%) [7]. Interestingly one-third of all strokes involved the posterior circulation [7]. Younger children (less than 5) accounted for almost one-half of cases (47%), suggesting that this may be a particularly vulnerable age. The majority of children had diffuse neurological signs (64%), with a large number presenting with a reduced level of consciousness and/or headache. Almost one-third (31%) had seizures at onset [7]. The majority of cases present with focal neurological

Pediatric Thrombotic Disorders, ed. Neil A. Goldenberg and Marilyn J. Manco-Johnson. Published by Cambridge University Press. © Cambridge University Press 2015.

signs (82%), including hemiparesis, visual disturbance or speech disturbance [7].

Despite the predominance of focal neurological signs and symptoms, childhood-onset AIS remains difficult to diagnose promptly. In a series of 88 children with AIS in Australia, the median time to diagnosis was just over 24 hours, with only six children (8%) being recognized within 3 hours (the standard time point for thrombolysis at time of publication – 2008) [8]. In response to the delayed identification of childhood AIS patients, many centers within the IPSS have initiated acute stroke protocols and acute stroke teams [9,10]. These protocols have demonstrated an ability to decrease the time from admission to head imaging [10]. In addition, the alerts appear to have a high specificity for childhood AIS, as one series from Children's Hospital of Philadelphia reported that 113 (79%) of 143 consecutive consults for possible stroke consults were diagnosed with AIS. The most common mimickers in this series were migraine, psychogenic diagnoses and reversible posterior leukoencephalopathy [9].

Thrombotic risk factors

Genetic thrombophilias

Genetic thrombophilias have been associated with both incident and recurrent AIS (Tables 17.1 and 17.2), although their association with childhood AIS in not fully understood. In a case–control study of 148 German children with AIS and 296 age-matched controls, 6% of childhood AIS patients possessed the prothrombin G20210A polymorphism, as compared to only 1% of controls [11]. The same study found the factor V Leiden (FVL) polymorphism in 20% of patients as compared to 4% of controls (OR: 6, 95% CI: 2.97–12.1) [11]. Several studies have demonstrated heterozygous FVL occurs more often in incident childhood-onset AIS case as compared to healthy controls [11–13]. Protein C deficiency has been evaluated as a risk factor for incident childhood AIS in multiple case–control studies [11,14–16], and in one German cohort of 310 German children, protein C deficiency was associated with a relative risk of recurrent childhood AIS of 3.5 (95% CI: 1·1–10.9) [17]. The same series reported an even higher relative risk of recurrent stroke for elevated lipoprotein(a) (RR = 4.4, 95% CI: 1.9–10.5), but no association between recurrence and protein S deficiency in childhood AIS (OR = 0.6, 95%

Table 17.1 Reported, statistically significant associations between incident childhood AIS and thrombophilic abnormalities

Genetic thrombophilia	
Factor V Leiden polymorphism	OR = 9.7 (95% CI: 1.1–84.7)* [12] OR = 4.8 (95% CI: 1.4–16.5) [13] OR = 6.0 (95% CI: 3.0–12.1) [11]
Factor II G20210A polymorphism	OR = 4.7 (95% CI: 1.4–15.6) [11]
Protein C deficiency	OR = 18.5 (95% CI: 2.2–160.0)† [14] OR = 9.5 (95% CI: 2.0–44.6) [11] OR = 6.5 (95% CI: 3.0–14.3)§ [16]
Lipoprotein(a) elevation	OR = 7.2 (95% CI: 3.8–13.8) [11] OR = 4.3 (95% CI: 1.3–14.4)† [14]
Homocysteine elevation	OR = 2.4 (95% CI: 1.5–4.5) [11] OR = 1.7 (95% CI: 1.2–2.3)§ [16]
Acquired thrombophilia	
Antiphospholipid antibodies	OR = 6.1 (95% CI: 1.5–24.3) [13]
Genetic and/or acquired thrombophilia	
ADAMTS13 below 10th percentile	OR = 6.70 (95% CI: 2.58–17.38) [26]
Activated protein C resistance	OR = 9.7 (95% CI: 1.1–84.7)* [12]

* Data calculated by the present authors based upon data provided in the original report. † Cases included cardiac patients only. § Data obtained by systematic review of observational studies.

CI: 0.1–6.4) [17]. The association between lipoprotein(a) and recurrent stroke has recently been confirmed in a prospective cohort of 46 children with AIS [18]. Lipoprotein(a) elevation has also been associated with cardioembolic AIS (for more details on AIS subtypes, see below) [11,14].

In a recent meta-analysis performed by Kenet and colleagues – which included both childhood and neonatal AIS – many of the aforementioned findings were substantiated. The analysis demonstrated a significant association with incident pediatric (childhood and neonatal) AIS and FVL (OR 3.70, CI: 2.82–4.85), factor II G20210A (OR 2.60, 95% CI: 1.66–4.08), protein C deficiency (OR 11.0, 95% CI: 5.13–23.59), elevated lipoprotein(a) (OR 6.53, 95% CI: 4.46–9.55) and MTHFR C677T mutation (OR 1.58, 95% CI: 1.20–2.08) [19]. Neither protein S deficiency nor antithrombin deficiency was significantly associated with incident pediatric AIS [19].

Table 17.2 Reported, statistically significant associations between recurrent childhood AIS and genetic thrombophilias or markers of endothelial activation

Genetic thrombophilia	
Protein C deficiency	RR = 10.7 (95% CI: 2.5–45.8)[17]
Lipoprotein(a) elevation	RR = 2.8 (95% CI: 1.1–7.5)[17]
Markers of endothelial activation/injury	
Endothelial cell-derived microparticles*	OR = 1.4 (95% CI: 1.1–1.5)[25]
Circulating endothelial cells*	OR = 2.4 (95% CI: 2.1–2.6)[25]

* Among children with AIS with cerebral arteriopathy.

Acquired thrombophilias

Acquired thrombophilia has been poorly studied in childhood AIS, with a few studies investigating factor VIII (FVIII) activity and antiphospholipid antibodies (APA). While evidence suggests that familial FVIII elevation may contribute to childhood AIS [20], most cases appear to be acquired. The FVIII activity was elevated in 65% of childhood AIS patients tested 4 months post-stroke as compared to 12.5% of control in one retrospective case–control study [21].

Early studies suggest that APAs are a risk factor for incident childhood AIS. Kenet and colleagues' meta-analysis in 2009 demonstrated a significant association between persistent APAs and incident pediatric AIS (neonates included – OR 6.95, CI: 3.67–13.14) [19]. A single case–control analysis of 58 children with AIS as compared to healthy controls, in 2000, demonstrated elevated anticardiolipin antibodies (defined by an IgG or IgM level > 18 or > 10 μ/ml, respectively) in nine AIS patients, for an odds ratio of OR = 6.1 (95%CI: 1.5–24.3) [13]. The APA syndrome is defined via international consensus as any patient with a history of arterial or venous clot and persistence of any of a variety of anti-phospholipid antibodies for at least 12 weeks [22]. Early studies likely do not reflect the true prevalence of APA syndrome in childhood AIS, as patients were tested for a single APA (as opposed to all three common APAs), and/or not tested sequentially for persistent antibodies. When systematically evaluating patients using current criteria (and evaluating all three major APAs including lupus anticoagulant, anticardiolipin IgG and IgM and beta-2-glycoprotein IgG and IgM), a recent single-center cohort study disclosed APA syndrome in 16% of 46 patients [23].

Other hematological biomarkers have been proposed as putative prognostic factors in childhood-onset AIS. These include markers of coagulation activation, endothelial specific markers and components of the fibrinolytic system. Recent work in a small cohort study in Colorado has demonstrated that D-dimer is acutely elevated in patients with childhood-onset AIS, especially patients with cardioembolic stroke [24]. Evidence from this center also suggested that D-dimer may be a predictor of adverse neurological outcome in childhood AIS [23]. These findings suggest that ongoing coagulation activation may be a marker of adverse outcomes in these patients. Markers of endothelial activation/injury may also be informative in childhood AIS, as a recent European study demonstrated that levels of circulating endothelial cells and microparticles are elevated in childhood AIS, and markedly elevated in the children with recurrent stroke [25]. Similarly, Lambers and colleagues demonstrated reduced ADAMTS13 levels in children with childhood AIS as compared to controls, a thrombophilia state that may suggest impaired endothelial regulation of von Willebrand factor (vWF) in these patients [26]. However, activity levels of PAI-1 (a protein stored in endothelial cells that functions as an inhibitor of fibrinolysis) have been shown to be increased in childhood AIS, which may indicate that this component of the endothelial response is not impaired [27].

Childhood AIS stroke subtypes and associated treatments

Multiple risk factors have been identified in childhood AIS, including congenital heart defects, cervical dissection, head trauma, intracranial dissection, intracranial arteriopathy, sickle cell disease (SCD) and multiple thrombotic disorders. In many cases, such as a child with intracranial arteriopathy, the mechanism of stroke remains uncertain. Recent efforts within the IPSS to simplify and codify classification and nomenclature have resulted in a consensus-based classification [28]. The Childhood AIS Standardized Classification and Diagnostic Evaluation (CASCADE) criteria classify patients within seven categories: small-vessel arteriopathy (SVA), unilateral focal cerebral arteriopathy of childhood (FCA), bilateral cerebral arteriopathy, aortic/cervical arteriopathy, cardioembolic, multifactorial and other [28].

Small-vessel arteriopathy (SVA) of childhood

The cause of SVA in childhood is usually an inflammatory process (arteritis). The role of inflammation in childhood AIS remains poorly characterized, and likely under-diagnosed due to the invasive nature of catheter angiography and brain biopsy, as well as the rarity of this diagnosis. According to the CASCADE criteria, confirmation of the definitive diagnosis of small-vessel arteriopathy of childhood requires multifocal arterial narrowing of small-caliber vessels on conventional angiogram and evidence of small-vessel vascular lesions on biopsy, including evidence of intramural/vasocentric inflammation of the small muscular arteries, capillaries, and/or venules on brain biopsy. Supportive evidence can be obtained from electron microscopy demonstrating endothelial cell activations and/or tubular reticular inclusions. Perivascular demyelination and/or gliosis can be found; however, specific histological features of other inflammatory brain diseases of childhood must be absent (i.e., diffuse parenchymal demyelination) [28].

Isolated small-vessel angiitis appears rare, as one series of 102 children with primary angiitis of the central nervous system found that the majority of patients had large- or medium-vessel disease that could be diagnosed via routine magnetic resonance angiography (MRA) [29]. Of 65 patients studied in a Canadian series, 95% had vascular anomalies identified on MRA [29]. Small-vessel disease (or distal stenosis) was identified on initial MRA in 40% of patients and on conventional angiography in 55%. In this series, progressive vasculitis was marked by non-specific neurological symptoms such as headaches (95%), cognitive dysfunction (75%), mood/personality change (60%) and constitutional changes such as fever or fatigue (25%). These symptoms, as well as elevated inflammatory markers, positive antinuclear antibody, white blood cells in cerebrospinal fluid and atypical presentations are essential clues to the diagnosis [29]. Small-vessel disease confirmation often requires conventional angiogram, and definitive diagnosis requires biopsy, as in some cases conventional angiography is normal, while biopsy confirms the disease [30].

The mainstay of treatment of SVA remains antithrombotic or anti-inflammatory medications. In the Canadian series described above, one-fifth of patients with non-progressive disease were treated with dual immunosuppression therapy and antithrombotic therapy, while two-thirds of children with progressive disease were treated with dual therapy [29].

Unilateral focal cerebral arteriopathy of childhood

Focal cerebral arteriopathy (FCA) encompasses multiple previously utilized terms that depict a focal stenosis of a large artery in children with AIS including: some types of moyamoya, transient cerebral arteriopathy, post-varicella arteriopathy, large-vessel childhood primary angiitis and basilar stenosis [28]. Confirmation of FCA in accordance with CASCADE criteria requires MRA, computed tomography angiography (CTA), or computed angiography (CA) displaying unilateral stenosis or irregularity of a large intracranial artery (internal carotid artery, middle cerebral artery, anterior cerebral artery) supplying the territory of infarct [28]. The condition of FCA is common in childhood AIS, present in 25% of cases in a large multicenter series of childhood AIS [31], and up to 80% of previously healthy children who have non-moyamoya arteriopathic AIS [32].

The etiology of FCA remains uncertain, with evidence that inflammatory or infectious etiologies play a role in pathophysiology. Askalan and colleagues first described the association between recent varicella infection and transient FCA, demonstrating that 31% of 70 childhood AIS cases in a Canadian series had a varicella infection within 1 year of stroke, as compared to 9% of healthy age-matched controls [33]. The influence of varicella vaccination upon this association remains uncertain, although a retrospective cohort of 3 million children in the USA demonstrated no association between the vaccination and subsequent AIS [34]. Post-varicella arteriopathy accounts for a minority of cases of FCA in childhood AIS. A recent study by Amlie-Lefond et al. describes an association between upper respiratory infection and FCA in a cohort of 667 patients from the International Pediatric Stroke Study (IPSS) [35]. Similarly, Hillis and colleagues demonstrated that an office visit for minor acute infection within 4 weeks of childhood AIS was an independent risk factor (OR: 4.6, 95% CI: 2.6–8.2) for patients as compared to controls. International multicenter cohort studies are ongoing to further evaluate the association between infection and childhood AIS [36].

The majority of FCA of childhood is non-progressive. Braun *et al.* published a series of 79 cases of unilateral intracranial arteriopathy, demonstrating that at a median follow-up of 1.4 years, only 6% of the children had progressive narrowing beyond the first 6 months after stroke. Of those without progressive arteriopathy, 23% had complete normalization, 45% slight improvement and 32% mildly progressive narrowing subacutely (0–6 months post-AIS) and then stabilization [37]. Similarly, in 43 children with arteriopathy in a European cohort, 12 had progressive disease (28%), seven stable disease (16%), and 24 had improved on follow-up imaging (56%) [32].

Although the majority of FCA appears to be non-progressive, and associated with an inflammatory/infectious condition, alternative etiologies have been identified in rare cases. Patients with PHACES syndrome (posterior fossa malformations, facial hemangioma, arterial cerebrovascular anomalies, cardiovascular anomalies and eye anomalies) can have unilateral vascular anomalies that are sometimes progressive and sometimes stable. In addition, intracranial dissection can initially appear to be FCA of inflammatory origin, but can progress extensively, often leading to death or severe disability [38]. Identifying patients with atypical causes/cases of FCA (such as dissection) early in their course may eventually rely upon enhanced imaging techniques such as vascular wall imaging [38].

The risk of recurrent AIS in FCA appears to be particularly high. In a nested case–control study of 97 children with AIS from within a California population-based (Kaiser Permanente) cohort, the 5-year recurrence risk for patients with FCA was 64%, as compared to 0% of those without vascular anomalies [39]. Importantly, recurrence usually occurred with the first year of incident stroke, and many of these patients were not treated with antithrombotic therapies. Other series have demonstrated a lower recurrence risk in this group, with only 18% of 79 children with FCA (variably treated with anticoagulation, aspirin or no antithrombotic therapy) developing recurrent events at a median follow-up of 1.4 years in a European series [37].

The mainstay of treatment for FCA and childhood stroke is antithrombotic therapy, with either anticoagulant or antiplatelet agents [40]. Recommendations for specific treatment of arteriopathy are not made in AHA guidelines, so most clinicians follow the recommendations for idiopathic patients outlined below – largely advising first-line therapy with aspirin. Recent evidence from a two-center prospective cohort,

however, suggests that anticoagulation may be safe in this setting [41], but confirmation is needed in larger series. While the use of immune-modulatory therapy such as steroid or azathioprine has been established for cases of obvious progressive CNS angiitis [42], the role for these therapies in FCA without inflammatory indicators and/or vascular progression is much less certain, and likely requires further study prior to widespread use.

Bilateral cerebral arteriopathy of childhood

Confirmation of bilateral cerebral arteriopathy of childhood via CASCADE criteria requires MRA, CTA or conventional cerebral arteriography (CA) showing bilateral stenosis or irregularity of a large intracranial artery (internal carotid artery, middle cerebral artery, anterior cerebral artery, posterior cerebral artery) supplying the territory of infarct [28]. Most bilateral cases are progressive, and thereby termed moyamoya. Moyamoya disease is associated with progressive narrowing of the intracranial internal carotid arteries and its proximate branches without an identifiable cause, while moyamoya syndrome is secondary to an alternative diagnosis such as sickle cell disease, trisomy 21, neurofibromatosis type 1, radiation injury or atherosclerosis [43]. Recent genetic advances have identified syndromes and/or specific genes associated with moyamoya [44–48].

Unless associated with sickle cell disease (see below), the treatment of choice for moyamoya is revascularization. Although multiple surgical techniques are utilized, they can be separated into two main categories: indirect and direct revascularization. The direct technique usually involves creating a direct microvascular anastomosis between the superficial temporal artery and a distal branch of the middle cerebral artery (MCA), allowing immediate recanalization of this territory [49]. Although this approach works faster than the indirect techniques, it remains technically challenging, and (according to AHA guidelines [50] should be reserved for patients with crescendo symptoms and/or "older" children [49]). Indirect revascularization typically involves redirecting the course of the superficial temporal artery to overlay the surface of the brain in the injured MCA territory, in the common scenario of MCA stroke [49]). Endogenous angiogenic factors – stimulated by hypoxia – induce angiogenesis of the superficial temporal artery into the MCA territory over 3–6 months [49]. The advantage of this technique is its relative

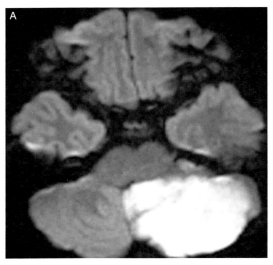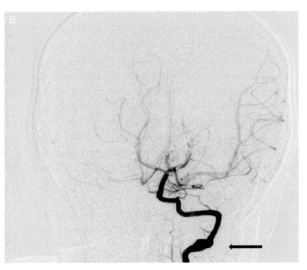

Figure 17.1 A 4-year-old male presents with acute-onset ataxia and headaches. MRI demonstrates restricted diffusion on diffusion-weighted sequence (panel A) in the left cerebellum. Follow-up conventional angiogram illustrates a dissecting aneurysm within the left vertebral artery (panel B, black arrow). After interventional coiling of the left vertebral artery, patient remains symptom-free for over 3 years.

simplicity, as compared to the direct technique, presumably reducing complications. In one series of 143 patients treated with the indirect technique, 4% of surgically repaired hemispheres were complicated by stroke during the acute (less than 30 days from operation) timeframe of recovery [51]. At a mean of 5.1 years' follow-up, less than 5% developed additional vascular events [51].

Aortic/cervical arteriopathy

The majority of aortic/cervical arteriopathic strokes in children consist of extracranial arterial dissection, although pseudoaneurysm, Takayasu arteritis and congenital anomalies can also account for thrombus formation in this region. Confirmation of the diagnosis of Takayasu arteritis via CASCADE criteria requires angiographic abnormalities (CA, CTA or MRA) of the aorta or its major branches (mandatory criterion) plus at least one of the following four features: (1) decreased peripheral artery pulse(s) and/or claudication of the extremities, (2) blood pressure difference >/= 10 mmHg, (3) bruits over aorta or its major branches or (4) hypertension (relative to childhood normative data) [28]. The diagnosis of extracranial dissection requires CTA, magnetic resonance imaging/MRA or CA with one of the following three patterns [1]: (1) angiographic findings of a double-lumen, intimal flap, or pseudoaneurysm, or, on axial T1 fat-saturation magnetic resonance imaging, a

"bright crescent sign" in the arterial wall [2]; (2) the sequence of cervical or cranial trauma, or neck pain, or head pain less than 6 weeks preceding angiographic findings of segmental arterial stenosis (or occlusion) located in the cervical arteries [3]; (3) angiographic segmental stenosis (or occlusion) of the vertebral artery at the level of the C2 vertebral body, even without known traumatic history [28].

Extracranial dissection occurs when intimal layers of the vessel wall tear, creating areas of injured endothelium. Exposure of blood to subendothelial collagen and tissue factor, uncoiled von Willebrand factor and activated platelets initiates and propagates thrombosis. Clot embolization and secondary vessel occlusion creates brain ischemia [52]. Acutely or chronically, aneurysmal dilation of a weakened vessel can create a pseudoaneurysm secondary to impaired vessel wall integrity (see Figure 17.1). Hence, follow-up imaging is necessary to assess for development of a pseudoaneurysm. Development of a pseudoaneursym is particularly common in the C1-C2 vertebral circulation in children [52,53]. Risk factors for dissection in children include head and neck trauma, connective tissue disorders (such as Ehlers–Danlos syndrome) and male gender [54–56].

Extracranial dissections account for 5–25% of childhood AIS [54,57,58], and are often preceded by head or neck injury [54–56]. Cervical bone anomalies can contribute to dissection and should be evaluated for in any case of suspected or confirmed extracranial dissection. [59,60] European cohort studies suggest that extracranial dissection in children is more prevalent in the posterior than anterior circulation [57]. As compared to adults – where neck pain is a hallmark of extracranial dissection – diffuse headache is a more common sign in children [54,56].

Treatment of adult and childhood extracranial dissection has become increasingly controversial, with some experts advocating for less aggressive management such as antiplatelet monotherapy, and others utilizing more aggressive therapies such as anticoagulation. Indeed, within the IPSS, acute treatment of extracranial dissection varies greatly with 66% of patients receiving anticoagulation therapy alone and 34% receiving antiplatelet therapy, combination therapy or no therapy [58]. There are no published randomized controlled trials comparing antiplatelet therapy to anticoagulation in adult or childhood patients with extracranial dissection and AIS. Recent adult studies suggest that antiplatelet therapy may be as efficacious as anticoagulation for the prevention of recurrent stroke in extracranial dissection of the carotid. A 2012 Cochrane meta-analysis of 36 observational studies concluded that there was no statistically significant difference in recurrent stroke risk in adults when comparing anticoagulation to conventional antiplatelet therapy (OR 0.63, 95% CI: 0.21–1.86) [61]. In a subanalysis of 26 studies, there was a strong nonsignificant trend favoring the use of anticoagulation in preventing death or disability, however (OR 1.77, 95% CI: 0.98–3.22, p = 0.06) [61]. Applicability of this meta-analysis to childhood AIS is unclear, as posterior circulation dissections predominate in the pediatric population [57]. The AHA recommendations in childhood extracranial dissection with AIS suggest acute treatment with either UFH or LMWH as a bridge to oral anticoagulation [50]. These recommendations also advocate treating with low molecular weight heparin or warfarin for 3 to 6 months [50]. The American College of Chest Physicians suggests for AIS secondary to dissection anticoagulant therapy with LMWH or vitamin K antagonists for at least 6 weeks, with ongoing treatment dependent on radiologic assessment [62]. Acknowledging the recent trend toward antiplatelet therapy in extracranial dissection, the AHA recommendations allow for substitution of an antiplatelet therapy for LMWH or warfarin [50]. Surgical options should be reserved for those with recurrent disease [50].

Cardioembolism

According to CASCADE criteria, *definitive* cardioembolic AIS is established by (1) a high risk for cardiac source of cerebral embolism (such as congenital heart disease with abnormal cardiac function, arrhythmia or endocarditis) or cardiac procedure within 30 days of stroke; AND (2) a territory of large/medium-sized cerebral artery or > 1 arterial territory (which may be large and/or hemorrhagic) [63]. *Probable* cardioembolic disease is established by a stroke in greater than one arterial territory (which may be large and/or hemorrhagic) in a child without another identifiable etiology and one of the following: (1) patent foramen ovale with right-to-left shunt or other subtle cardiac anomaly; or (2) occlusion: a discrete and abrupt blockage of an artery consistent with a clot, without any surrounding irregularity or stenosis suggestive of arteriopathy [63].

Commonly, definitive cardioembolic AIS in children is associated with congenital heart disease such as transposition of the great arteries or hypoplastic left heart. Multiple studies have demonstrated that white mater injury (WMI) is exceedingly common in CHD. Injury is likely a combination of hypoperfusion injury and embolic events. Interestingly, WMI is prevalent prior to any intervention, as 43% of newborns with CHD have WMI on preoperative MRI [64]. Postoperative injuries are also common, with 40% of children with CHD demonstrating new WMI on postoperative MRI [64]. In the IPSS cohort, 20% of 667 strokes were cardioembolic in origin, with an association between cardioembolic stroke subtype and treatment with anticoagulation (OR = 1·87, CI: 1.20–2.92, p = 0·01) [40].

The AHA guidelines suggest the following approach to cardioembolic AIS:

> For children with a cardiac embolism unrelated to a PFO who are judged to have a high risk of recurrent embolism, it is reasonable to initially introduce UFH or LMWH while warfarin therapy is initiated and adjusted. Alternatively, it is reasonable to use LMWH initially in this situation and to continue it instead of warfarin. In children with a risk of cardiac embolism, it is reasonable to continue either LMWH or warfarin for at least 1 year or until the lesion responsible for the risk has been corrected (class IIa, level of evidence C). If the risk of recurrent embolism is judged to be high, it is reasonable to continue anticoagulation indefinitely as long as it is well tolerated. For children

with a suspected cardiac embolism unrelated to a PFO with a lower or unknown risk of stroke, it is reasonable to begin aspirin and to continue it for at least 1 year. [50]

Idiopathic/other

Despite a large number of identified etiologies for childhood AIS, many cases remain without an identifiable cause. In addition, there remain rare causes of the disease such as metabolic anomalies. Patients with atypical stroke patterns or recurrent stroke should be screened for metabolic anomalies such as homocysteinuria, organic acidemias, amino acidemias and urea cycle defects [65]. Recent evidence suggests that subclinical Fabry disease is a rare cause (0.65%) of stroke in young males [66]. Despite extensive evaluation, idiopathic stroke represents a large percentage of childhood AIS, with one IPSS series demonstrating 9% of childhood AIS patients had no associated risk factors [7].

The AHA guidelines suggest that the mainstay of treatment for idiopathic AIS is antithrombotic therapy. No randomized controlled trials exist to inform treatment decisions in this population. One multicenter, non-randomized, prospective German cohort study demonstrated equivalent rates of recurrent stroke in children with idiopathic AIS treated with aspirin and LMWH [67]. Once dissection, sickle cell disease and/or cardioembolic AIS are ruled out, AHA guidelines recommend that aspirin 3–5 mg/kg/day be initiated as long-term secondary prevention [50].

Thrombolytic therapy for non-sickle cell-associated childhood AIS

Acute therapy for patients with childhood AIS is controversial, with only 1.6% of childhood AIS patients in the USA receiving thrombolytic therapy [68]. The AHA guidelines comment that: "Until there are additional published safety and efficacy data, tPA generally is not recommended for children with AIS outside a clinical trial. However, there was no consensus about the use of tPA in older adolescents who otherwise meet standard adult tPA eligibility criteria."[50]

Sickle cell disease

Sickle cell disease (SCD)-associated AIS is the only subtype of childhood AIS with class 1 data by which to inform treatment strategies. Vascular occlusion in SCD is a multistep process involving endothelial activation, white blood cell adhesion, red blood cell–white blood cell interactions and heterocellular aggregates [69]. Patients with SCD are at increased risk for development of moyamoya disease and associated infarcts. In patients with hemoglobin SS the age-adjusted prevalence of stroke is 4.01%, with lower rates in hemoglobin S-β^0 (2.43%), S-β^+ (1.29%) and hemoglobin SC (0.84%) [70].

Prevention of SCD-associated AIS is achieved through a regular exchange transfusion program in patients with large artery stenosis as identified by increased flow velocity transcranial Doppler (TCD) or those with incident stroke off therapy. The transfusion program is designed to reduce hemoglobin S to less than 30% of total hemoglobin [50]. The AHA guidelines suggest screening children older than 2 years of age annually with TCD as long as the blood velocity remains within the normal range (≤ 170 cm/s) [50]. In patients with abnormal TCD results (≥ 200 cm/s), chronic transfusion is recommended [50]. Borderline TCDs need to be monitored closely for consideration of therapy. This recommendation is based upon the Stroke Prevention Trial in Sickle Cell Anemia. In this trial, patients randomized to this screening and treatment had a yearly stroke risk of less than 1% as compared to controls without intervention, where the rate remained at 10% [71].

Acute treatment for AIS in SCD patients includes exchange transfusion designed to reduce sickle hemoglobin to less than 30% total hemoglobin. Secondary prevention for first-time untreated AIS is also chronic transfusion [50]. For patients with AIS while being treated with exchange therapy and/or repeated events, bone marrow transplant or revascularization should be considered [50].

Outcomes

Recurrent stroke risks and associations of recurrent AIS with clinical and laboratory factors have been discussed above. As for other clinical outcomes, the risk of symptomatic hemorrhagic transformation in childhood AIS appears low. In one series of 63 patients with childhood AIS, only 3% of patients had symptomatic hemorrhage within the first 30 days of stroke [72]. Other series have demonstrated similar rates in children with arteriopathy (0%) and those treated with anticoagulation (0–4%) [41,73]. Mortality is not insignificant, at 2–11% [39,67,74,75]. However, death from underlying disease (non-stroke) is most common, and death from ICH is rare.

With regard to neurological outcomes, the majority of patients with childhood AIS have long-term morbidity, with 68% to 73% of patients suffering persistent neurological deficit [75–77]. Arteriopathic subtype has been associated with both short-term and long-term adverse neurological outcomes [23,23,23,23,58]. While biomarkers, such as D-dimer and endothelial microparticles, show potential for a role in predicting adverse outcomes and/or recurrent stroke events, more data are needed in this area [25].

Conclusions

Childhood AIS affects over 25,000 children worldwide each year. While significant progress has been made in understanding the epidemiology, standard of care and natural history generally in this disease, further work is needed to understand subtype-specific etiologies and outcomes. With the exception of sickle cell disease, treatment recommendations are largely based upon consensus and vary considerably worldwide. As in adult AIS, improvement in outcomes will likely rely upon risk-stratified therapies directed by subtypes. The role of thrombotic risk factors in childhood AIS remains largely understudied, although recent studies suggest endothelial and coagulation activation biomarkers are of interest. Given high risks for recurrent AIS and long-term neurological deficit, clinical trials remain a very high priority for advancing the field.

References

1. Schoenberg BS, Mellinger JF, Schoenberg DG. Cerebrovascular disease in infants and children: a study of incidence, clinical features, and survival. Neurology 1978 Aug;**28**(8):763–8.

2. Broderick J, Talbot GT, Prenger E, Leach A, Brott T. Stroke in children within a major metropolitan area: the surprising importance of intracerebral hemorrhage. J Child Neurol 1993 Jul;**8**(3):250–5.

3. http://www.census.gov/popest/data/national/asrh/2011/index.html.

4. http://www.census.gov/population/international/data/idb/worldpop.php.

5. Golomb MR, Fullerton HJ, Nowak-Gottl U, DeVeber G. Male predominance in childhood ischemic stroke: findings from the International Pediatric Stroke Study. Stroke 2009 Jan;**40**(1):52–7.

6. Fullerton HJ, Wu YW, Zhao S, Johnston SC. Risk of stroke in children: ethnic and gender disparities. Neurology 2003 Jul 22;**61**(2):189–94.

7. Mackay MT, Wiznitzer M, Benedict SL, Lee KJ, deVeber GA, Ganesan V. Arterial ischemic stroke risk factors: the International Pediatric Stroke Study. Ann Neurol 2011 Jan;**69**(1):130–40.

8. Srinivasan J, Miller SP, Phan TG, Mackay MT. Delayed recognition of initial stroke in children: need for increased awareness. Pediatrics 2009 Aug;**124**(2):e227–34.

9. Shellhaas RA, Smith SE, O'Tool E, Licht DJ, Ichord RN. Mimics of childhood stroke: characteristics of a prospective cohort. Pediatrics 2006 Aug;**118**(2):704–9.

10. Fenton LZ, Stence N, Strain J, Carrol E, Calhooh M, Hollatz A., et al. Development of a pediatric stroke imaging pathway. Abstract presentation. The Society for Pediatric Radiology. 4-1-2012.

11. Nowak-Gottl U, Strater R, Heinecke A, Junker R, Koch HG, Schuierer G, et al. Lipoprotein (a) and genetic polymorphisms of clotting factor V, prothrombin, and methylenetetrahydrofolate reductase are risk factors of spontaneous ischemic stroke in childhood. Blood 1999 Dec 1;**94**(11):3678–82.

12. Duran R, Biner B, Demir M, Celtik C, Karasalihoglu S. Factor V Leiden mutation and other thrombophilia markers in childhood ischemic stroke. Clin Appl Thromb Hemost 2005 Jan;**11**(1):83–8.

13. Kenet G, Sadetzki S, Murad H, Martinowitz U, Rosenberg N, Gitel S, et al. Factor V Leiden and antiphospholipid antibodies are significant risk factors for ischemic stroke in children. Stroke 2000 Jun;**31**(6):1283–8.

14. Strater R, Vielhaber H, Kassenbohmer R, von Kries R, Gobel U, Nowak-Gottl U. Genetic risk factors of thrombophilia in ischaemic childhood stroke of cardiac origin. A prospective ESPED survey. Eur J Pediatr 1999 Dec;**158**(Suppl 3):S122–5.

15. Brown DC, Livingston JH, Minns RA, Eden OB. Protein C and S deficiency causing childhood stroke. Scott Med J 1993 Aug;**38**(4):114–15.

16. Haywood S, Liesner R, Pindora S, Ganesan V. Thrombophilia and first arterial ischaemic stroke: a systematic review. Arch Dis Child 2005 Apr;**90**(4):402–5.

17. Strater R, Becker S, von Eckardstein A, Heinecke A, Gutsche S, Junker R, et al. Prospective assessment of risk factors for recurrent stroke during childhood – a 5-year follow-up study. Lancet 2002 Nov 16;**360**(9345):1540–5.

18. Goldenberg NA, Bernard TJ, Hillhouse J, Armstrong-Wells J, Galinkin J, Knapp-Clevenger R, et al. Elevated lipoprotein (a), small apolipoprotein (a), and the risk of arterial ischemic stroke in North American children. Haematologica 2013;**98**(5): 802–7.

19. Kenet G, Lutkhoff LK, Albisetti M, Bernard T, Bonduel M, Brandao L, et al. Impact of thrombophilia on risk of arterial ischemic stroke or cerebral sinovenous

thrombosis in neonates and children: a systematic review and meta-analysis of observational studies. Circulation 2010 Apr 27;**121**(16):1838–47.

20. Kreuz W, Stoll M, Junker R, Heinecke A, Schobess R, Kurnik K, et al. Familial elevated factor VIII in children with symptomatic venous thrombosis and post-thrombotic syndrome: results of a multicenter study. Arterioscler Thromb Vasc Biol 2006 Aug;**26**(8):1901–6.

21. Cangoz E, Deda G, Akar N. Effect of factor VIIIc levels in pediatric stroke patients. Pediatr Hematol Oncol 2004 Apr;**21**(3):255–60.

22. Miyakis S, Lockshin MD, Atsumi T, Branch DW, Brey RL, Cervera R, et al. International consensus statement on an update of the classification criteria for definite antiphospholipid syndrome (APS). J Thromb Haemost 2006 Feb;**4**(2):295–306.

23. Goldenberg NA, Jenkins S, Jack J, Armstrong-Wells J, Fenton LZ, Stence NV, et al. Arteriopathy, D-dimer, and risk of poor neurologic outcome in childhood-onset arterial ischemic stroke. J Pediatr 2013;**162**(5):1041–6.

24. Bernard TJ, Fenton LZ, Apkon SD, Boada R, Wilkening GN, Wilkinson CC, et al. Biomarkers of hypercoagulability and inflammation in childhood-onset arterial ischemic stroke. J Pediatr 2010;**156**:651–6.

25. Eleftheriou D, Ganesan V, Hong Y, Klein NJ, Brogan PA. Endothelial injury in childhood stroke with cerebral arteriopathy: A cross-sectional study. Neurology 2012 Nov 20;**79**(21):2089–96.

26. Lambers M, Goldenberg NA, Kenet G, Kirkham FJ, Manner D, Bernard T, et al. Role of reduced ADAMTS13 in arterial ischemic stroke: A Pediatric Cohort Study. Epub: Ann Neurol 2012 Aug 25.

27. Nowak-Gottl U, Strater R, Kosch A, von EA, Schobess R, Luigs P, et al. The plasminogen activator inhibitor (PAI)-1 promoter 4G/4G genotype is not associated with ischemic stroke in a population of German children. Childhood Stroke Study Group. Eur J Haematol 2001 Jan;**66**(1):57–62.

28. Bernard TJ, Manco-Johnson MJ, Lo W, Mackay MT, Ganesan V, DeVeber G, et al. Towards a consensus-based classification of childhood arterial ischemic stroke. Stroke 2012 Feb;**43**(2):371–7.

29. Benseler SM, Silverman E, Aviv RI, Schneider R, Armstrong D, Tyrrell PN, et al. Primary central nervous system vasculitis in children. Arthritis Rheum 2006 Apr;**54**(4):1291–7.

30. Benseler SM, DeVeber G, Hawkins C, Schneider R, Tyrrell PN, Aviv RI, et al. Angiography-negative primary central nervous system vasculitis in children: a newly recognized inflammatory central nervous system disease. Arthritis Rheum 2005 Jul;**52**(7):2159–67.

31. Amlie-Lefond C, Bernard TJ, Sebire G, Friedman NR, Heyer GL, Lerner NB, et al. Predictors of cerebral arteriopathy in children with arterial ischemic stroke: results of the International Pediatric Stroke Study. Circulation 2009 Mar 17;**119**(10):1417–23.

32. Danchaivijitr N, Cox TC, Saunders DE, Ganesan V. Evolution of cerebral arteriopathies in childhood arterial ischemic stroke. Ann Neurol 2006 Apr;**59**(4):620–6.

33. Askalan R, Laughlin S, Mayank S, Chan A, MacGregor D, Andrew M, et al. Chickenpox and stroke in childhood: a study of frequency and causation. Stroke 2001 Jun;**32**(6):1257–62.

34. Donahue JG, Kieke BA, Yih WK, Berger NR, McCauley JS, Baggs J, et al. Varicella vaccination and ischemic stroke in children: is there an association? Pediatrics 2009 Feb;**123**(2):e228–234.

35. Amlie-Lefond C, Bernard TJ, Sebire G, Friedman NR, Heyer GL, Lerner NB, et al. Predictors of cerebral arteriopathy in children with arterial ischemic stroke: results of the International Pediatric Stroke Study. Circulation 2009 Mar 17;**119**(10):1417–23.

36. Fullerton HJ, Elkind MS, Barkovich AJ, Glaser C, Glidden D, Hills NK, et al. The vascular effects of infection in Pediatric Stroke (VIPS) Study. J Child Neurol 2011 Sep;**26**(9):1101–10.

37. Braun KP, Bulder MM, Chabrier S, Kirkham FJ, Uiterwaal CS, Tardieu M, et al. The course and outcome of unilateral intracranial arteriopathy in 79 children with ischaemic stroke. Brain 2009 Feb;**132**(Pt 2):544–57.

38. Dlamini N, Freeman JL, Mackay MT, Hawkins C, Shroff M, Fullerton HJ, et al. Intracranial dissection mimicking transient cerebral arteriopathy in childhood arterial ischemic stroke. J Child Neurol 2011 Sep;**26**(9):1203–6.

39. Fullerton HJ, Wu YW, Sidney S, Johnston SC. Risk of recurrent childhood arterial ischemic stroke in a population-based cohort: the importance of cerebrovascular imaging. Pediatrics 2007 Mar;**119**(3):495–501.

40. Goldenberg NA, Bernard TJ, Gordon A, Fullerton H, DeVeber G. Acute treatments and early outcomes of childhood arterial ischemic stroke: first analysis of the International Pediatric Stroke Study. Blood 2008;**112**:1978A.

41. Bernard TJ, Goldenberg NA, Tripputi M, Manco-Johnson MJ, Niederstadt T, Nowak-Gottl U. Anticoagulation in childhood-onset arterial ischemic stroke with Nonmoyamoya arteriopathy: findings from the C`olorado and German (COAG) collaboration. Stroke 2009 Aug;**40**(8):2869–71.

42. Cantez S, Benseler SM. Childhood CNS vasculitis: a treatable cause of new neurological deficit in children. Nat Clin Pract Rheumatol 2008 Sep;**4**(9):460–1.

43. Sebire G, Fullerton H, Riou E, deVeber G. Toward the definition of cerebral arteriopathies of childhood. Curr Opin Pediatr 2004 Dec;**16**(6):617–22.

44. Roder C, Nayak NR, Khan N, Tatagiba M, Inoue I, Krischek B. Genetics of Moyamoya disease. J Hum Genet 2010 Nov;**55**(11):711–16.

45. Dougu N, Takashima S, Sasahara E, Taguchi Y, Toyoda S, Hirai T, et al. Differential diagnosis of cerebral infarction using an algorithm combining atrial fibrillation and D-dimer level. Eur J Neurol 2008 Mar;**15**(3):295–300.

46. Mineharu Y, Liu W, Inoue K, Matsuura N, Inoue S, Takenaka K, et al. Autosomal dominant moyamoya disease maps to chromosome 17q25.3. Neurology 2008 Jun;**70**(24 Pt 2): 2357–63.

47. Mineharu Y, Takenaka K, Yamakawa H, Inoue K, Ikeda H, Kikuta KI, et al. Inheritance pattern of familial moyamoya disease: autosomal dominant mode and genomic imprinting. J Neurol Neurosurg Psychiatry 2006 Sep;**77**(9):1025–9.

48. Matsushima T, Inoue T, Ikezaki K, Matsukado K, Natori Y, Inamura T, et al. Multiple combined indirect procedure for the surgical treatment of children with moyamoya disease. A comparison with single indirect anastomosis and direct anastomosis. Neurosurg Focus 1998 Nov;**5**(5):e4.

49. Smith ER. Moyamoya arteriopathy. Curr Treat Options Neurol 2012 Dec;**14**(6):549–56.

50. Roach ES, Golomb MR, Adams R, Biller J, Daniels S, deVeber G, et al. Management of stroke in infants and children: a scientific statement from a Special Writing Group of the American Heart Association Stroke Council and the Council on Cardiovascular Disease in the Young. Stroke 2008 Sep;**39**(9):2644–91.

51. Scott RM, Smith JL, Robertson RL, Madsen JR, Soriano SG, Rockoff MA. Long-term outcome in children with moyamoya syndrome after cranial revascularization by pial synangiosis. J Neurosurg 2004 Feb;**100**(2 Suppl Pediatrics):142–9.

52. Tan MA, Armstrong D, MacGregor DL, Kirton A. Late complications of vertebral artery dissection in children: pseudoaneurysm, thrombosis, and recurrent stroke. J Child Neurol 2009 Mar;**24**(3):354–60.

53. Fusco MR, Harrigan MR. Cerebrovascular dissections – a review part I: Spontaneous dissections. Neurosurgery 2011 Jan;**68**(1):242–57.

54. Rafay MF, Armstrong D, deVeber G, Domi T, Chan A, MacGregor DL. Craniocervical arterial dissection in children: clinical and radiographic presentation and outcome. J Child Neurol 2006 Jan;**21**(1):8–16.

55. Brandt T, Orberk E, Weber R, Werner I, Busse O, Muller BT, et al. Pathogenesis of cervical artery dissections: association with connective tissue abnormalities. Neurology 2001 Jul 10;**57**(1):24–30.

56. Tan MA, deVeber G, Kirton A, Vidarsson L, MacGregor D, Shroff M. Low detection rate of craniocervical arterial dissection in children using time-of-flight magnetic resonance angiography: causes and strategies to improve diagnosis. J Child Neurol 2009 Oct;**24**(10):1250–7.

57. Ganesan V, Cox TC, Gunny R. Abnormalities of cervical arteries in children with arterial ischemic stroke. Neurology 2011 Jan;**76**(2):166–71.

58. Goldenberg NA, Bernard TJ, Fullerton HJ, Gordon A, deVeber G. Antithrombotic treatments, outcomes, and prognostic factors in acute childhood-onset arterial ischaemic stroke: a multicentre, observational, cohort study. Lancet Neurol 2009 Dec;**8**(12):1120–7.

59. Dirik E, Yis U, Dirik MA, Cakmakci H, Men S. Vertebral artery dissection in a patient with Wildervanck syndrome. Pediatr Neurol 2008 Sep;**39**(3):218–20.

60. Sedney CL, Rosen CL. Cervical abnormalities causing vertebral artery dissection in children. J Neurosurg Pediatr 2011 Mar;**7**(3):272–5.

61. Lyrer P, Engelter S. Antithrombotic drugs for carotid artery dissection. Cochrane Database Syst Rev 2010; (**10**):CD000255.

62. Monagle P, Chalmers E, Chan A, deVeber G, Kirkham F, Massicotte P, et al. Antithrombotic therapy in neonates and children: American College of Chest Physicians Evidence-Based Clinical Practice Guidelines (8th Edn). Chest 2008 Jun;**133**(6 Suppl):887S–968S.

63. Bernard TJ, Manco-Johnson MJ, Lo W, Mackay MT, Ganesan V, deVeber G, et al. Towards a consensus-based classification of childhood arterial ischemic stroke. Stroke 2012 Feb;**43**(2):371–7.

64. Block AJ, McQuillen PS, Chau V, Glass H, Poskitt KJ, Barkovich AJ, et al. Clinically silent preoperative brain injuries do not worsen with surgery in neonates with congenital heart disease. J Thorac Cardiovasc Surg 2010 Sep;**140**(3):550–7.

65. Pavlakis SG, Kingsley PB, Bialer MG. Stroke in children: genetic and metabolic issues. J Child Neurol 2000 May;**15**(5):308–15.

66. Wozniak MA, Kittner SJ, Tuhrim S, Cole JW, Stern B, Dobbins M, et al. Frequency of unrecognized Fabry disease among young European-American and African-American men with first ischemic stroke. Stroke 2010 Jan;**41**(1):78–81.

67. Strater R, Kurnik K, Heller C, Schobess R, Luigs P, Nowak-Gottl U. Aspirin versus low-dose low-molecular-weight heparin: antithrombotic therapy in pediatric ischemic stroke patients: a prospective follow-up study. Stroke 2001 Nov;**32**(11):2554–8.

68. Janjua N, Nasar A, Lynch JK, Qureshi AI. Thrombolysis for ischemic stroke in children: data from the nationwide inpatient sample. Stroke 2007 Jun;**38**(6):1850–4.

69. Kassim AA, Debaun MR. Sickle cell disease, vasculopathy, and therapeutics. Annu Review Med 2013;**64**:451-66.

70. Ohene-Frempong K, Weiner SJ, Sleeper LA, Miller ST, Embury S, Moohr JW, et al. Cerebrovascular accidents in sickle cell disease: rates and risk factors. Blood 1998 Jan 1;**91**(1):288–94.

71. Adams RJ, McKie VC, Hsu L, Files B, Vichinsky E, Pegelow C, et al. Prevention of a first stroke by transfusions in children with sickle cell anemia and abnormal results on transcranial Doppler ultrasonography. N Engl J Med 1998 Jul;**339**(1):5–11.

72. Beslow LA, Smith SE, Vossough A, Licht DJ, Kasner SE, Favilla CG, et al. Hemorrhagic transformation of childhood arterial ischemic stroke. Stroke 2011 Apr;**42**(4):941–6.

73. Schechter T, Kirton A, Laughlin S, Pontigon AM, Finkelstein Y, MacGregor D, et al. Safety of anticoagulants in children with arterial ischemic stroke. Blood 2012 Jan 26;**119**(4):949–56.

74. Ganesan V, Prengler M, Wade A, Kirkham FJ. Clinical and radiological recurrence after childhood arterial ischemic stroke. Circulation 2006 Nov 14;**114**(20):2170–7.

75. Steinlin M, Pfister I, Pavlovic J, Everts R, Boltshauser E, Capone MA, et al. The first three years of the Swiss Neuropaediatric Stroke Registry (SNPSR): a population-based study of incidence, symptoms and risk factors. Neuropediatrics 2005 Apr;**36**(2):90–7.

76. Chabrier S, Husson B, Lasjaunias P, Landrieu P, Tardieu M. Stroke in childhood: outcome and recurrence risk by mechanism in 59 patients. J Child Neurol 2000 May;**15**(5):290–4.

77. deVeber GA, MacGregor D, Curtis R, Mayank S. Neurologic outcome in survivors of childhood arterial ischemic stroke and sinovenous thrombosis. J Child Neurol 2000 May;**15**(5):316–24.

Index